# WHO YOU GONNA CALL?

# Who You Gonna Call?

## Emergency Medical Services in Winnipeg, Canada and Beyond

Halldor K. Bjarnason

Second Edition—2025



On the cover: (center image): 1910s-era Winnipeg police call-box (Courtesy of WPS Archives). (From top left, clockwise): WFD first aid team using pulmotor in 1930 (Courtesy of FFHSW); Veterans-Prince 1962 Eureka-Cadilac Ambulance (Courtesy of Ken Burdyny Collection); Winnipeg Police 1966 Plymouth ambulance (Courtesy of WPS Archives); WFPS Advanced Care Paramedic Practitioner chase car (Courtesy of WFPS); WGH's 1911 Waverley electric ambulance (Courtesy of HSC Archives); WFD's 1949 Diamond T combination rescue squad/ambulance (Courtesy of FFHSW).

ISBN 978-1-0694500-1-2 Paperback
ISBN 978-1-0694500-0-5 Electronic book

4008-13495 Central Avenue
Surrey, BC V3T 0K2
Halldor@accesslaw.ca
www.HalldorBjarnason.com

Design & Layout: self-publish.ca

Printed in Canada.

# Contents

# Acknowledgements

In researching and writing this book, I have received amazing help from a squadron of people: EMS mangers, paramedics, firefighters, historians, archivists, photographers, writers, editors, beta readers, and folks who wanted to support me "because." Each of the following has played a role in ensuring that this story's details are accurate. However, despite their guidance, sometimes I have still have gotten it wrong—and for these mistakes, I take full responsibility.

Thanks to the following amazing people. If I've missed anyone (which I know I have—having visited many EMS/Fire stations, and interviewed dozens of frontline staff—I simply didn't catch each name), I apologize profusely; not intended:

Winnipeg's Fire and Paramedic Chief, Christian Schmidt, for his unwavering support—and acknowledgement of the need—of this project.

Sandy Shoofs, Derric Boles, Stan Stone, Barry Guttormson, retired paramedics extraordinaire. No matter what early part of Winnipeg Ambulance I was trying to understand, each contributed their knowledge, experience, and resources to help me find the answer.

Jennifer Lundin, Marty, Caitlin, Russ McKenzie, Jeremiah MacKenzie-Willner, Jaspar, Chris Bruce-Smith, Lori Bruce-Smith, Jeff Sippel, Lynea Finn—Ottawa Paramedics, Bruce Newton—Toronto Paramedics, Erin Massen, Jim McKinley, Kevin Moniz—Winnipeg Fleet Management, Terryn Shiells, Terry Lange, Sean Frain, Donna Perry and Christopher McCreery—St. John Ambulance, Stuart Hay—Manitoba Legislative Library, Patricia Sweryd—Bardel Funeral Home, Dr. Ryan Corbett Bell, Brent Crighton, Ryan Sneath, Peter Adsten, Jim McKinley,

Ralph Essinger, and Edward Burgener. Each, along the way, helped to find the needed information to fill gaps.

Ted Kuryluk, Jim Brennan, Barrie Lough, Jack Coulter, Bill Sandison, and Ken Sim, for their help in understanding the evolution of Winnipeg's fire department first responders.

Nick Kasper and Alex Forrest, for their help in explaining the UFFW's perspective.

Brett Lougheed and Tanya Wiegand, of the Western Canadian Pictorial Index, Nadya—*Winnipeg Free Press*, and James Kominowski—UM Archives, for their help in chasing down vintage pictures.

Peter Adsten, Ken Burdyny, Bryan Leach, Brian Schuff, Sandy Shoofs, Dave Stewardson, and Stan Stone for sharing their fabulous photo collections.

Scott Sawatsky, from Crestline Coach, for sharing a plethora of information and photos of Winnipeg's ambulances.

Lynn Klein, of BC Ambulance Service, for his help in understanding the "bigger picture" of EMS delivery.

Mary Agnes Welch, formerly of the *Winnipeg Free Press*, for her insightful research and writing on the politics of Winnipeg's fire and ambulance services.

Wayne Farmer, Garry Leach and John Wylie, for their in-depth explanations of pre-WAS private ambulance companies.

Louise Stitt and Susan Thompson, for their insights on women in Winnipeg's EMS.

Shane Cooke—WPS tactical officer extraordinaire—for his help in enhancing my understanding of Winnipeg's TEMS.

Emma Prescott, HSC archivist, for her fabulous research on Winnipeg's first ambulances, and Tammy Skrabek and Rod Hutter, WPS archivists, for their assistance with tracing Winnipeg Police's ambulance service.

My beta readers: Toni Armanno, Lise Bjarnason, JJ Lee, Joys Chow, Katie Bowring, and Shanga Karim, whom surprisingly were happy to tell me, in the kindest way possible, when the writing was "boring crap"—and then provide suggestions on how to fix it.

My editors, Eileen Velthuis and Amanda Bidnall, who managed to get these words into a readable format, and designer Michal Kozlowski for getting the words into the right places.

To Dorothy and Berni Plett, for being such gracious hosts on my many "digging expeditions" to Winnipeg.

To my parents, Ken and Mildred, and my son, Elliot, who somehow have managed to keep from rolling their eyes as they have been subjected to my unbridled enthusiasm for EMS since time immortal.

Finally, thanks to Bill Whitehead and Dr. Glen Bergeron, for their amazing inspiration on why we need to care for others when they're hurt or sick.

# Preface

Strange as it may sound, the most common question I got when writing this book was *Why; Why bother writing a book on the history of emergency care in Winnipeg?*

At first blush, it may seem a bit odd. Why would a guy with cerebral palsy (a lifelong condition characterized by an uneven walking pattern and a wacky speech impediment) who has been a lawyer for thirty-odd years, write about a bunch of often unknown heroes who spend their days doing a stressful, mostly thankless job where they regularly meet strangers who are having their worst days ever?

I usually respond with: "Well, I already wrote a book about the history of the Winnipeg Fire Department (WFD), and realized that there's a much bigger human story to be told."

Strange, but true.

Most people are familiar with other key community first responders, such as firefighters and police officers, and fortunately understand what they do. While these groups serve our communities well, paramedics—as part of our emergency medical services (EMS)—and their equipment are often overlooked; going unnoticed by the bulk of society until needed.

In Winnipeg—as well as many other Canadian cities—the police and/or fire departments have provided the ambulance services at different times during history. In Winnipeg, this list of providers has expanded to include the city, provincial government, the federal government, the Canadian Army (and the Royal Canadian Air Force), the Department of Veterans Affairs, funeral homes, the municipal hospitals, Winnipeg General Hospital, taxi companies, private ambulance companies, a private insurance company, local auto racing tracks, a horse race track, towing companies…

When you stop to catch your breath, you sometimes wonder who, at one time or another, *hasn't* provided ambulance and/or emergency care to Winnipeggers over the past 140-odd years. At some points during Winnipeg's history, when there was a medical emergency, "Who You Gonna Call?" became the response to "get an ambulance." At times in the past, there were many options, some bad and some not-too-bad, none great, but no central location to contact for help. At other times, the options for emergency medical transportation were minimal at best. Fortunately, this has evolved to today's Winnipeg Fire Paramedic Service, a modern, effective, one-stop emergency medical service provider.

Despite the wide range of ambulance providers over the past century and a half, often using different equipment and with a varied range of skill levels, two factors have remained constant: the history of EMS in Winnipeg, as with many regions in Canada, has been so full of obstacles, so constant and formidable, that the service should have collapsed long ago. What has consistently helped with the progression has been the unstinting commitment of devoted emergency care workers on the ground, keeping Winnipeggers safe every day. Ultimately, it's the stories of people who provide emergency care to the sick and injured that drew me to write this book.

My own story started as a kid in Cub Scouts, where I had an amazing leader named Bill Whitehead. The timing was perfect, as this culminated with the exact time period that the paramedic profession was being born. Mr. Whitehead began to share his fascination of how, using your bare hands and just a few basic tools, you can keep dying people alive and the sick or injured comfortable. This interest blossomed into my life-long fascination with emergency care.

Fast forward a decade, and I met the University of Winnipeg's head athletic therapist (at the time) Dr. Glen Bergeron, who also picked up on my fascination of helping injured people. Through Dr. Bergeron, I acquired more knowledge of emergency care, and how, in the sport setting, it can be the difference between a minor inconvenience and the end of a promising sport career.

As I did emergency care as a volunteer, I quickly realized that there were people in the community, working fulltime, keeping people—often complete strangers—alive and in the game as their job, often with more compassion in an hour than most of us can muster in a month!

I was in awe and have been ever since.

When I started researching the history of the WFD in the late 1990s, I was amazed to discover that there was little recorded about the history of Winnipeg's Emergency Medical System (EMS). I felt it was important to cover the evolution of both services, fire and emergency medical. While there was a significant overlap of the two services for much of Winnipeg's history, the city was in the midst of the arduous task of combining its EMS and firefighting services. Given the lack of historical information on EMS, this component was left out of the original WFD history book.

Twenty years later, through both my own and other historians' digging, I feel that I can finally capture this lost part of Winnipeg's history. Further, by giving context to Winnipeg's EMS with comparisons to the rest of Canada, this book will hopefully provide insight as to the evolution of EMS from coast-to-coast.

You might be asking, what does writing EMS history have to do with being a lawyer with cerebral palsy? Absolutely nothing, except that my life experiences have enabled me to sometimes spot good stories. My cerebral palsy, especially as I've gotten older, has given me numerous direct experiences of using EMS. My interest in the emergency services industry combined with my experience as a lawyer has allowed me to compare the operations in different jurisdictions as I've helped to write policies and procedures. Not being in the industry (except as a volunteer), I can write about these amazing public servants with accuracy but without self-promotion.

Popular media—movies and television—captures part of the true spirit of the modern paramedic; we often see dramatic images of paramedics doing phenomenal saves. Reviving heart attack victims, stopping deadly bleeds, successfully extricating drivers from horrific car accidents, or intervening with complex, out-of-hospital child births, are but a few of these examples. While important, and crucial for the people involved, these are only a small part of the paramedic's job. It's when they lend their skills and compassion to less dramatic medical complexities that paramedics shine the most.

If you think about it, human bodies are weird! While it's fairly simple to find the protocols to stop a deadly bleed or to resuscitate a non-breathing casualty, it's the billions of other odd, irregular things that a human body can do that paramedics have to try and figure out how to treat that create some of the biggest challenges.

At the receiving end of my personal experiences in the EMS field, a number of years ago, I woke up one morning to find that I couldn't stand up, and my brain had somehow switched to two different parts: One half was perfectly logical, and assessing what was going on, and the other half was having completely wacky hallucinations; including my visualizing a herd of cows dancing around in grass hula-skirts. At the same time, my body was starting to have convulsions; something with which the rational side of my brain was not happy. My son was off on a school camping trip, so I was stuck trying to figure out how to get help on my own.

Rolling out of bed, I crawled to the front door, got it unlocked and opened, and then called 911. The irrational part of my brain began explaining to the call-taker about the dancing cows, while the rational part outlined the inability to walk and the convulsions.

Within two and a half minutes, I had a pair of firefighter first responders in my living room, doing a primary assessment, and three minutes later, two primary care paramedics arrived and began doing their job.

What do you do when a guy whom you've never met before is lying on the floor, talking about cows doing the hula dance? Start looking for clues and asking questions. A quick search of my home showed no signs of drugs or alcohol, with an assortment of law books, firefighting and emergency care books, and a bunch of projects that a devoted dad would be doing with a pre-teenage son. Not a scenario that would suggest a drug-induced reaction.

Using the tests that were available to them, the paramedics were coming up blank. While there are dozens of tests that can be run in a hospital emergency ward, with the equipment carried in a well-stocked ambulance, the types of blood tests needed in this scenario were limited to three or four.

In the end, the paramedics decided that getting me to the hospital as quickly as possible would be the wisest move. Subsequent hospital lab tests showed that I had acquired a serious bout of pneumonia, and the toxins were seeping into my brain, making it do all kinds of funky things. A couple of days of heavy antibiotic treatment brought the pneumonia and my hallucinations under control, and me on my way to recovery.

Without the tests or an in-depth knowledge of cerebral palsy and its relationship to pneumonia, despite being life threatening, paramedics likely would never have specifically recognized it, as it's one of hundreds of conditions that are just too obscure. However, their value came in recognizing that advanced medical help was needed, and ensuring I got it safely and quickly.

The part of their treatment that remains as vivid to today as at the time was, after arriving at the hospital, instead of just handing me over to staff, the young female paramedic, noticing my fear and increased convulsions, sat down beside me, held my hand, and spoke quietly and reassuringly. For almost half an hour, she kept me calm until the hospital ER staff was ready to start work on me. Not a dramatic, life-saving action, but for a guy who had no comprehension of what was happening to his body but knew it wasn't good—and was terrified—the paramedics couldn't have picked a more meaningful way to provide support.

In the end, this example captures what EMS is and has always been about—caring people trying to figure out how to help others on what is often the casualty's *worst day ever.* Whether it be a life-threatening emergency, an emergency for that recipient (and perhaps a few others), or somewhere in between, Winnipeg's emergency medical crews, as their colleagues across the country, seem to rise to the occasion, and do their best to care for others, despite limited resources. It's these people, and the resources they've acquired, that this book celebrates.

# Pre-Winnipeg History

The evolution of Emergency Medical Services (EMS), be it in Winnipeg or elsewhere, is wonky!

When we look at modern ambulances, chase cars, paramedical equipment, advanced life skills, and paramedics themselves, the need for each piece of equipment and skill set makes sense. History, on the other hand, paints a different picture and is by no means linear—there's no simple moving from Point A to Point B. The overarching questions of whether EMS is better run by the private or public sector, should be financed by the community or by the user, whether it is a public health service or an emergency response service (or even a glorified taxi service), as well as how war, disease, and private enterprise all affect its evolution provide a tapestry which is beyond the scope of this book. However, these issues have all affected the development of Winnipeg's EMS.

While this book is about the history of Winnipeg's (and Canada's) Emergency Medical Services, it's worth having a quick look at how prehospital care and transportation evolved before Winnipeg's creation. There are several reliable, written histories of EMS, so the following is a quick overview of some of the developments that have affected modern prehospital care.

## Prehospital Care: A Global Concern

Throughout history, different entities have tried developing systems for both the proper transportation of casualties and prehospital care. The path has not been linear, new innovations have not always been for the better, but over time, experiments have created the system we now have. It has typically been a case of two steps forward, one step, (sometimes three steps) back. As historians have different opinions as to what advances were vital in the evolution of prehospital emergency care, I provide but a few examples of key EMS developments. Nevertheless, several key milestones are found throughout the western world, thus they also affect Winnipeg.

The first effort to provide organized emergency care seems to have arisen during the eleventh century with the Knights Hospitaller of Saint John of Jerusalem; a very early version of the St. John Ambulance organization that exists today. With the First Crusades, a group of Catholic monks noticed that many pilgrims were being beaten and robbed as they made their way to Jerusalem. Seeing a need, Blessed Gerard, a monk, set up an aid station to assist injured pilgrims. It got a bit complicated when the same people who were beating and robbing the pilgrims started beating and robbing the monks and acquiring their supplies. After a few robberies—which greatly defeated their abilities to assist—the monks adjusted their strategy and recruited a new branch, essentially *warrior knights* to provide security and keep the riffraff at bay. They did a great job of protecting the monks and their supplies but created a whole new class of casualties.

As with most early attempts at providing emergency care or ambulance-type services, the Knights Hospitallers' efforts were task-specific and fairly short-lived. Being a Catholic organization, after the Islamic reconquest of the Holy Land in 1291, they were chased from Jerusalem to Rhodes, and later Malta. After being kicked out of Malta by, what will turn out to be somewhat ironic, French Commander Napoleon Bonaparte—more on him in a few paragraphs—the Knights Hospitallers were dispersed throughout Europe, losing most of their assets and becoming more of a military than an emergency care organization.

In 1240, in Florence, Italy, a porter named Pietro di Luca Borsi collected coins from his drinking buddies as fines for swearing. The collection provided funding for the *Compagnia della Misericordia* or "Brothers of Mercy," a primitive ambulance service where the drinking buddies transported the sick and injured on a crimson litter (a hand-propelled vehicle used to carry people) to the hospital. It was primarily a transportation service. While not offering much in the way of care. it provided teams of dedicated volunteers who got the injured to medical care. The volunteers wore heavy robes to ensure the stretcher-bearers could not be identified, ensuring their efforts remained charitable.

The service operated for a couple of hundred years, but as with many charities, it became a victim of its own success. After becoming an affluent organization—thanks to significant public support—it became susceptible to plundering by other alleged charities. By 1475, penniless, *Compagnia della Misericordia* faded into oblivion. While the need remained, the service died.

For the next few hundred years, various temporary solutions—improvisations to fill an immediate need—were made to provide emergency transport during plagues and wars. Ryan Corbett Bell's book *The Ambulance: A History* (McFarland & Company, 2012) provides a superb compendium of efforts made throughout the ages to develop reliable prehospital emergency care and transport.

An effort to create a more permanent model for EMS emerged in the late 1700s. In 1797, French Commander Napoleon Bonaparte's chief surgeon, Dominique Jean Larrey, tired of seeing thousands of soldiers slaughtered on the battlefields while surgeons stood in the distance watching, proposed an effective solution. By equipping surgeons with quick, artillery-type carriages and medical supplies, and developing a system of triage (determining which injuries, based on seriousness, would be treated first), Larrey created a system for soldiers to be treated as they fell, before being transported to a field hospital.

Napoleon liked the idea. Keeping soldiers alive was cost-efficient, and Napoleon immediately approved Larrey's proposal. Thus, the first dedicated military ambulance corps was formed, and triage was used for the first time. Ultimately, many soldiers would be kept alive thanks to these measures.

Until the 1850s, most successful prehospital emergency care/transport systems were military-based. As with Larrey's ambulances, they were created to deal with injured soldiers. However, there were exceptions. In 1817, the infamous cholera pandemic began, eventually killing millions worldwide. It ravaged much of civilization until 1832 when the cities of Manchester and London (both in England) decided to tackle it. While apparent today, at the time, isolating infected patients was a novel concept. In London and Manchester, the cities' hospitals acquired carriages—the world's first infectious disease ambulances—and at the first sign of a person being affected, the hospital dispatched a carriage to bring them to the isolation hospital. While treatment was debatable, and survival not assured, the system of isolating casualties reduced the spread of diseases. It also marked the creation of the world's first hospital-based ambulance services. Coincidentally, York,

Ontario (present day Toronto) also developed an infectious disease ambulance in 1832.

A few cities created ambulance services for specific purposes, such as those for infectious diseases and for transporting returning, injured Civil War soldiers in the US. However, municipal emergency ambulance services took longer to evolve. While Bellevue Hospital in New York City claims to have started the first city-wide ambulance system in 1869, Commercial Hospital in Cincinnati beat them by four years.

At Commercial Hospital, in 1865, there was a perfect storm. Cincinnati was a major producer of military ambulances, but with the American Civil War winding down, there was already an over-supply in the city. To try to reduce some of its significant economic problems, Commercial Hospital hired a new medical director, Robert Bartholow, whose varied experience included setting up several military hospitals with ambulance services. With a need to increase revenues at Commercial Hospital and an abundance of new ambulances in the city, Dr. Bartholow devised a perfect solution. He created an ambulance service that would deliver casualties from all over Cincinnati to the hospital's front door. It was more or less a delivery service where, based on American military design, Cincinnati's ambulances transported casualties to the hospital without providing much additional service. Bartholow's ambulance service would be the model followed, more or less, for the next hundred years.

Four years later, in 1869, New York City's Bellevue Hospital took Commercial Hospital's ambulance service design a few steps further.

Bellevue Hospital's emergency ambulance service was also created out of financial need. When the New York Hospital wasn't making enough money, the landlord closed the building and razed it, leaving no hospital south of Central Park. Losing access to the busy, industrialized southern neighbourhoods, where factories and docks created a significant range of injuries to keep hospitals busy, it became apparent that a means was needed to bring unharnessed business to the remaining hospitals. Dr. Edward Dalton, who had already designed New York's cholera ambulance service and had managed field hospitals during the Civil War, was recruited to build Bellevue Hospital's city-wide emergency ambulance service.

Dalton incorporated his past experiences and created a sophisticated system that responded to requests by police officers with first aid training. The on-call system used light, maneuverable horse-drawn wagons carrying significant medical supplies, including tourniquets, splints, blankets, bandages, and the ultimate cure-all: a quart of brandy. Of particular benefit was the addition of medical staffing: A doctor rode in the ambulance, starting medical care immediately upon arrival. While Cincinnati's system modeled the "you call, we haul, that's all" form of ambulance service that was typical for much of the twentieth century, New York's system had many characteristics of modern paramedic ambulances.

The problem was, and still is, that running an ambulance service is not cost-effective. While there was and is a recognized need for the service, the question remains: Who will pay for it?

For hospitals needing "customers," particularly from other neighbourhoods, ambulances were a cost of doing business. In other cities, as the concept of ambulance services became established, the role was either accepted by or assigned to different bodies: typically, funeral homes, fire departments, police departments, and/or municipal health departments.

As will be discussed, Winnipeg's various ambulance services over the past 140 years epitomize the range of ambulance providers. We have seen an everchanging, ever-evolving, but somehow always quirky development of emergency care in Winnipeg. With that history, we celebrate the amazing people who have made—and continue to make—it happen.

## 1874-1910

# Winnipeg Gets an Ambulance

On October 1, 1875, Winnipeg General Hospital (WGH) moved into its new Bannatyne and Sherbrook location; a building which, for the first time, the hospital could call its own. Unfortunately, the building's location, in a swamp, was less than ideal. In the springtime, planks were needed to enter the building, making it inaccessible to most patients. Unless the patient was agile enough to climb across the planks, getting medical assistance was a non-starter.

By 1882, the Canadian Pacific Railway had reached Winnipeg, and with it came a rapid increase in population, going from 7,995 in 1881 to roughly 25,000 in 1891. While the population growth increased the need for improved (and accessible) medical care, the smallpox epidemic in 1882–1883 highlighted the limited medical resources existing in Winnipeg. The introduction of the railway industry in Winnipeg, with its related trauma and high level of injuries, created an unprecedented need for medical care prior to arriving at a hospital.

The issue of proper health care was finally addressed in 1884 when WGH opened its new facility (on the same spot as the old building) on Sherbrook Street. Besides being accessible, with planks no longer needed for access, the new facility had a specific ward dedicated to the care of "accident victims."[1] While it would be many decades before the term "Emergency Ward" came into being, and even more, about 80 years, before emergency medicine became a recognized medical specialty, it's both interesting and remarkable that Winnipeg had a facility devoted to trauma. When Winnipeg's railyards opened in 1882, making it an

1 *Healing & Hope: A History of Health Sciences Centre.* Health Sciences Centre, Winnipeg, 2009: 4.

essential railway terminus for Western Canada, the railway became one of Winnipeg's biggest industries; associated with significant numbers of injuries. As a result, it makes sense that there would be an "accident ward" at Winnipeg's hospital.

While WGH had the new accident ward, getting there was still a significant challenge. The injured typically arrived by horseback, wagon, sleigh, Red River cart (a large, two-wheeled oxen-drawn wooden cart used extensively by the Metis to assist with the prairie buffalo hunt), blanket stretcher, the occasional dog sled, or were just brought by friends in whatever manner was possible. The CPR shops kept a covered spring wagon on hand as a make-shift ambulance.[2] Whatever the means of transport, it tended to do more harm than good for the casualty. With no ambulance service in Winnipeg, getting to WGH remained an enigma for another five years.

It reached a head in 1886, as the "National Dream" (as Canada's cross-country railway system was described) came to fruition and the Canadian Pacific Railway reached Vancouver. Winnipeg's rail yards became a key part of Canada's national transportation system. With thousands of people employed in the industry, railway-related injuries skyrocketed, as noted in the 1887 WGH Annual Report.

## Hospital Ambulances

With an increased need to figure out transport to medical care, in 1888 the hospital's board of directors decided to find a solution. Noting that the Toronto General Hospital had already found a solution eight years before by acquiring Canada's first ambulance,[3] they decided to follow suit. Through networking, the idea of an ambulance was communicated to Charles S. Hoare, the Manager of the Imperial Bank. Mr. Hoare canvassed his friends and colleagues and raised more than $500 to purchase a new ambulance.

As explained in WGH's 1888 Annual Report:

> Great difficulty has very often been experienced in getting patients sent into the Hospital for the want of a properly constructed ambulance. In accident cases it is most serious, as well as in cases

2 Edward O'Reilly. "Hospital Reminiscences." *WGH Nurses Alumni Journal.* 1929: 22.
3 Hanna (1982): 15.

of infectious disease. A few friends of the Hospital have raised a subscription to provide an ambulance.[4]

Under the direction of Edward O'Reilly, the hospital's first Medical Superintendent, the hospital's new horse-drawn ambulance, and the first ambulance in Manitoba, was built by Armstrong & Dougall, a local carriage-maker.

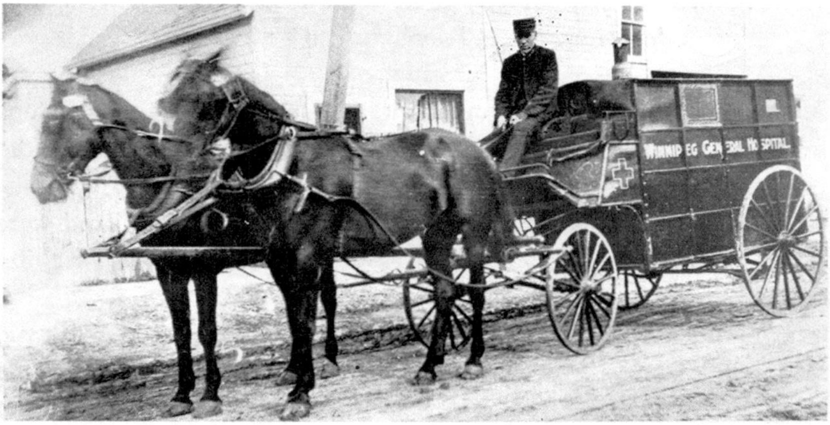

*Winnipeg's First Ambulance, built in 1889 by Armstrong & Dougall for WGH. (Courtesy of HSC Archives)*

In a January 28, 1889 report to the WGH Board, Secretary-Treasurer Charles John Brydges noted:

> An ambulance is now ready for use at any hour, night or day, at the following charges: From 8 a.m. to 8 p.m., 75 cents. From 8 p.m. to 8 a.m., $1.25. It will be sent on telephone call 477. It is supplied with medical appliances." To promote the new service, Red Cross cards were posted in prominent places around the city, citing the: "Winnipeg General Hospital Ambulance Service.[5]

The *Manitoba Daily Free Press* expanded on the report, providing front-page coverage of the new rig. At the time, it was the latest in technology. While primarily acquired for responding to accidents and illness, the ambulance also helped in preventing the spread of infection; a common problem when using regular cabs to transport patients. The paper reported:

4 Winnipeg General Hospital. *Annual Report*, 1888: 11.
5 Edward B. O'Reilly. "Hospital Reminiscences." *Nurses' Alumnae Annual*. 1937: 51.

> The ambulance has lockers, in which medical appliances are kept, and in cases of emergency, a medical man can, if necessary, accompany the patient to the hospital. As it is important, to very many cases, that no delay should occur in getting patients into the hospital, a gong will be sounded on the ambulance, similar to the fire engine gongs, and it is earnestly hoped that when the gong is heard right of way may be freely given to the ambulance so that no stopping or delay may occur. Telephone call 477.[6]

As the Winnipeg General Hospital's budget did not include provisions for the ambulance, Winnipeg pharmacist John F. Howard donated the medicines and surgical appliances (i.e., the first aid supplies). The ambulance came with stretchers made of "first growth hickory" and were tested by having WGH's secretary-treasurer, Charles Brydges, weighing 210 pounds, lie on them.

Winnipeg General Hospital's ambulance had its first call on February 4, 1889.[7] While unclear whether the traffic conditions warranted an audible warning device, driver Arinbjorn S. Bardal (more about Mr. Bardal in a bit) used the ambulance's gong as it raced along Main Street. Two days later, this incident led to an angry editorial in the *Manitoba Daily Free Press* about using the ambulance's warning device. The paper expressed concerns about the gong, suggesting that the ambulance might be confused with fire apparatus and fool people into believing that there was a fire.[8] This raised interesting issues, including what constituted an "emergency vehicle," whether an ambulance was such, and when a siren or other audible warning was needed. Despite city councillors raising the issue at the next WGH board meeting, it didn't get settled. Even as late as the mid-1960s, there was still public debate as to whether it was appropriate for Winnipeg's privately run ambulances to use audible warning devices like sirens.

A couple of weeks after the WGH ambulance's first run, on February 16, 1889, the rig had its official public demonstration, with Mr. Brydges becoming the first "patient" to use the stretcher. As the rig did not have a heater, and it being in the midst of winter, it seems that Mr. Brydges had a frigid ride. Given that Mr. Brydges died a few hours after

6 "The New Ambulance", *Manitoba Daily Free Press*, January 28, 1889.

7 *Manitoba Daily Free Press*, February 5, 1889.

8 "Suppress the Gong", *Manitoba Daily Free Press*, February 7, 1889.

giving the demonstration,[9] one can't help but wonder if the ride was a bit too cold (there was a blizzard in Winnipeg the day the new ambulance was tested). After the official demonstration, 290 other patients utilized the ambulance in the first year.[10]

As noted in WGH's Annual Report for that year:

> The ambulance, which was presented to the Hospital in January last by the kindness of a few friends in Winnipeg, has been found to be of great benefit in comfortably conveying patients who come from a distance from the trains to the Hospital, as well as in conveying those who live in the city from their homes.[11].

It is debatable whether the patients were truly *comfortable.* Still, a vehicle that could carry them in a reclined position on a cot had definite benefits over being tossed onto the back of a donkey for a sauntering, bumpy ride to the hospital.

While it may seem strange today, in the 1880s, it was a reasonable question as to whether an ambulance was an emergency vehicle. From the 1880s through to the 1960s, when a person was sick or injured, the first person contacted was often the local physician. He (or occasionally, she) provided immediate care. The physician then determined whether the patient should be transported to the hospital, or more often, the patient's home for further care. With physicians of that period doing most of their work via house calls and hospital care facilities being rudimentary, and perhaps germ infested, an injured or sick person could often get the same (or better) care at home with family support. In the early 1930s, 40 percent of doctor-patient meetings were made via house calls. By contrast, in 1980, only 0.6 percent of a doctor's work was done in a patient's home.[12]

WGH internists and surgeons accompanied the ambulance as required, and in 1903, it became standardized practice to have a physician riding in

---

9 Manitoba Historical Society Archives: Memorable Manitobans: Charles John Brydges (1827-1889), https://www.mhs.mb.ca/docs/people/brydges_cj.shtml, accessed July 3, 2024; Edward O'Reilly. "Hospital Reminiscences", *Nurses' Alumnae Annual.* 1929. 23.

10 "Hospital Work." *Manitoba Daily Free Press.* February 7, 1890.

11 Winnipeg General Hospital. *Annual Report,* 1889. 8.

12 Helen Kao; Conant, Rebecca; Soriano, Theresa; McCormick, Wayne (February 2009). "The Past, Present, and Future of House Calls." *Clinics in Geriatric Medicine.* 25 (1): 19–34.

WGH's ambulance. As noted in WGH's 1903 Annual Report: "A radical change was made in [the Ambulance] service during the year. A medical man now invariably accompanies the ambulance and the intelligent treatment of patients while being conveyed to the Hospital is thus assured."[13] However, given that the ambulance was usually requested by the onsite local physician, it's likely that using an "ambulance surgeon" was more of an exception than the rule. This gives more credibility to the question as to whether ambulances of this era were true "emergency vehicles." With the exception of railway-related trauma calls, it is more likely than not that the WGH hospital ambulance was used as a non-emergency transport vehicle.

There is another, more interesting explanation for the addition of an ambulance surgeon on WGH ambulances. As outlined in the hospital's 1904 Annual Report, there were 1,461 trips made by the ambulance that year, an increase from 1,296 trips in 1903. The "increase would have been much greater but for the fact that several private ambulances are now assisting in this work."[14] With a committee appointed to manage the hospital's ambulance business, and increased competition from private ambulance providers, there may have been a concerted effort to generate more business. The addition of an onboard physician seems like a reasonable attempt to increase the level of service and draw in more customers; providing a level of service with which funeral homes couldn't compete. However, as will be shown, the mass education of Winnipeggers in first aid didn't start for another seven years. Further, the recognition of the need for medically based, onsite emergency care didn't start for another sixty years. Hence, it's debatable how effective the onboard physician was. Quite possibly it was a means of justifying the $1 increase (up to $2 per trip) for an ambulance ride.

What was particularly interesting was that the 1895 report highlighted the need for a separate, "infectious case" ambulance to deal with the ongoing stream of patients with scarlet fever, typhoid fever, measles, whooping cough, and diphtheria.[15] With typhoid outbreaks being an annual occurrence, the 1882-1883 smallpox epidemic in recent memory, and the understanding of "germ transmission" being a relatively new

13 WGH Annual Report 1903: 12.

14 WGH Annual Report 1903: 12.

15 "The Hospital." *Manitoba Daily Free Press.* August 8, 1895.

area of medical science, this was a progressive recommendation. Unfortunately, as funds for medical care were scarce in Winnipeg at the time, and the *germ theory* was still reasonably controversial, it would take another nine years to get a designated infectious case ambulance.

By 1897, things had reached the stage, and perhaps medical knowledge had expanded to understand how disease spreads, that an ambulance exclusively for patients with infectious diseases was required. Alice Sprague, wife of WGH director Daniel Sprague, and a Mrs. H. Bell, president of the Women's Hospital Aid Society, took up the torch.[16] It is not clear what vehicle was acquired as an infectious disease ambulance. Three years later, after WGH acquired a new (third) ambulance, the *Manitoba Daily Free Press* was critical of the hospital for still using "an old covered-in milk or delivery wagon" as its infectious disease ambulance instead of repurposing its older ambulance.[17]

With the new infectious disease unit, assuming it was a reconstituted milk wagon, parked beside the eight-year-old original ambulance, the WGH's ambulance hospital fleet left something to be desired. As a result, the WGH board immediately began a fundraising campaign for a new ambulance.

In December 1897, the Board hosted an art exhibition at the Masonic Temple, raising $331.15.[18] Falling significantly short of what was needed, Mesdames Bell and Sprague immediately started fundraising for a new, state-of-the-art horse-drawn ambulance. By December 1898, after raising $840 toward the new ambulance, the two women gave the funds to WGH as a Christmas offering.[19] Ordering it in April 1899, the ambulance's September arrival coincided with the October opening of the WGH's new Jubilee Wing.[20]

Of interest, the unit was purchased from the Studebaker Company in Chicago.[21] At the time, before Studebaker began building motor cars, they were one of North America's premier ambulance manufacturers.

---

16 Marion Bryce. "Historical Sketch of the Charitable Institutions of Winnipeg", *Manitoba Historical Society Archives.* Series 1, No. 54. https://www.mhs.mb.ca/docs/transactions/1/charitableinstitutions.shtml, accessed July 6, 2024.

17 "The Smallpox Cases." *Manitoba Daily Free Press.* April 29, 1900.

18 "The General Hospital." *Manitoba Daily Free Press.* March 10, 1899.

19 "New Hospital Ambulance." *Manitoba Daily Free Press.* December 10, 1898.

20 "The Jubilee Addition." *Winnipeg Daily Tribune*". October 6, 1899.

21 "The Hospital Contracts." *Manitoba Morning Free Press.* April 18, 1899.

With WGH now operating three ambulances, it seems that medical transportation was becoming more of an ongoing concern. According to WGH's Annual Reports, an Ambulance Committee was listed as one of the standing committees of the Board of Directors between 1900 and 1911. The timing is interesting in that in 1911, Bardal ceased to contract with WGH to provide ambulance drivers. It may be that after 1911, with ambulance services being brought fully inhouse, they became more of a day-to-day hospital management issue, avoiding the need for a separate committee.

At the time, the most significant types of ambulance responses were for typhoid and railway injuries. In 1886, when the Canadian Pacific Railway reached the West Coast, Winnipeg became the "Gateway to the West." All rail traffic between Eastern Canada, the Prairies, and the West Coast moved through Winnipeg. By the mid-1890s, Winnipeg had the largest railyards in the world.[22]

Railways were also inherently dangerous; history shows that more than 600 Chinese labourers died while building the western section of the Canadian Pacific Railway[23]. Once completed, the railway system remained a constant source of casualties. A look through the *Manitoba Daily Free Press* from the 1880s and 1890s shows almost weekly reports of persons being injured or killed in or around Winnipeg's railway facilities.

As this new form of mass transit evolved across North America, railway-related injuries were rampant. In 1888, Johnson & Johnson Company founder Robert Wood Johnson, while on vacation, had a chance conversation with the Denver & Rio Grande Railway's medical officer. After hearing about the dangers and serious injuries related to the railway industry, often combined with a lack of immediate access to hospitals, Johnson saw a fabulous opportunity: a chance to help others by improving health care while at the same time creating a product that would help his business grow exponentially. Responding to this need, the Johnson & Johnson Company introduced a novel invention: The prepackaged, commercial first aid kit.[24]

---

22 "The CP Rail yards over the years", *Winnipeg Free Press.* July 6, 2012. https://www.winnipegfreepress.com/multimedia/2012/07/06/the-cp-rail-yards-over-the-years. Accessed October 2022.

23 Asian Heritage Society of New Brunswick. "Chinese Labour on the Canadian Pacific Railway", at www.ahsnd.org. Accessed July 3, 2024.

24 "The Birth of the First Aid Kit": Johnson & Johnson Company website: https://ourstory.jnj.com/birth-first-aid-kit. Accessed October 2020.

In the United States, at the time, approximately 12,000 railway workers and operators died each year. It immediately occurred to Johnson that if he began packaging his company's newly invented sterile surgical supplies into a portable wooden or metal case, it would be an ideal device for railways. He put Johnson & Johnson's scientific director, Fred Kilmer, to work, and within months, they had developed a marketable first aid kit.

With the introduction of the commercial first aid kit, it became possible for people onsite to provide immediate medical aid. As a result, an interest in emergency first aid, particularly in the railway industry, evolved. In Winnipeg, this interest seems to have been first highlighted in 1891 when a *Manitoba Daily Free Press* editorial noted that railway company employees, policemen, and firemen needed to learn first aid, as moving people after catastrophic accidents often did more damage than the accident itself.[25] The Canadian Pacific Railway acted on this suggestion, and in 1893, the Company's medical officer began providing free first aid lectures to CPR employees each Tuesday.[26]

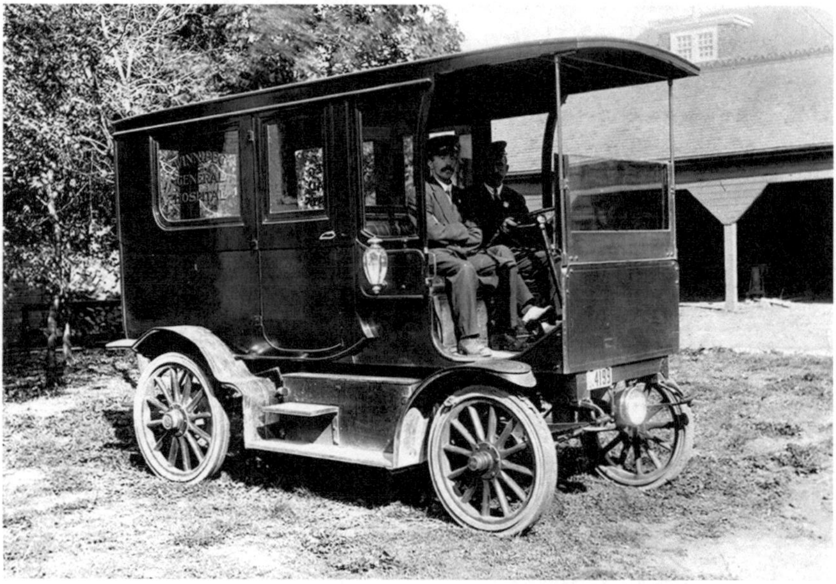


*WGH's first motorized ambulance; a 1911 Waverley electric unit. (Courtesy of HSC Archives)*

25 "In Case of Accident." *Manitoba Daily Free Press.* June 10, 1891.
26 "Lecture to the CPR Employees." *Manitoba Daily Free Press.* February 8, 1893.

Back to Winnipeg General Hospital; In 1911, the hospital entered the motorized world. Through the T. Eaton Company it purchased a "Waverley" electric ambulance. According to the WGH's Annual Report, this vehicle: "was to be kept at the hospital and was to be entirely under the control of the hospital."[27] It seems that this may have been a means of preventing Arinbjorn Bardel from using the hospital's ambulance for his own business purposes (more on this in a moment). As electric vehicles were in their infancy, like many other electric vehicles of the period the Waverley was not very successful. The Pope-Waverley Motor Car Company itself went out of business in 1914. At this point, even though the hospital's Waverley was only three years old, WGH purchased a gasoline-powered vehicle. While gasoline-powered commercial vehicles were also in their infancy, they were already proving themselves to be significantly more efficient, both cost-wise and operationally, than either electric or horse-drawn vehicles.

To give context to motorized ambulances, the first mass-production automobile-based ambulance (rather than the one-off models) was produced in the United States in 1909 by James Cunningham, Son & Company of Rochester, New York, a manufacturer of carriages and Hearses. This ambulance, appropriately named the *Model 774 Automobile Ambulance*, featured a 32 horsepower (24 kW), 4-cylinder engine. The chassis rode on pneumatic tires, while the body featured electric lights, a suspended cot with two attendant seats, and a side-mounted gong.

## Private Ambulances

With emergency medical services, there is a distinction between public and private provision. Public ambulances are those provided entirely or primarily using funding generated through taxes and/or government contributions. Private ambulances, on the other hand, are a for-profit operation, utilized, at least in theory, to make an income for the owner.

If we think of WGH as providing a semi-public ambulance service, it gets a bit confusing in that from 1886 to 1894, its driver, Arinbjorn Bardal also operated a livery stable and transport business near Sherbrook and

27 Winnipeg General Hospital. *Annual Report*, 1911: 14.

William. This is the same period, starting in 1889, that he was the driver for WGH's ambulance. During the time he was running his transport business, one of his main sources of revenue was assisting with construction of the Canadian Pacific Railway.

In 1894, Mr. Bardal opened a funeral home and by 1906, he was providing ambulance services as an offshoot of his funeral service. The provision of private ambulance services corresponds with Mr. Bardal opening a new funeral home at 843 Sherbrook Street (across the street from WGH). He and his family lived on the second and third floors, allowing him to respond immediately to calls, day or night.

It remains unclear as to whether the service he provided to WGH in 1889 was as an employee of the hospital or as a contractor as part of his transport business.

It gets murkier in 1901, when Frank McKague, WGH's staff ambulance driver, was arrested for keeping the $1 ambulance fees for himself. He was also charged with defrauding and/or over-charging patrons. Ultimately, McKague was fined $25.[28] As a result, it appears that WGH switched back to utilizing Bardal's services. This was clarified in 1907 when WGH acquired a new ambulance, confirming in its 1911 annual report that it was being operated by Mr. Bardal.

In competition with Mr. Bardal, other Winnipeg funeral homes began getting into the ambulance business. With Hearses already existing to transport bodies in a horizontal position, it seemed a good fit. In 1905, Gardiner Funeral Home purchased a horse-drawn ambulance. Newspaper reports note that it had seating for both a doctor and nurse, suggesting it was used for non-emergency or transfer services. As a bonus for Winnipeg winters, it had a charcoal furnace which kept it warm.[29] It's not entirely clear how the ambulance was able to have an internal charcoal furnace without giving the patients carbon monoxide poisoning, but supposedly it worked.

As of 1911, for the two horse-drawn ambulances owned and operated by WGH, Bardal was still providing drivers and horse teams to the hospital on a fee-for-service arrangement. At the same time, he was also running his own ambulance service. Company record books show that

28 "City and General." *Manitoba Morning Free Press.* November 11, 1901.
29 "A New Ambulance." *Winnipeg Free Press.* November 27, 1905.

between 1916 and 1923[30], one of his main clients for ambulance calls was his former employer, the Canadian Pacific Railway.[31]

While the details of the business relationship have been lost over time, it raises interesting questions as to how Mr. Bardal could be legitimately providing services to WGH's ambulance service, which was losing money, while at the same time, be running his own ambulance to service the CPR; one of the most accident-prone industries in Winnipeg. The logistics of a contractor for WGH, running a parallel business and taking the most profitable aspects of the business for his own could use some further inquiry.

As noted, it appears that the hospital was aware of the conflict, in that when the motorized ambulance was acquired in 1911, the forementioned board regulation was passed that only hospital staff could drive the ambulance. This partially ended Bardal's involvement with WGH's ambulance service, with Bardal only operating WGH's horse-drawn ambulances.

## Changes in the City and Worldwide Affecting Ambulance Services

As will be discussed in the next chapter, the opening of the Panama Canal in 1914 resulted in the decimation of Winnipeg's rail industry after the end of World War I. This resulted in businesses dependent on the railway, such as Bardal's ambulance service, to suddenly become unprofitable.

According to WGH's newsletter, which ran a series of historical articles in 1972, the WGH ambulance service showed a deficit every year. In 1902 the ambulance service cost the hospital $505.92 but only $255.25 was collected in fees. By 1939 the service appears to have declined, or perhaps became too unprofitable, and ceased operations during the Second World War. There is no further mention of a WGH ambulance service in the Annual Reports after 1939.[32]

Between the construction of the Canadian Pacific Railway's Royal Alexandra Hotel in 1904-06, and the Hotel Fort Garry in 1911-13, approximately

---

30 Between 1916 and 1923, Bardal was listed in Winnipeg's *Henderson Directory* as providing ambulance services.

31 Online interview with Patricia Sweryd. Vice-President, Bardal Funeral Home. September 10-11, 2020.

32 *The Generator.* Volume 14, Number 9, October 1972.

sixty hotels were established along Main Street. Between the gambling, prostitution, and significant alcohol consumption, the area gained significant notoriety, giving the city the moniker of "Winnipeg the Wicked." Not surprisingly, this particular area also had a high incidence of beatings, stabbings, and shootings; the kind of trauma that requires immediate medical attention.

Also related to this period was the introduction of the automobile. Winnipeg's first automobile arrived in June 1901, and by 1904, there were enough motor vehicles around to warrant the opening of the city's first automobile garage and creation of the Winnipeg Automobile Club. In 1912, the provincial government introduced the first *Manitoba Highway Act.*[33] Since the first North American automobile-attributed death in 1899, when New Yorker Henry Hale Bliss was hit by a motorized taxi, automobiles became a significant cause of trauma and often death or serious injury in the urban setting.

By the early 1900s, between the increase in violence related to the hotel strip, the booming (and dangerous) rail industry, and the introduction and rapid growth of the automobile (and related trauma), Winnipeg's existing ambulance services were falling short of meeting the city's needs for prehospital emergency transport and care.

33 Karen Nicholson. "Manitoba History: A.C. Emmett and the Development of Good Roads in Manitoba." *Manitoba History*, Manitoba Historical Society, Number 27, Spring 1994.

## 1910-1950

# Quest for a Municipal Ambulance Service

On August 15, 1914, 6500 kilometres away from Winnipeg's windy corner of Portage and Main, the Panama Canal opened. This was a faraway event that, after the end of World War I, would permanently decimate Winnipeg's economy and negatively affect its emergency medical services for the next 110 years.

While it seemed like a non-event to an emerging industrial hub in central Canada, it soon became a financial catastrophe for the city. From 1882 until 1914, Winnipeg's economy was based almost exclusively on the railway. Every commodity, from wheat to lumber to parts for new-fangled telephones, travelling across Canada needed to pass through Winnipeg. The railway and related industries kept Winnipeg's economy booming.

The newly-built Panama Canal shortened the distance ships travelled between the Atlantic and Pacific Oceans. It enabled shippers to transport goods across the North American continent faster and at less expense. Before the construction of the Panama Canal, a ship moving goods between San Francisco and New York had to cover 12,000 miles. After the canal was complete, the ship only traveled 4,000 miles[34]. Translated into Canadian terms, it was now cheaper to ship goods from Montreal to Vancouver (or vice versa) and then use regional rail services to transport the goods to a closer destination. A new demand for post-war consumer goods emerged after the war ended. Despite this increased demand, Winnipeg's rail services were not needed by Canada's transportation industry to the same degree to ensure supply. This decreased

34 WorldAtlas.com, "Why the Panama Canal was Built." https://www.worldatlas.com/articles/why-was-the-panama-canal-built.html. Accessed September 25, 2021.

need resulted in an implosion of Winnipeg's rail industry, causing thousands of jobs (and related businesses) within the city to evaporate almost overnight.

With a significant decrease in its formerly its robust rail industry, Winnipeg's economy plummeted. Besides the immediate loss of jobs in the rail sector, almost every other industry in Winnipeg—public and private—suffered job losses. When mixed with the addition of thousands of returning soldiers seeking employment, the ravishment of the city by the 1918 Spanish flu pandemic, and labour unrest demonstrated by the 1918 and 1919 Winnipeg General Strikes, the city's economy was in tatters. The Winnipeg Fire Department's closure of stations, Winnipeg Police Department's reduction of staff, and Bardal Funeral Home—a key supplier of private ambulance services in the city—ceasing its ambulance business, aptly illustrates the situation.

In a nutshell, Winnipeg's economy was a mess!

## Police Ambulances

In July 1890, not even a year after the Winnipeg General Hospital's ambulance service began operations, a new area of controversy emerged—one that is still ongoing 140 years later—the cost of using an ambulance. As reported in the *Manitoba Daily Free Press*, police typically took street accident sufferers to the nearest office of a "medical man" (a physician) and then subsequently to the hospital by ambulance—if the injured could afford the $0.75.[35] It is crucial to keep in mind that with the vast railway industry, Winnipeg was home to a large number of typically underpaid immigrant workers. The average worker in the early 1900s made $200 to $400 per year, so a $0.75 charge could represent a couple of days' wages; an expense that was well beyond the means of most labourers of the era.

In the early 1880s, many American municipal police departments acquired "patrol wagons" for carrying prisoners. The wagons were also often used to transport drunk prisoners, and the drunk prisoners were frequently lying down. It quickly became evident that the wagons could also transport injured citizens who were neither drunk nor prisoners.

In 1885, Toronto's police chief, Frank Draper travelled to several American cites to examine the new concept of a combination police

35 "The Hospital Ambulance." *Manitoba Daily Free Press.* July 11, 1890.

patrol wagon and ambulance.[36] Intrigued by the idea of an ambulance service provided to citizens for free, he began lobbying Toronto's city council for a similar system. As in Winnipeg, Toronto's General Hospital had already established a fee-for-service ambulance, but collecting payment was a problem.

Toronto Police's ambulance service was finally introduced three years later, in 1888, with a donation to the city of two horse-drawn ambulances/patrol wagons. A designated police driver staffed each unit. The Toronto police ambulances were provided on an optional payment system, enabling users to pay as they could. Toronto became the first city in Canada to have a free, publicly funded ambulance service. The following year, Toronto Police introduced first aid training for all of its officers, providing a first responder-type system throughout the city.

Winnipeg's police chief, John McRae saw the benefit of Toronto's system and started campaigning to get a police ambulance for the *Windy City*. In early 1895, he asked City Council for an ambulance and call box system.[37] Telephones had been introduced in Manitoba twenty years before and were rapidly gaining acceptance as a practical communication device. The idea was that with police call boxes on street corners throughout the city, a beat patrol officer could call into the police headquarters and request an ambulance or other assistance. In many ways, it was similar to a two-way radio or a cell phone today, albeit not as portable.

Unfortunately, Winnipeg council's response was not as positive as that of their counterparts in Toronto. It took sixteen years for a public ambulance and call box system to arrive in Winnipeg. Professor Alan Artibise's elitist analysis of Winnipeg's politics provides a compelling explanation for this delay.[38] From 1874 to 1914, Winnipeg's city council was comprised exclusively of business owners; citizens focused on promoting the city's commerce. While there is no evidence of "evil intent" on the part of Council, councillors saw little purpose in spending municipal funds unless it would directly benefit Winnipeg's growth and economy.

36 Bruce Newton. *Accidents, Illness and Sirens – The History of Toronto's Ambulance Services.* City of Toronto Paramedic Services. 2015: 101.

37 "Police Signal Service." *Manitoba Daily Free Press.* January 11, 1895.

38 Alan Artibise. *Winnipeg: A Social History of Urban Growth 1874-1914.* McGill-Queen's University Press. 1975.

## Health Issues Spur Change

Winnipeg had to deal with many serious health issues at the time, including regular epidemics of typhoid fever, smallpox, tuberculosis, venereal disease, scarlet fever, and diphtheria. However, as these conditions were seemingly, at least initially, restricted to the immigrants living in the North End, Council's attitude was that conditions were attributable to the "ignorance, laziness, and immorality of the North End's foreign population" and hence, were not the city's problem.[39]

At the time, health was not seen as a "public issue," resulting in nominal municipal expenditures in the area. For example, in 1898, Council budgeted $17,000 for the police department and $2,000 for the health department—of which $1200 was the salary of the health officer.[40] It seems that protecting the commercial elite's property was crucial, but addressing health conditions in the North End, where no councillors lived, was ignored.

In many ways, the mindset was understandable. People tend to view the world through their own experiences. If doctors were the primary health care providers at the time, and councillors had quick access to doctors—typically their neighbours—why would they believe it necessary to spend money on services that were already close at hand?

Serious typhoid outbreaks occurred each year, as evidenced by Winnipeg General Hospital's repeated requests, and eventual acquisition, of an infectious disease ambulance. The problem was routinely ignored by City Council until 1904, when there was a massive typhoid outbreak in the city. For the first time, the epidemic jumped the social barriers. Residents living in Point Douglas and Armstrong Point, the main living quarters of the city's economic elite, started dying. The issue was no longer viewed as a "foreigner problem" and was affecting members of City Council directly. Funny how when your own family members, and especially your children, start getting sick or dying, your perspective changes!

As a result, in 1905, the city councillors realized that an improved public health system might benefit them personally. This started the flow of funds for the city's health department and related facilities. They spent significant amounts of money upgrading the water system (which had been a key factor in the typhoid outbreak). Unfortunately, the funds were

39 Artibise (1975): 225.
40 Artibise (1975): 225.

used primarily to build a separate high-pressure water system for firefighting. While this took some of the strain off the domestic water system, it only supported firefighting efforts in the central business district.

After installing the high-pressure water system, City Council imposed a moratorium on further expenditures to improve the city's water supply until 1910. In fact, during this period, the city closed its water softening plant as a cost saving measure, and with the city's increasing population, the amount of fresh water supplied to the public significantly decreased per capita. With a city council disinterested in addressing such basic health issues as adequate water supply, it is of little wonder that a municipal ambulance service received minimal attention.

However, the door to funding *some* public health-related services had opened. Despite the moratorium on water supply expenditures, the city continued to fund the health department. In 1904, it had a budget of $36,000. This almost doubled in 1905 to $65,000 and doubled again in 1906 to $130,000. With the increased budget, the health department's staff almost tripled, going from fourteen in 1905 to thirty-four in 1906.[41] While the role of many of the new staff was the enforcement of health bylaws, the reality was, the increased concern about Winnipeg's health had a significant educational impact on the city. As Artibise points out, this led to a significant interest in preventative medicine, and to an even greater degree, a general response to health concerns within the city.

With Winnipeg's interest in public health evolving, another factor contributed to the growth of Winnipeg's emergency health care development—Winnipeg's main industry, the railway. With the Canadian Pacific Railway reaching Winnipeg in 1882 and Vancouver in 1886, Winnipeg had become the transportation hub for Western Canada. As the railway was an inherently dangerous industry, rail-related injuries skyrocketed as Western Canada's reliance on the railway increased.

## The Railway and St. John Ambulance

In 1893, St. John Ambulance—the British non-profit society which teaches first aid—set up its new "Dominion Branch" in Toronto. As a result, given the previously mentioned high incidence of injuries in the railway industry, the CPR started utilizing St. John's services to teach its employees first aid. Unfortunately, the Dominion Branch's influence never expanded

41 Artibise (1975): 225.

much beyond the Toronto-area. The teachings expanded nationally in 1910 when the Canadian Branch of St. John Ambulance received its charter, and provincial chapters began forming.

St. John set-up shop in Winnipeg in 1910 when the Canadian Pacific Railway's Weston Shops established the initial Manitoba chapter. The Weston Shops were a logical place for a first aid team. Employing several thousand workers, the Weston Shops repaired and maintained most of the CPR's engines, as well as repairing and building much of the company's rolling stock—injuries were plentiful and often significant. The CPR evidently saw a benefit to first aid training, as by July 1910, it gave the sixty-member club an hour a week to practice first aid skills.[42] As many of CPR's employees were British immigrants, they already had training with St. John Ambulance before immigrating to Canada. The CPR Chapter, in turn, recruited two Winnipeg physicians: Dr. Ernest Moorehead (also spelled Muirhead) and Dr. Robert Blanchard (the CPR's Chief Physician) to assist in giving team's training[43]. With the CPR's interest in first aid, the Weston Shops Chapter of St. John Ambulance began teaching first aid to other interested citizens, albeit, mainly railway employees, at the former Western Canada Railway Club; a social club for CPR employees.

As a result of the developing interest in first aid within Winnipeg's railway industry, in January 1911, Captain R.J. Birdwhistle, the General Secretary for St. John Ambulance Canada, arrived in Winnipeg to set up the official Manitoba chapter[44]. After its inaugural meeting on January 6, 1911, St. John began running first aid courses for the general public. The City of Winnipeg quickly jumped on board, and shortly after the Winnipeg chapter's February 5, 1911 inauguration, arranged for a first aid course for fifteen employees of the city's electrical department[45]. It likely seemed urgent as the recent electrocution of a Winnipeg citizen was negatively impacting the city's conversion to electricity, giving incentive for civic electrical employees to know first aid.

A further unit was established in Elmwood, shortly after Birdwhistle's visit. During this period, St. John Ambulance did a phenomenal job of marketing first aid training. Their senior members were visiting each

---

42 *Manitoba Free Press.* January 5, 1911.

43 "Firemen Win." *Manitoba Free Press Winnipeg,* December 11, 1911.

44 "St. John Ambulance Branch is Formed." *Manitoba Free Press.* January 7, 1911.

45 "Work of the St. John Ambulance Association in Winnipeg." *Manitoba Free Press: Winnipeg.* January 13, 1912.

province, they would recruit high profile members of the community to act as ambassadors, and the organization was very efficient at updating the local press of first aid training activities within their communities.[46]

Almost immediately after the city's electrical department received their training, the fire department's Chief Buchanan authorized a course for firefighters, and thirty-three firefighters subsequently received their first aid certificates. Despite Toronto Police's twenty-year involvement with first aid training, once Manitoba's St. John chapter was established, it took Winnipeg Police almost another year to organize training for its members.

## Combination Police Patrol Wagon and Ambulance

Even before Winnipeg police officers got first aid training, the Winnipeg Police Commission began the process of getting a police/public ambulance. While the original idea for Winnipeg's police ambulance was floated in 1895, it's not clear why the decision was finally made in 1911. Vancouver Police acquired their motorized ambulance in 1906, and Winnipeg Fire Department acquired their first motorized apparatus in 1910, so the motor-vehicle era was starting.

With Winnipeg needing a new police patrol wagon, combination patrol wagons/ambulances being popular with American police departments, and Winnipeg investing in public health, it may be that the stars aligned. In any event, the decision to purchase a motorized combination ambulance captured the uncertainty of the transportation industry at that time. According to its April 7, 1911 minutes, after approving the issuance of tenders for a Motor Police Patrol Wagon and Ambulance—combination vehicle, of 50 to 60 horsepower, the police commission also approved the purchase of two, two-horse hitch (horse-drawn) patrol wagons. Interestingly, the tender for the combination ambulance was published a few days earlier, on April 4, 1911,[47] suggesting that the recording of the decision in the police commission's minutes was more of an afterthought or formality.

A month later, on May 6, 1911, the police commission approved the purchase of a 1911 Speedwell chassised truck from Winnipeg's Breen Automobile Company for $5950.

---

46 McCreery (2008): 55.
47 *Manitoba Free Press*, April 4, 1911.

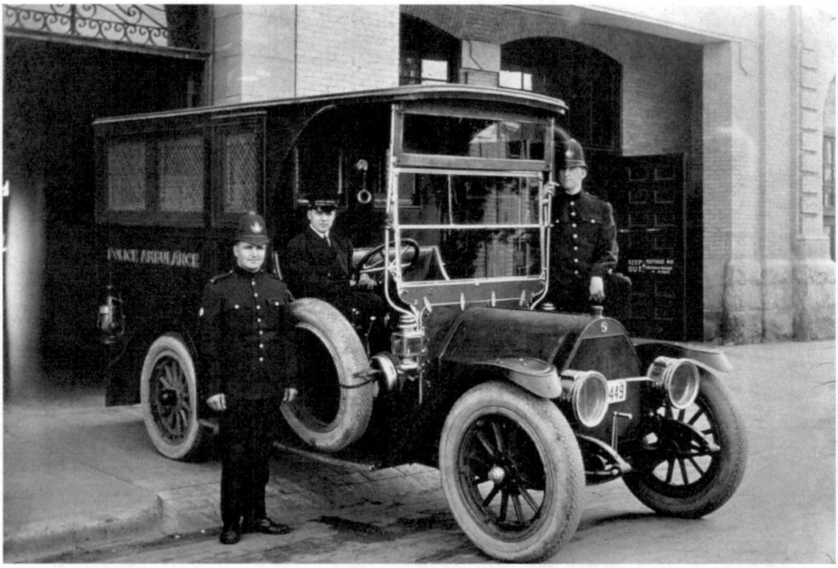


*Original 1911 Speedwell-chassied Winnipeg Police Ambulance. (Courtesy of WPS Archives)*

In preparation for the ambulance, in October, 1911, Alderman Herbert Gray went on a trip to Vancouver, British Columbia to examine the Vancouver Police Department's operations. As reported in the *Manitoba Free Press*: "The police ambulance attached to the department in Vancouver is also something which Winnipeg must have and which Ald Gray understands will shortly be added to Winnipeg's police department."[48] It seems that Alderman Gray's October 1911 assessment of Vancouver's police ambulance was more of an inquiry into procedure than assessing its necessity, given that the decision to purchase was made six months before. At the same time, the city began installing the long-awaited police signal/patrol box system, which, as noted by the *Manitoba Free Press*, would greatly speed up ambulance dispatch.[49]

The first newspaper reference to the ambulance's use is on January 19, 1912, when, as a result of a Logan Avenue collision between two streetcars, the police ambulance was needed to transport the injured to Winnipeg General Hospital.[50] There were subsequent reports of it being used on January 26, 1912 and January 27, 1912, with a local

48 "Nothing Better than Winnipeg." *Manitoba Free Press Winnipeg*. October 16, 1911.
49 "Signal System for Winnipeg Police." *Manitoba Free Press Winnipeg*. October 20, 1911.
50 "Motorman hurt in Head-on Collision." *Manitoba Free Press Winnipeg*. January 19, 1912.

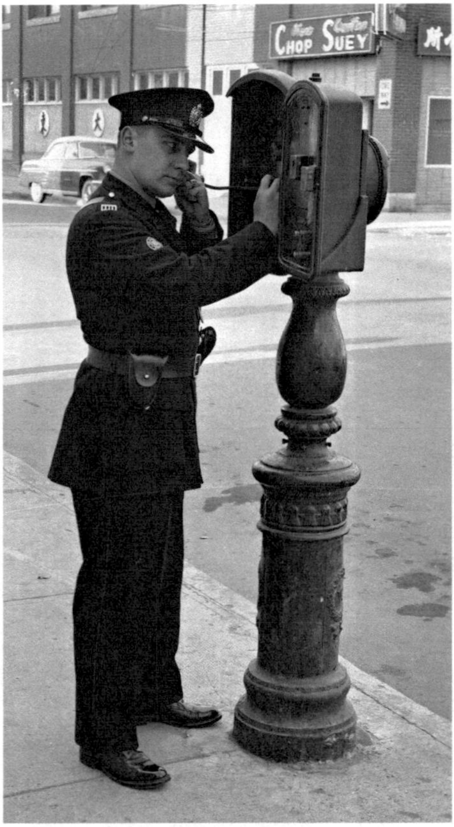


*Early 1910s-era Winnipeg Police street-corner call-box being used in the early 1960s. Instrumental in ensuring quick police ambulance response. (Courtesy of WPS Archives)*

doctor authorizing transport, as per procedure.

There was some delay in police officers receiving first aid training, but by February 22, 1912, shortly after WPD received its ambulance, the chief, deputy chief, two sergeants, four detectives, and forty-six constables had received first aid certificates.[51] As the first officers received their certificates, Sergeant Instructor John Patrick of WPD was running classes every day with the goal of having every one of Winnipeg's officers trained within a few months.[52] With the acquisition of the ambulance and first aid training, the WPD began providing public ambulance services to the community.

When looking at Winnipeg today, and most of North America, it may seem odd to have the police providing emergency care. This is more commonly tied to the fire service. However, at the turn of the twentieth century, Winnipeg Police were seen as the "go-to guys" for almost any problem. Officers were continually on the street, responding to whatever distress calls Winnipeggers could throw at them; providing aid for medical emergencies was a natural fit. It would not be until 1929 that Winnipeg's fire department started taking an active role in responding to non-fire-related emergencies.

Even as the new police ambulance was delivered, there was some debate as to who was better equipped to provide an emergency ambulance service.

51 "Constables Ambulance Men." *Manitoba Free Press Winnipeg.* February 22, 1912.
52 "Constables Ambulance Men." *Manitoba Free Press Winnipeg.* February 22, 1912.

In January, 1912, about the time that the new police ambulance arrived, there was an article in the *Manitoba Free Press, Winnipeg,* suggesting that a "major ambulance wagon" be established within the fire department, with emergency calls being directed to the fire stations.[53] Part of this is related to the already general mess that existed within Winnipeg's emerging ambulance industry.

At the time the above *Manitoba Free Press* article was written, Winnipeg firefighters had first aid training, but no ambulance. Winnipeg police had an ambulance, but police officers had no first aid training.

## Funeral Home Ambulances

Shortly after the turn of the century, and continuing into the 1910s, a number of Winnipeg's funeral homes began acquiring ambulances. J. Thomson and Company funeral home acquired the city's first automobile ambulance in June 1911. It was "to be used for accidents and other matters that demand speed as the essential factor."[54] Staff had no training except that acquired in handling corpses. Winnipeg's original ambulance provider, Winnipeg General Hospital, was operating two horse-drawn ambulances, and as noted below, acquired its first motorized unit in the spring of 1912. This service had been contracted out to Bardal's Funeral Home, until the motorized unit arrived. WPD's first motorized unit was delivered in December 1911/January 1912.

While there were numerous ambulances and some first aid training around Winnipeg, no one was equipped to provide proper on-call emergency transport to injured Winnipeggers. To be clear, by emergency transport, it is meant an ambulance equipped with the current first aid/emergency care equipment, and staffed on a full-time, twenty-four hour basis, with personnel with basic medical or advanced first aid training.

The acquisition of WGH's electric ambulance captured the state of the automobile industry at the time. There was fairly stiff competition between gasoline and electric vehicles, with a few manufacturers, such as White, using steam. WGH's new electric ambulance was an Indianapolis-built Waverley, ordered through the T. Eaton Company in August 1911, which finally arrived in the Spring of 1912. Capable of doing 20

53 "Work of the St. John Ambulance Association in Winnipeg." *Manitoba Free Press Winnipeg,* January 13, 1912.

54 "Automobile Ambulance for Winnipeg." *Manitoba Free Press.* June 3, 1911.

km/h, it came with electric heat; a bonus for Winnipeg's frigid climate. To aid during winter, WGH also built a garage beside the hospital's ambulance/casualty entrance.[55] As with most electric vehicles, it did not last long and was replaced by a gasoline-powered unit three years later. An interesting commentary of the times, the electric ambulance was used for paying patients, and the horse drawn unit (with coal-powered heat) was used for "public ward" patients[56]—many of whom lived in the city's poorer North End.

While not a very positive picture, it is important to appreciate the state of emergency care in the early 1900s. In a nutshell, emergency medicine didn't exist. The need for emergency intervention for trauma wasn't fully understood until the Korean War in the 1950s, and the specialty of emergency medicine was not recognized until the late 1960s. Ambulances until the early 1960s were a form of transportation which enabled the casualty to be transported lying down, and little else. When an injury occurred, the nearest doctor was usually summoned, and he (or on a very rare occasion, she) would patch the casualty up and with the help of whatever ambulance could be located, and order the casualty transported to either their own home or the hospital, as resources allowed, for a slow recovery.

While the need for a dedicated "emergency" ambulance system in Winnipeg had been acknowledged for fifteen years, the serious pitfalls in the existing system were not totally appreciated until March 7, 1912. During the Saturday night blaze at the Radford-Wright warehouse at 776 Main Street, six people, including two firefighters, died and nine people were injured. With five people being buried under a falling wall, it was Winnipeg's first recorded mass casualty event. Fortunately, the police department had started training its officers in first aid two weeks before the fire. As a result, the WPD's Sergeant Instructor Patrick and other officers were able to administer rudimentary medical care to the injured before the physicians arrived.[57] Nevertheless, in part because of limited emergency ambulance services, with no central coordination, there was a significant death toll.

---

55 "Modern Electric Ambulance for General Hospital." *Winnipeg Tribune.* January 20, 1912.

56 "Want Pay for Ambulance." *Winnipeg Tribune.* October 17, 1912.

57 "Six Lives Lost in Saturday Night Fire – Five of Victims Buried Under Falling Walls." *Manitoba Free Press Winnipeg,* March 11, 1912.

The Radford-Wright blaze helped to propel the WPD, with financial assistance from City Council, into providing a more reliable ambulance service. Two weeks after the blaze, WPD's Sergeant Instructor Patrick opened first aid classes at North and South police stations with the goal of training every officer in first aid.[58] A month later, Patrick recruited Dr. Alexander Douglas, the city's medical health officer, to give five lectures in advanced first aid, the "Medallion Course," to thirty six constables from all three stations.[59] This created a nucleus of officers who were competent to run an ambulance service. The training continued for the next ten months, and by February 1913, the final forty eight police constables received their first aid training. All Winnipeg police officers were now trained in first aid.[60] As the Department proudly announced, in the newest class, there wasn't a single failure.[61] At the 1913 Canadian police chiefs' convention, Toronto, Winnipeg, and Vancouver were recognized as the only cities where police officers were trained in first aid.[62]

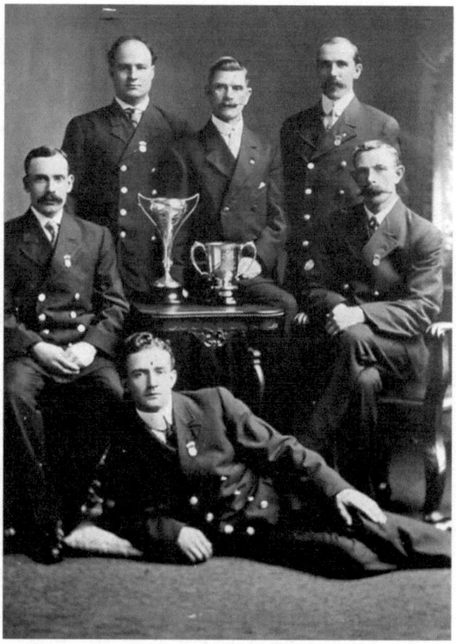

*Winnipeg Fire Department's first St. John Ambulance first aid team–1910. (Courtesy of FFHSW)*

## The Question: Who's Funding It?

While the Radford-Wright fire stimulated first aid training for all Winnipeg's police officers, there was also mounting public pressure, directed at City Council, emphasizing the need to properly fund a public ambulance service. On April 5, 1912, Winnipeg's Trades and Labour Council

58 *Manitoba Free Press.* Match 19, 1912.

59 *Manitoba Free Press.* April 17, 1912.

60 "Exceptional Result in Examinations." *Manitoba Free Press.* February 22, 1913.

61 "Exceptional Result in Examinations." *Manitoba Free Press.* February 22, 1913.

62 "More Barriers in the Path of Criminals." *Manitoba Free Press.* July 4, 1913.

passed a resolution asking the city to provide a public ambulance for immediate service for accidents. The resolution also stipulated that it be provided for free.[63]

Then, in September 1912, the *Winnipeg Tribune* began running a string of articles outlining the cost of ambulance services. It reported that Winnipeg General Hospital had racked up $800 in uncollectable contract ambulance fees for "charity patients."[64] This was followed up by an article a month later, noting that Winnipeg General Hospital had two ambulances: a horse-drawn ambulance and an electric. The electric ambulance was charged at $3 per trip, while the horse-drawn ambulance was free and used for public ward patients. The horse-drawn unit made 443 trips in 1912 and cost the hospital about $1,300. The article noted that the hospital board had asked the city again to pay the $2 fee for public ward patients.[65]

At a December 4, 1912 meeting of the city's Market, License, and Relief Committee,[66] a further complaint from the local plasterer's union was reviewed. In demanding a public ambulance service, similar criticisms to the earlier Winnipeg Trades and Labour Council complaint were raised. In a nutshell, the current private ambulance services were expensive, inefficient, and not readily available to people; the majority of the North End's population could not afford them.

The Committee also reviewed several complaints that the funeral homes, when sending ambulances, would not provide service unless paid. Bystanders had to contribute money before casualties were transported. The most extreme example reviewed was an accident at the Canadian Northern Railway (CNorR) railyards. After a three-hour wait and multiple follow-up calls, a private ambulance finally arrived. However, at this point, the attendant refused to treat or transport until one of the casualty's co-workers provided a guarantee of payment. As a final insult, the CNoR worker died enroute to the hospital.[67]

After investigating the issue, Mayor Richard Waugh reported to the Market, License, and Relief Committee that, from his inquiries,

---

63 "Wants Ambulance." *Manitoba Free Press Winnipeg*. April 6, 1912.
64 "Charity Ambulance Calls." *The Winnipeg Tribune*. September 12, 1912.
65 "Want Pay for Ambulance." The *Winnipeg Tribune*. October 17, 1912.
66 "Want Better Service." *Manitoba Free Press*. December 5, 1912.
67 "Want Better Service", *Manitoba Free Press*, December 5, 1912.

equipping public ambulances would cost about $18,000 per year.[68] He further indicated that he believed it made more sense to work out a better arrangement with the current roster of private ambulances. At the time, the city guaranteed the fees if either the police or a doctor authorized the ambulance. As Winnipeggers often requested an ambulance by calling the WGH or other service directly, the reimbursement system needed adjustments.

Two days later, on December 6, 1912, the Market, License, and Relief Committee met with owners of private ambulances, including Bardal Funeral Home, Clarke-Leatherdale Funeral Home, Clark Bros. and Hughes Funeral Home, Gardiner's Funeral Home, Kerr's Invalid Ambulance Service, J. Thomson Company—Undertaker, and Winnipeg General Hospital, Police Chief MacPherson, Fire Chief Buchanan, and various city physicians. Following City Council's past practices, the Committee confirmed that spending money on public ambulances was not appropriate. Instead, the Council continued promoting the city's business sector by guaranteeing the ambulance fees of all private operators when they responded to "accident cases" where the patient was unable to pay.[69] By making this commitment, City Council failed to address the real issue: how to provide adequate emergency ambulance services within the city. This decision exemplified the ongoing disconnect between Winnipeg's council and the realities of the city. Councillors were primarily focused on business development. For the most part Council was comprised almost exclusively of wealthier business/property owners. As a result, the need for an effective, cost-efficient ambulance service was not apparent to them.

This discussion would arise again in the 1960s, as private ambulance operators wanted to ensure that they were paid, and City Council did not want the police and fire services to provide ambulance services because of the cost.

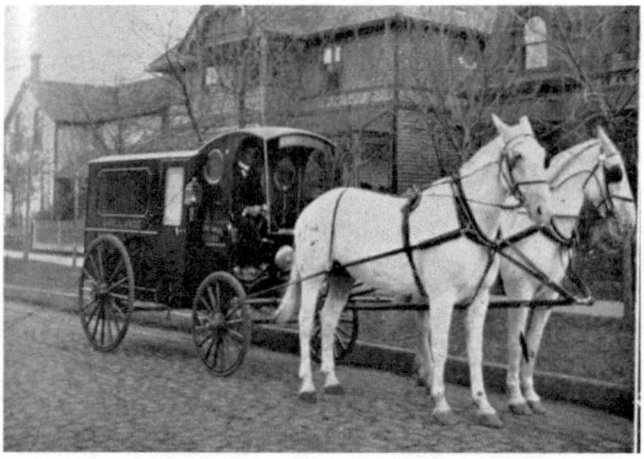

*Typical funeral home-run ambulance of the early 1900s. This unit was operated by Mordue Bros Ltd Funeral Home in 1903. (Courtesy of WCPI)*

68 "Want Better Service." *Manitoba Free Press*, December 5, 1912.
69 "City to Guarantee Fees." *Manitoba Free Press*. December 7, 1912.

City Council effectively avoided the establishment of an emergency ambulance service—a need that seemed apparent to everyone except Council. In response, the police department used creativity to partially address the need—at least for the short term. Given that the WPD had already acquired the Speedwell combination ambulance/patrol wagon in 1911, had officers trained in first aid, and as per City Council's directive was responding to injuries and accidents "on public property," it was not a significant step to adapt internally to accommodate the unmet need for an emergency ambulance.

With Vancouver and Toronto as templates for a police-based ambulance service, a month after having the request for a public ambulance service was shot down, on January 10, 1913, the city's police commission decided to reconfigure the WPD's motorized vehicles. It ordered the conversion of the chief's large 1906 Studebaker automobile into a patrol wagon for routine drunk transport. The Commission then delegated the larger 1911 Speedwell, now painted red, for ambulance duty and police raids.[70] With a prisoner transport body mounted on the Studebaker chassis, it enabled the police ambulance to be available for patient transport as needed and the patrol wagon to be used as a back-up ambulance on busy days.

While unwilling to support a municipal ambulance service, City Council appreciated the need for speedy emergency services. A few weeks after the WPD established its ambulance service, on February 4, 1913, the city passed a traffic bylaw giving fire apparatus, ambulances, and police vehicles the right of way over other traffic.[71]

The WPD formalized its "Patrol Wagon and Ambulance Service," once the police department's first aid training was completed, Three chauffeurs (two on the day shift, and one at night), three "wagon men," (attendants, or "police ambulance officers," with training in "first class" first aid) provided staffing for the service.[72] At the time, a police ambulance responded to all fires in the city and any injury which occurred on public property. However, the name of the service reinforced the overall view of ambulances at the time, with priority being on prisoner transport.

It's worth recognizing that while the WPD ambulance service was not an "emergency" ambulance service, *per se*, it was better than anything

---

70 *Manitoba Free Press.* January 11, 1913.

71 *Manitoba Free Press.* February 5, 1913.

72 E.C. Cleaver. *City of Winnipeg Police Department.* Winnipeg, 1920.

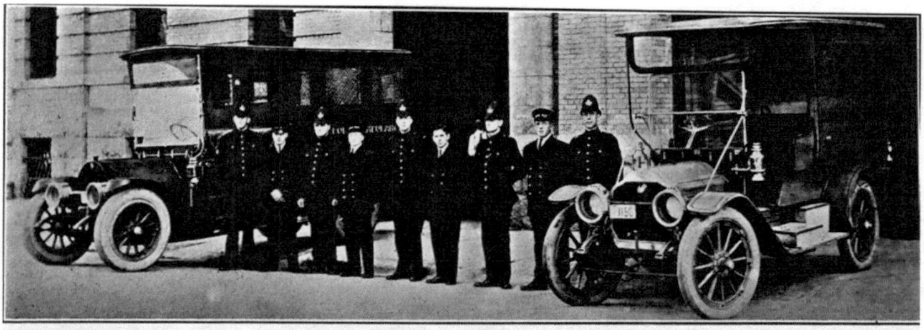

AMBULANCE AND PATROL WAGON MEN, 1913

*Winnipeg Police's Patrol Wagon and Ambulance Service – 1913; 1911 Speedwell on the left and 1906 Studebaker on the right. (Courtesy of WPS Archives)*

existing in Winnipeg at the time. To be an emergency service, it needed to have a dedicated driver and attendant who were assigned exclusively to respond immediately to emergency medical calls. With WPD's service, the staff were also assigned prisoner transport duties. With only one dedicated ambulance, WPD had neither the personnel nor the equipment to provide a proper emergency response.

The "Patrol Wagon and Ambulance Service" eventually evolved into the police department's chauffeur service. Wars and the Great Depression reduced personnel, and management's demands changed the role of drivers within the police ambulance service. It gradually became even less of an emergency response service and more of an "as time permits" responder.

As it turned out, the Speedwell chassis didn't last that long. In 1915, the police ambulance was involved in a significant mishap. On July 26 of that year, the police ambulance was taking nine-year-old Lottie Farquahar to WGH after a street car crushed her foot. Swerving to avoid a cyclist, the ambulance drove over the sidewalk at Sargeant and Sherbrook, hitting a cyclist and a tree, and then driving into McComb's restaurant where it drove over a pedestrian. Despite breaking all windows in the ambulance and bending the front axle, driver George Fogg and attendant J. Curtis loaded the additional casualties into the damaged ambulance and continued to the hospital. Fred Bowles, who was riding the bicycle, subsequently died. The pedestrian, Paulo Gails (or Gawlo—both names are used by the *Manitoba Free Press*), died at the scene.[73] While

73 "One Man Killed, Another May Die." *Manitoba Free Press*. July 27, 1915; "Fresh Feature to Monday's Fatality." *Manitoba Free Press*. July 28, 1915: "Jury on Double Killing." *Manitoba Free Press*. July 29, 1915.

Fogg was ultimately found blameless by the coroner's jury, it nevertheless found that ambulances, police vehicles, and fire engines travel too quickly on Winnipeg's streets. Interestingly, the jury did not take issue with the ambulance driver making use of the gong,[74] a criticism that was regularly raised by the news media before and after the accident. While the coroner's jury found no liability, Manitoba's Court of Kings Bench eventually found the City of Winnipeg liable for wrongful death and ordered it to pay Bowles' widow $12,000. Even though Bowles cut in front of the ambulance on his bicycle, he was not found to be contributorily negligent.[75] It appears that in the early days of motoring, excessive speed was the main concern.

While the police ambulance was severely damaged, the WPD continued to provide the ambulance service. Whether using the damaged Speedwell, or the back-up Studebaker patrol wagon is unclear, as newspapers of the time only mention the "police ambulance". However, the runs by the General Hospital's ambulance doubled; there were 184 trips in December 1914 (before the accident) versus 367 trips in December 1915 (after the accident).[76] This suggests that the police ambulance was being used less, with the work passed on to WGH's unit. It's important to remember that this damage occurred to the ambulance during World War I. As a result, purchasing a new motor vehicle would have likely been difficult, due to wartime restrictions.

Unfortunately, the process of offloading some of the ambulance work to WGH ended abruptly on March 21, 1917, when WGH's motorized ambulance was hit by a streetcar and destroyed[77]. While there was no indication of injuries, this put the WGH in a difficult position as its coal-heated, horse-drawn ambulance was now only used for "charity cases." There were no longer the resources to handle both the paying patients and the extra work from the WPD.

Immediately, WGH ordered a new REO truck chassis from Joseph Maw & Company, with bodywork by the Lawrie Wagon and Carriage Company. It seems that without the WGH hospital ambulance available, the police commission quickly realized how dependent Winnipeg had become on the police ambulance service. The request for tenders for a

---

74 "Exonerate Driver Police Ambulance." *Manitoba Free Press.* July 30, 1915.
75 "Verdict of $12,000 for the Plaintiffs." *Manitoba Free Press, Winnipeg.* June 17, 1918.
76 "Big Increase in Hospital Patients." *Manitoba Free Press.* January 10, 1916.
77 WGH Financial Committee minutes. March 23, 1917.

new chassis for the police ambulance was issued on April 10, 1917, and on April 28, 1917, the Police Commission announced that it was also awarding the $1600 ($400 cheaper than the WGH unit) contract for a new chassis to Joseph Maw & Company.[78] With both of the city's primary ambulances needing immediate replacement, it would have been more straightforward for the city to get war-time permission to purchase the new trucks.

Two months later, two complete ambulances arrived from Joseph Maw & Company. It seems that during the interim, the police commission had revised its order and purchased a new ambulance body from Lawrie Wagon and Carriage Company.[79] One unit was labeled for the Winnipeg General Hospital and the other for the Winnipeg Police. While the explanation for the addition of the new body for the police ambulance has been lost, given that the original body was damaged in the 1915 accident, it seems likely that either the police commission came to its senses and decided the replace the entire unit, or it was advised that the original body couldn't be mounted on the new chassis. Despite being replaced in 1917, between January and April 1920, the police ambulance was again repaired, and then completely renovated with a fully enclosed body and new, lighter paint scheme by Joseph Maw & Company. A best guess is that the new work was done to access materials that were not available earlier due to wartime restrictions. While records are sketchy, the bodywork was likely subcontracted to Lawrie Wagon and Carriage Company.

With the WPD's and the WGH's respective ambulance services back in full operation with new vehicles, the timing was perfect, as the end of World War I brought a flux of returning veterans with new health issues.

The First World War's end in November 1918 brought many returning soldiers to Winnipeg. While the underlying reasons have been lost over time, the police commission recommended that patrol and ambulance constables be selected from returning soldiers who were previous members of the department.[80] While the Commission's direction doesn't give a reason, one can speculate that it was concerned with job creation; presumptions that soldiers had more experience in doing first aid, had experience driving trucks, and that soldiers were likely better at han-

78 "Buy Auto Chassis." *Winnipeg Tribune.* April 28, 1917; "Police Buy New Chassis." *Manitoba Free Press Winnipeg.* April 28, 1917.

79 "Police Ambulance on Reo Chassis sold to City." *Winnipeg Tribune.* June 30, 1917; *Manitoba Free Press.* June 30, 1917.

80 "Winnipeg Police Ambulance." *2020 Winnipeg Police Museum Annual Report:* 23.

dling rambunctious drunks (the ambulance chauffeur would also drive the patrol wagon). At the same time, the hiring of soldiers, for a brief time, gave the Patrol Wagon and Ambulance Service a full complement of staff. Providing that the ambulance and patrol wagon were not being used for prisoner transport and there was a driver available, the ambulance could respond quickly for medical transport.

While the failure to find a suitable ambulance replacement for two years reinforced the point that civic leaders did not consider the police ambulance an emergency unit, the 1918 Spanish flu pandemic provided a final confirmation. With returning soldiers and less-than-ideal housing conditions in Winnipeg's North End, between October 1918 and February 1919, the city experienced the pandemic, an event often compared to the COVID-19 pandemic one hundred years later, but with a lot more deaths. With over 1,200 deaths and thousands sick, the city's hospitals were over-run with patients. As a result, during the peak of the pandemic, Winnipeg Police leased its ambulance to the Winnipeg Municipal Hospital Commission for about sixty five days, charging the Hospital Commission $530; $5/day plus repairs.[81] While the WPD had its patrol wagon as a back-up ambulance, it's open to speculation how much of an ambulance service was provided during this period. The Municipal Hospital, comprised of the King Edward Hospital (1912), the King George Isolation Hospital (1914), and the Princess Elizabeth Hospital (1950), appears to have purchased its own ambulance in 1921 and continued to provide a transfer service until 1950 when inter-hospital transfers were contracted out. Given that the Municipal Hospital was a sanitorium and isolation hospital, it provided transfer ambulance services as opposed to emergency ambulance-type responses.

While the WPD's ambulance service was a compromise by the police commission to cover for City Council's ongoing refusal to provide a municipal emergency ambulance service, the police ambulance continued to attract controversy. It's important to acknowledge the criticism of the service was typically directed at the management and organization of the service, both departmentally and at City Council level, and not individual ambulance officers. Despite the poor management, the ambulance division attracted many devoted constables whose efforts saved lives. Unfortunately, for the entire sixty three years of the service,

81 Winnipeg Board of Police Commissioners minutes, March 7, 1919.

it was never operated as a dedicated emergency ambulance. Rather it was a secondary service with constables and drivers normally assigned to other police duties, such as handling drunks, transporting prisoners, directing traffic, driving senior officers to meetings, etc. As a result, it was never used to its fullest potential.

Almost immediately after creating the Patrol Wagon and Ambulance Service, a debate arose about casualty transport. From the beginning, the police ambulance could only be used when requested by a physician or beat constable and only for an injury that had occurred on public property or at a fire. This ensured that the ambulance wasn't overused—a necessity when the police only had one designated ambulance for Winnipeg's 180,000-odd people. The tried and true method in Winnipeg of having a doctor assess the casualty before authorizing transport to a hospital had some detractors.

In March 1913, a Winnipegger accidentally drank poison and died; a fairly regular occurrence during this period. A Dr. Grieveson publicly complained that the police ambulance does not take the patient to the hospital immediately, but rather waits for a physician's assessment. Grieveson argued that more people would be saved if a doctor could command the ambulance to take the patient to the hospital (presumably without the doctor first assessing them). The rationale was that a doctor could not carry his equipment to a residence, and so it would be better to get the patient to a hospital for the needed equipment.[82] This debate would rage for several decades, until doctors ceased routinely making house calls and hospitals became seen as the place to go for medical help. As emergency medicine was not recognized as a medical specialization until the 1970s, it was assumed that any (and every) doctor had the necessary skills and training to deal with trauma.

As Winnipeg grew and fewer doctors were willing to respond to street accidents, the police ambulance began transporting patients more often without a doctor's direction. It is unclear whether this came about as a specific policy change or simply a reflection of changes in the availability of doctors.

In November 1922, the WGH Ambulance, assisted by Clark-Leatherdale's ambulance, responded to the St. Boniface College fire.[83] With no

---

82 "Drank Carbolic Acid by Mistake." *Manitoba Free Press.* March 31, 1913.
83 "Coroner Announces Inquest Unnecessary." *Winnipeg Free Press.* December 1, 1922.

assistance from WPD's ambulance and no public ambulance in Winnipeg's neighbouring community, St. Boniface (St. Boniface Police did not acquire their ambulance until 1926), WGH's ambulance crew found themselves handling ten dead and multiple living casualties.

As a result of the St. Boniface College fire, the WGH Board debated whether to start a hospital-based emergency ambulance service. Given the increased dependency on the WGH ambulance by the WPD to handle emergencies, and WGH's recognition of the financial need to get more patients coming through the front door, the concept of an emergency ambulance had merit. In questioning whether to purchase one or two new ambulances, one was most likely a replacement for the aging horsedrawn unit, and one was needed if WGH was to provide the new emergency ambulance service.[84] The Board eventually settled on one replacement ambulance and scrapped the emergency ambulance plan. Given that the hospital was facing financial difficulties and by 1924 had acquired a $50,000 deficit,[85] it's likely that the Board was doing a cautious cost analysis. WGH purchased a second replacement ambulance in 1928 but never instituted the plan for a more expensive emergency ambulance service.

An emergency ambulance—with single-purpose, full-time staff—was an expensive proposition. It was one that no agency in Winnipeg: City Council, the WPD, nor the WGH seemed willing to pursue. For a privately run hospital, having an emergency ambulance with single-purpose staff, when the goal was to increase the number of patients coming in the front door, was not cost efficient. The hospital already had two ambulances which could bring in most patients, albeit at a slightly slower rate. Even with a true emergency ambulance service, only about ten percent of calls are medical emergencies: calls where a person's life is dependent on the speed of the response.

As noted in the 1922 WGH board debate, there really wasn't an emergency ambulance in Winnipeg, meaning an ambulance that was fully staffed, on standby, and ready to respond twenty-four hours a day. In this era in Winnipeg, when you called for an ambulance, whether it be one of the funeral homes, WGH, or WPD, unless there happened to be staff available, an ambulance typically took more than twenty minutes to arrive.

---

84 Winnipeg General Hospital Annual Report, 1922: 20.

85 "City Hospital at Parting of Ways Symington Says." *Winnipeg Tribune.* December 13, 1924.

## Effects of the Economy

With the end of the First World War, the opening of the Panama Canal, and the evaporation of Winnipeg's rail industry, Winnipeg's economy went into a serious tailspin. These occurrences had a significant impact on Winnipeg's prehospital transportation industry.

At the turn of the century, many of Winnipeg's funeral homes acquired ambulances and were providing either "accident" or "invalid/transfer" ambulance services—albeit, the distinction often wasn't made. By 1928, Clarke-Leatherdale Funeral Home, Clark Brothers and Hughes Funeral Home, Coutu Funeral Home, Gardiner's Funeral Home, Kerr's Invalid Ambulance Service, Mordue Bros Funeral Home, and J. Thomson Company were all operating ambulance services.

While the concept of running an ambulance service seemed appealing, providers discovered that business-wise, it wasn't cost-efficient, and in 1923, Bardal Funeral Home withdrew from the ambulance business. This started a gradual exodus of funeral home-based ambulance services.

Although Winnipeg General Hospital and Winnipeg Police also provided ambulance services, none of the providers were overly efficient in their response times when it came to emergencies.

## Winnipeg Fire Department Rescue Squad

While not speeding up ambulance response times, in 1928 the Winnipeg Fire Department (WFD) took steps to improve emergency medical response in the city. In addition to their fleet of engines and ladder trucks, the WFD followed a growing North American trend and added a "rescue squad" to their roster. While the primary purpose was to carry the recently developed self-breathing apparatus, a device which enabled firefighters to walk into smoke or chemical-filled rooms, the rescue squad also carried a variety of non-firefighting rescue equipment, including extrication gear, cutting tools, and first aid supplies, such as pulmotors/resuscitators (at the time, these were basically bicycle pump-like contraptions which forced air into a person's lungs) and inhalators (which provided a steady stream of oxygen or a mixture of carbon dioxide and oxygen) to help unconscious people breathe.

The rescue squad's equipment enabled a non-breathing casualty to get oxygen therapy before arriving at the hospital. Unfortunately, it was thirty-years before the introduction of Winnipeg's three-digit, all-encompassing emergency phone number. As a result, unless the caller knew to contact the WFD, or a doctor or police officer requested the WFD's response, this service wasn't utilized as often as it could or should have been.

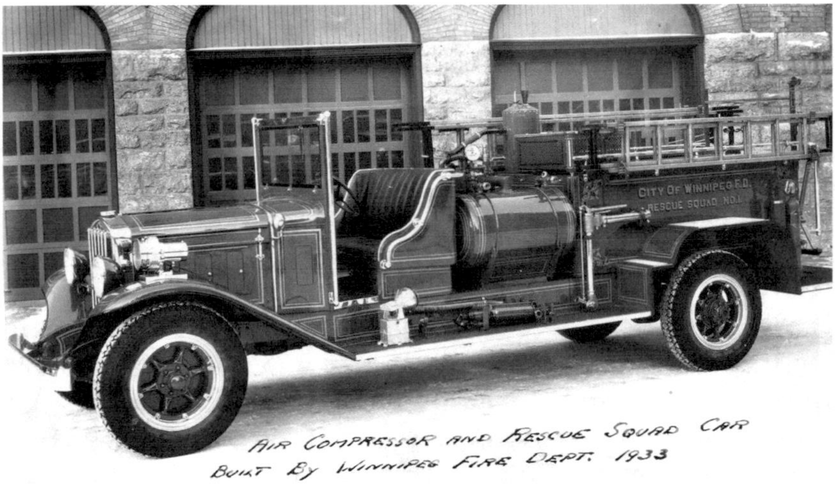


*Winnipeg Fire Department's 1933 Diamond T-chassised Rescue Squad, a replacement for the original 1928 unit. While not used for patient transport, it was instrumental for quickly delivering emergency first aid, including oxygen and pulmotors, throughout the city. (Courtesy of FFHSW)*

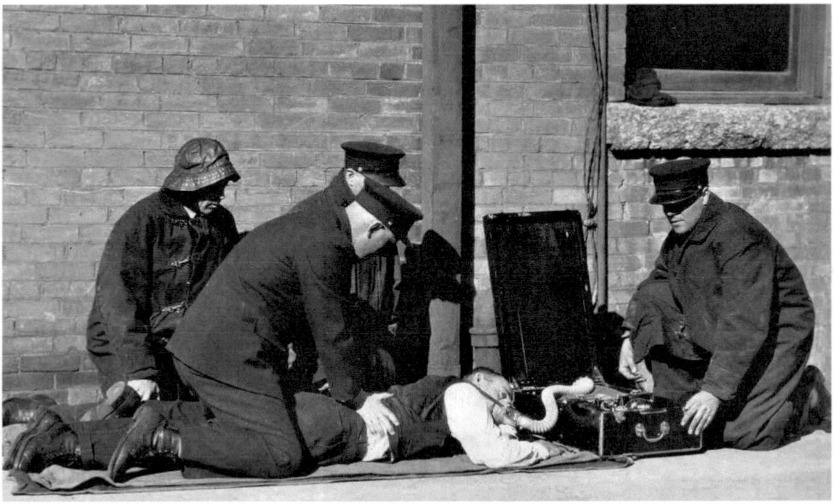

*Winnipeg firefighters in action in 1930, resuscitating a casualty using a pulmotor and the Shafer method of artificial respiration. The picture appears to have been staged. (Courtesy of FFHSW)*

Other than allegations of misuse within the WPD, little has been written about ambulances in Winnipeg from the late 1930s to the mid-1940s. Between the unfavourable economics of the Great Depression and the subsequent Second World War, there was a serious decrease in the number of ambulance providers in Winnipeg. To make matters worse, with the WPD's staffing cuts during the 1930s and the exodus of officers leaving for military service (so many that the WPD had to start rehiring retired and former members in order to maintain adequate service levels) the WPD ambulance service got short shrift. There were five drivers assigned for all vehicle-related assignments at headquarters, with no one specifically assigned to drive the ambulance and no ambulance attendants.[86]

Interestingly, when the department installed two-way radios in all of its police vehicles, it only installed a one-way system in the ambulance. As reported in the *Winnipeg Free Press*, the ambulance was used primarily for hauling bootleggers, gamblers, and drunks, indicating that even the ambulance was being used more often as a prisoner transport patrol wagon.[87] Even if partially correct, this observation raises concerns about the ongoing availability of the police ambulance.

At the same time, with 1,104 people injured in motor vehicle accidents in 1937, the WPD's accident prevention car, a Nash LaFayette sedan, was designed so that it could be converted into an ambulance as needed.[88] Unfortunately, it's debatable whether a convertible police vehicle, the driver of which was assigned to conducting vehicle inspections throughout the city, and an ambulance-turned-patrol wagon, without a designated driver except when hauling reprobates, could provide a particularly efficient ambulance service.

Nevertheless, the combination accident prevention car/ambulance was replaced in 1941 with a Nash Ambassador 600 Sedan.[89] It appears to have gotten a significant amount of use, in that in 1942, it was further replaced by an International Harvester K2 panel truck.[90]

---

86 "Winnipeg's Police Protection Among Best on Continent", *Winnipeg Free Press.* December 29, 1939.

87 C.E. Louth. "Winnipeg Police Force Growth Reflects Changing Times", Winnipeg Free Press, Feb 12, 1938.

88 "Slayers, Bank Robbers Give City Wide Berth; Fatality Toll is Lower." Winnipeg Free Press. February 28, 1938.

89 Winnipeg Police Commission Minutes, November 28, 1940.

90 Winnipeg Police Commission Minutes, March 6, 1942

This situation was ripe for investigation. When it allegedly took the police ambulance, driven by the department's assistant mechanic, two hours to arrive at an emergency call, City Council established the Donovan Commission under the Manitoba Evidence Act to investigate the misuse of police resources. Amongst other irregularities, with no specifically assigned ambulance drivers, it found that the Chief Constable (in addition to the forementioned reprobates) was often chauffeured in the police ambulance. Other police vehicles were used to chauffeur the police magistrate, deputy chief, detective inspectors, senior officers' children, and the maid of the deputy chief, leaving the ambulance without a driver for actual emergencies. This led to the assistant mechanic or other hastily recruited driver operating the ambulance.

The need to find a replacement driver in an emergency was a significant problem. In the late 1930s and 1940s, many people did not have driver's licences, including, ironically, the sergeant in charge of cruiser cars,[91] so any on-duty officer did not necessarily have the ability to drive the ambulance. This led to ambulance response calls routinely taking twenty five minutes.[92] While Justice Donovan ultimately did not find serious misconduct within the department, he did conclude that the use of police vehicles for private purposes was improper and detrimental to the operations of the WPD.[93]

With police chauffeurs relegated to only driving senior officers on official business, and not the management's kids or maids, it suggests that the ambulance became available for its intended use – when a driver was available. As a result, in 1941 the department acquired a new custom-built Seibert-Ford ambulance. This appears to be the first stretched, automobile-based single-purpose ambulance on the WPD roster, providing a much smoother, comfortable ride for patients. The design also ensured that it could not be used as a make-shift patrol wagon. Unfortunately, due to having no assigned driver, and the chauffer department often driving one of the two patrol wagons, it seems that often the WPD would pick up accident victims in the patrol wagon as opposed to returning to the garage to get the ambulance. While not ideal for the patients, except for perhaps providing a faster response time, it certainly reduced wear

91 "Police Probe." *Winnipeg Free Press.* March 5, 1940; "Probe Hears Police Cars Used Privately." *Winnipeg Free Press.* May 11, 1940.

92 "Police Probe." Winnipeg Free Press. March 5, 1940; "Probe Hears Police Cars Used Privately." *Winnipeg Free Press.* May 11, 1940.

93 "Probe Finds all Charges Not Proven." *Winnipeg Free Press.* October 1, 1940.

and tear on the ambulance. The WPD didn't have to replace it for thirteen years, despite there being a severe deficit of ambulances in the city.

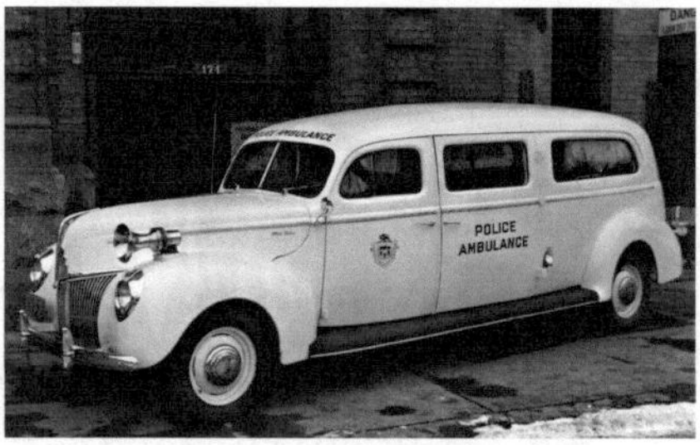

*Winnipeg Police's new 1941 Siebert-Ford ambulance. (Courtesy of Ford Motor Company Archives)*

It appears that by 1943, the only emergency-type ambulances in Winnipeg were the WPD's 1941 Siebert-Ford and the previously mentioned 1942 International Harvester K2 combination accident prevention/ambulance unit. In response to a major highway accident in October 1943 where nine people were injured, both police ambulances responded, as well as one of Kerr's Invalid Ambulance Service's transfer/non-emergency ambulances. Two additional ambulances had to be requested from the Canadian Army's depot in Winnipeg.[94]

In response to the Donovan Commission's findings, and the fact that WPD was now providing the only service that resembled an emergency ambulance in the city, at the end of 1942, the Police Commission introduced formal regulations for the police ambulances' use:

> 172. The patrol wagon and ambulance shall be under the direction of the Operator-Despatcher on duty, but the Constable in charge will not be restricted by the instructions of the Operator-Despatcher and will act in the interest of the public as may be necessary.
>
> 173. The ambulance is intended for the removal of sick and injured persons from the streets to their homes or a hospital. Infectious or contagious cases shall not be removed in the ambulance. The ambulance shall not be used for an emergency occurring outside the city. Except in cases of accident or emergency, the ambulance shall not be used to remove any person from his home to a hospital.
>
> …
>
> 176. The driver shall notify the Operator-Despatcher immediately of the return to the garage after answering a call.

94 "1 Dead, 8 Hurt in Car Crash On Smoky Road." *Winnipeg Tribune*. October 4, 1943.

177. Drivers of the patrol wagon and ambulance shall respond promptly to the instructions of the Operator-Despatcher.

178. Constables assigned to attend a patrol wagon or ambulance call shall be in command of the patrol wagon or ambulance and the drivers shall follow their instructions.

179. Constables on regular patrol wagon and ambulance duty will perform such duties as may be assigned to them by the officer in charge of the station. The Constable on first day relief shall be responsible that the equipment of the ambulance and patrol wagon is complete and in good order.

180. Except in cases of great emergency, drivers of the patrol wagon and ambulance shall obey the following instructions:

(a) The use of the siren is prohibited.

(b) The vehicle shall be driven within the speed limit prescribed by law.

(c) All traffic lights, stop signs and other traffic signs and regulations shall be obeyed.

Cases of great emergency include the pursuit of suspected offenders, calls to robberies, riots, murders and instances in which the officers have good reason to believe life is at stake.[95]

By January 1946, the issue of police patrol wagons transporting street accident victims to hospital in particular, and the state of ambulances in the city in general, was raised by City Council. The debate started with Alderman William Scraba expressing concerns about a personal friend receiving emergency transport in a patrol wagon, which led to a heated discussion about ambulance services in Winnipeg. As usual, the debate captured the spectrum of beliefs, ranging from Alderman Jack St. John stating that the city wasn't "in the ambulance business" to Alderman Brotman expressing concerns that only drunks, and not private individuals, were getting rides in ambulances.[96]

95 Winnipeg Police Commission Minutes, December 28, 1943.

96 "Ambulance Service Gets Aldermen In Argument." *Winnipeg Free Press.* January 31, 1946.

In an attempt the clarify, the city's medical health officer pointed out that there were two private ambulance services in Winnipeg – Kerr's Invalid Ambulance Service, and J. Thomson Company, and two in St. Boniface – Coutu Funeral Home (which had bought up both Clarke-Leatherdale and Mordue Brothers Ltd.) and Desjardin Funeral Home, and the police ambulance service; which often used the patrol wagons for patient transport. After Alderman Scraba raised concerns about street accident victims waiting twenty minutes in sub-zero temperatures, council agreed to get an opinion from the Winnipeg Medical Association as to whether Winnipeg had a sufficient number of ambulances.[97]

Six months later, Council received a response from the Winnipeg Medical Association, confirming that in its opinion, given Winnipeg's size, the number of ambulances was adequate.[98] The problem was that at the time, few people in Winnipeg understood the difference between an "emergency ambulance" and a "transfer ambulance". In the Winnipeg Medical Association's assessment, they counted four privately-run transfer ambulances and one partially staffed police ambulance and came up with five ambulances. This seems to suggest that the WPD's combination accident prevention car/ambulance was no longer being used as an ambulance – bringing the number of quasi-emergency ambulances in the city down to one.

It is likely that Winnipeg was compared to Toronto, with its three full-time, city-run emergency ambulances (with medically trained crews), one spare/infectious disease unit, plus several private ambulances that did transfer work and contract emergency response.[99] The Winnipeg Medical Association also likely considered Edmonton, which had the city ambulance service, operating out of Royal Alexandra Hospital, where a driver and an intern would respond, and three private ambulance companies: one with one ambulance, one with two (but often neither worked), and one had four units. While Edmonton, like Winnipeg. had no dedicated emergency ambulance, it technically had eight ambulances.[100]

The Winnipeg Medical Association report was "filed" by the city council, but the issue was far from settled. If members of city council believed that the police ambulance service was substandard, and the

97 "Ambulance Service Gets Aldermen In Argument." *Winnipeg Free Press.* January 31, 1946.

98 "Aldermen Who Quit Early Draw Blast." *Winnipeg Free Press.* June 6, 1946.

99 Newton (2017): 136.

100 Plumbtree (2011): 205.

WPD wouldn't change the way it operated the service, it was only a matter of time until the issue arose again.

In August 1948, one of Alderman John Blumberg's friends died as a result of a traffic accident, a death that potentially could have been prevented had there been a proper ambulance response. As a result, Blumberg recommended to the Civic Finance Committee that they budget for a municipal emergency ambulance; something more effective than the police ambulance for accident calls. Before making a decision, the committee referred the matter to the police commission.[101]

Little happened, as the police commission wasn't in a position to change how the police ambulance was managed. Things changed on August 21, 1949, when eleven people were injured in a motor vehicle – train accident at Nairn and Eaton. Using the ambulance, patrol cars, and unmarked detectives' cars to transport casualties, it was clear that with the absence of ambulances in the city, both Winnipeg and the WPD were unequipped to handle multiple casualty events.[102]

A month later, the front page of the Winnipeg Tribune described how the police ambulance had taken half an hour to respond to a sixteen-year-old boy whose friend had accidentally blasted him with a shotgun.[103] As the police only requested the fire department's rescue when there was a respiratory problem, there was a significant delay in getting help for the badly bleeding teen. These incidents, combined with the fact that despite it being part of its defined mandate, the police ambulance hadn't been responding to structure fires within Winnipeg for years, was enough to show the change was necessary.

As will be discussed below, in 1946-47, private ambulance services began making their appearances on Winnipeg streets, and were responding to some emergency calls. However, these services were mainly created to respond to the increased medical needs of returning World War II veterans, and were not a substitute for a publicly operated emergency ambulance service.

It appears that a growing number of aldermen were in support of an emergency ambulance for the city. This, combined with a new fire chief, David Clawson, who proposed minimizing cost by creating a new fire

101 "Ald. Blumberg Urges Better System of Caring For Accident Victims." *Winnipeg Free Press.* August 27, 1948.

102 "Head-On Collision Injures 11 Persons." *Winnipeg Free Press.* August 22, 1949.

103 "Boy Critically Wounded in Play Duel." *The Winnipeg Tribune.* September 22, 1949.

department vehicle that combined a needed replacement rescue squad with an ambulance, finally gave Council a solution that it could accept. Like many other Canadian fire departments, for example Toronto[104], and Vancouver[105] providing first aid/inhalator service at a doctor's (or police) request, the WFD had already established a record of fast responses to medical emergencies with their non-transport rescue squad. Given the discontent amongst council members with the WPD's ambulance service, a patient transport-capable rescue squad to augment the WFD's twelve-year-old open rescue unit was a fairly easy sell.

During this period, there was no criticism directed at the individual officers who worked on the police ambulances. Nothing suggests that they were anything besides dedicated, committed, and effective. As noted in the *Winnipeg Tribune* at the time, in an article about WGH's Casualty Ward: "Dr. Govan praised the city police ambulance service which brings most of the serious accident victims to the hospital. 'They do a very good job,' he said."[106] The issue was how the police ambulance service's resources were utilized.

Respecting the new rescue squad, prior to Clawson being appointed as the new fire chief, he had been the department's master mechanic. In that role, he had gained a reputation for building inhouse, creative, multi-purpose fire apparatus. This background gave him the skills to design a rig that both met the fire department's needs and addressed City Council's concerns respecting the acquisition of a fully staffed emergency ambulance.

After becoming Chief and inheriting the quest for a department ambulance, Clawson immediately saw a solution in American "disaster wagons." These units were being built by numerous American fire departments as the Cold War-era evolved, which combined rescue gear transport with medical treatment/transport in the same vehicle.

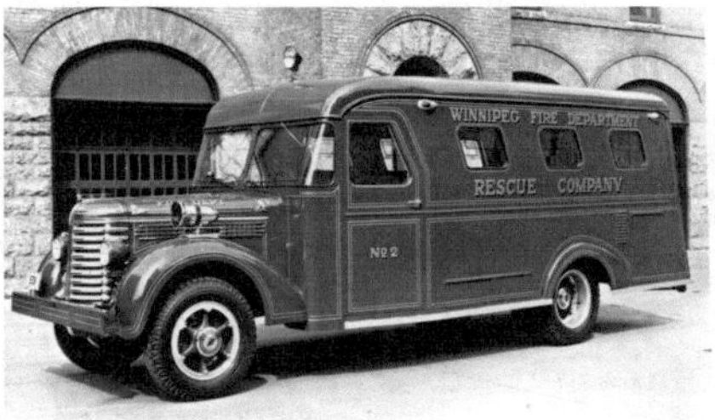


*In 1949, after a twenty-year fight with city council, the Winnipeg Fire Department finally got its enclosed combination rescue squad/ambulance approved; a 1949 Diamond T/WFD shop built commercial van. (Courtesy of FFHSW)*

104 Newton (2017): 144.

105 Matches (2016): 190.

106 Glenn McDougall. "Doctors See Death Drama, Urge Need of City Safety." *Winnipeg Tribune.* October 24, 1949.

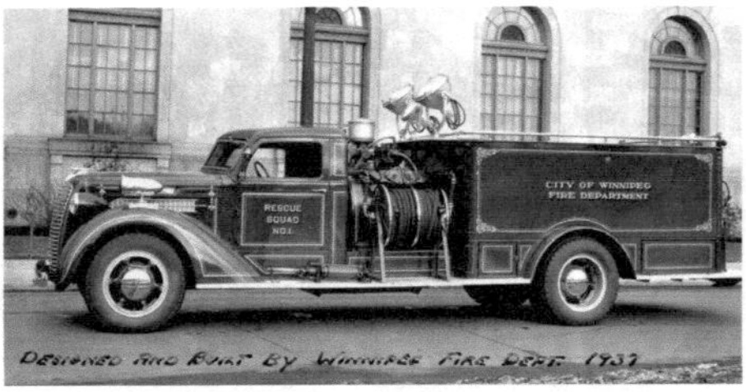


*Winnipeg Fire Department's Rescue 1, a 1937 Diamond T-chassised rescue squad, used for carrying the heavy rescue gear so that Rescue 2 could be used as an ambulance. (Courtesy of FFHSW)*

With Council's blessing, in late 1949 the WFD purchased a Diamond T commercial van and converted it into a rescue/ambulance ("Rescue 2"). It formally went into service in March 1950.[107] Normally, this design would create a problem at accident scenes. After removing the rescue tools needed for an extrication, the casualty couldn't be transported immediately because the gear had to be reloaded into the truck. Winnipeg Fire Department got around this problem by keeping its 1937 rescue squad ("Rescue 1") in operation as an "equipment transporter," carrying heavy gear like the generator, air compressor, etc. When responding to a situation where crews needed extensive rescue equipment, they could rely on the equipment from Rescue 1 and then transport the patient in Rescue 2.

Rescue 1 could also provide independent initial response, allowing the WFD to provide inhalator/first aid services to two medical calls at once. All firefighters were trained to use the equipment[108], so it was easy to interchange crews. Winnipeg finally had an ambulance that could respond, day or night, immediately to serious medical emergencies. While it was not a perfect system – one fire department emergency ambulance that could respond immediately, and a police ambulance (and a patrol wagon that doubled as an ambulance) that could respond as staffing permitted – it provided a means for Winnipeg's seriously sick and injured to get help quickly.

## Veterans Return and the Canadian Taxi Wars

As Winnipeg's City Council was wrestling with what to do about municipal emergency ambulances, thanks to the taxicab industry, an odd solution arose to the address the lack of private ambulances in the city; an absence created when Winnipeg funeral homes vacated the quasi-emergency medical transport industry.

---

107 "Fire Dept. Life Savers." *Winnipeg Tribune.* March 20, 1950.
108 "Fire Rescue Wagon Proves Life Saver." *Winnipeg Tribune.* March 16, 1950.

The end of World War II brought the challenge of reintegrating thousands of returning soldiers into the workforce. Many of the cab owners/drivers who left the taxi industry for military service came home expecting to take up their old profession. Also, the industry's prosperity, thanks to the post-wartime economy, attracted newcomers to apply for cab licences. The sudden glut of licence applicants presented the industry with a significant problem. Governments were understandably not keen to deny veterans access to cab licences, but there needed to be some control. Winnipeg's Transit Control – responsible for licensing taxis – began relaxing quotas on taxi licenses as early as 1944. In 1946 the Manitoba Taxicab Board approved 60 new licences.[109] However, a problem arose in December 1946, when Transit Control set the maximum number of taxi licences in the city at 400. This number remained frozen for the next three decades.[110]

Despite the freeze, there was a loophole. While taxis were heavily regulated, there were no restrictions for running an ambulance; a taxi for people lying down. Winnipeg didn't introduce its first ambulance bylaws until January 1, 1962.[111] This enabled people who wanted to get into the taxi-related industry but who couldn't get one of the exclusive taxi licences to still compete… sort of.

There was a second, corresponding issue that needed an immediate solution. As part of the services provided by the Department of Veterans Affairs (DVA) was free health care, including ambulance services, to all veterans for the first year after their release from service. In a city like Winnipeg, where there was a serious void in the number of ambulances, this created an interesting business opportunity; especially when there were no regulations.

The first to take advantage of this opportunity, in March 1946, were Maurice Prince and Napoleon "Johnny" Prince, two brothers from St. Boniface. As they were both Second World War veterans, and the DVA was in need of ambulances, the DVA was anxious to help them develop their new business venture – a win-win for everyone involved. The Prince brothers rebuilt a 1939, seven-passenger Buick sedan into an ambulance and began marketing themselves as Prince Brothers Ambulance Ser-

---

109 "60 Veterans Allowed Taxi Cab Licenses." *Winnipeg Tribune.* July 30, 1946.

110 Donald F. Davis. "The Canadian Taxi Wars, 1925-1950." *Urban History Review.* 27(1) (1998): 17.

111 "Licensed Men Behind the Siren." *Winnipeg Tribune.* August 22, 1961.

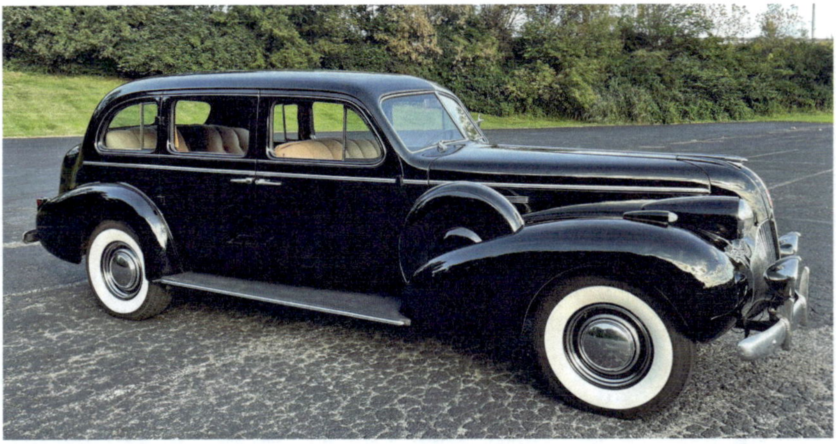

*While not the actual Prince Brothers' ambulance, this 1939 Buick Limited nine-passenger sedan appears to be an identical model. By cutting out the "B" pillar (the roof support between the front and rear passenger-side doors), and removing the seats, the sedan could neatly carry a sideloaded stretcher. (Courtesy of Connors Motorcar Company)*

vice. While Maurice had previously worked for an undertaker,[112] neither seems to have had any specific medical training. DVA assisted by giving them a significant amount of contract work – transporting veterans to and from Deer Lodge Hospital. With its first advertisement appearing in the Winnipeg Free Press on June 17, 1946, Prince Brothers Ambulance Service appears to be the first stand-alone ambulance business in the city. It lasted until being amalgamated into the second generation of Winnipeg's private ambulance services in the early/mid 1950s.

## More Independents

The following year, in 1947, Veterans Taxi, a consortium of independent taxi owners (all or most of whom were World War II veterans), took advantage of the same factors: a definite need, not enough taxi licenses, and no ambulance regulations. They incorporated the "Greater Winnipeg Veterans Ambulance Service." While it employed eight veterans to staff its two ambulances, despite the need, it soon became obvious that the problem faced by ambulance services in Winnipeg for the previous sixty years remained the same; It wasn't profitable!

---

112 James C. Anderson. "Prince Brothers Open Ambulance Service." *Winnipeg Tribune.* July 27, 1946.

At first blush, it seemed like an astute move. If Winnipeggers were already calling for taxi rides to the hospital, and the DVA was paying for veterans' ambulance services, providing ambulances at a slightly higher rate than taxis made good business sense. However, by 1948, Veterans Ambulance was already seeking financial assistance from the City of Winnipeg to keep its operations running.[113]

While it is not clear whether the city provided Veterans Ambulance with a grant, things went from bad to worse for both Veterans Ambulance and Prince Ambulance in 1949 when the DVA set up its own ambulance service to transport veterans. This took away significant business from the two private companies. The DVA's ambulance, a 1949 Chevrolet sedan, was painted either black or dark blue with limited warning devices. As a result, the two private ambulances providers got a slight reprieve in January 1951 when the DVA's ambulance was hit and wrapped around a telephone pole while transporting patients to Deer Lodge Hospital.[114] The DVA's ambulance was eventually replaced, and Deer Lodge Hospital/DVA continued providing ambulance services for veterans until the early 1970s.

Unlike taxi cabs, which on a busy day or by parking on the right street corner seemed to attract an endless supply of customers, private ambulances were stuck waiting until someone got sick or injured. While repeat customers needing help with patient transfers, such as Deer Lodge Hospital, helped to a degree, it soon became evident that running an ambulance service was very different than a taxi company. With minimal possibilities of breaking even financially, in North America, many operators subsidized the service with some other commercial enterprise or went out of business entirely. As a startling example of this reality, of 425 ambulance operators identified in Ontario in 1964, 345 or 81 percent were no longer in business in 1981 – just seventeen years later.[115]

Veterans Ambulance, like the Prince Brothers Ambulance Service, hobbled along until 1954, when they were both purchased and absorbed into the second generation of Winnipeg's private ambulance services.

(I will cover more of the private ambulance wars in the next chapter.)

113 "Vet Ambulance Seeking Grant." *Winnipeg Tribune.* December 31, 1948.

114 "Veteran Dead, Two Hurt In Car-Ambulance Crash." *Winnipeg Free Press.* January 20, 1951.

115 Hanna (1982): 64.

## Changes in 1950

Through the fire department, Winnipeg finally established a public ambulance that could respond quickly to emergencies. Whether efficient in the long run with one unit and its crew of five (later reduced to four firefighters), is another issue. While the city also had an emerging private ambulance industry, the 1950 flood firmly captured the state of Winnipeg's ambulance services.

In early May 1950, the run-off from the previous winter's heavy snow was invading Winnipeg and the Red and Assiniboine Rivers were rising at an astronomical rate. Thousands of volunteers and soldiers helped build sandbag dikes around vulnerable infrastructures. Unfortunately, the human-built dykes were no match for the forces of nature. By May 6, the dykes started to collapse, making ambulances an absolute necessity for evacuating patients.

On Saturday, May 6, 1950, the dikes around Winnipeg's Municipal Hospital collapsed. Fortunately, the new Princess Elizabeth Hospital had not admitted patients yet, so the staff was already evacuated. Coordinated by the Canadian Army's Prairie Command,[116] between 2:00 and 3:30 a.m., a squadron of three army ambulances, one Royal Canadian Air Force (RCAF) ambulance, and various private ambulances, including Kerr's Invalid Ambulance Service, J. Thomson Company, Coutu Funeral Home, Desjardin Funeral Home, Veterans Ambulance, and Prince Brothers Ambulance descended on King Edward Hospital and moved 170 patients to Deer Lodge Hospital. At 5:00 a.m., the same ambulance team descended on King George Hospital and moved 50 patients to Deer Lodge Hospital.

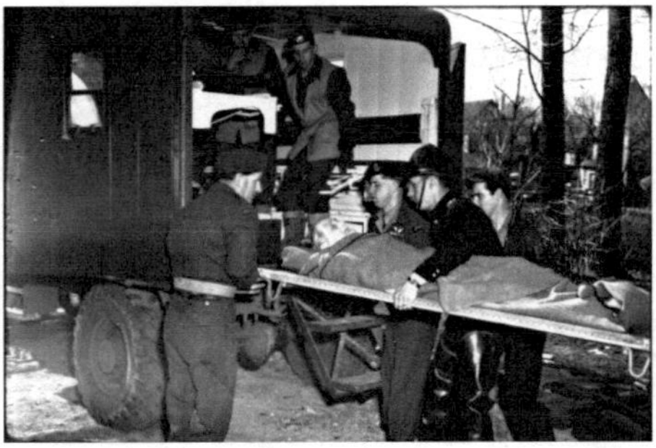

*Canadian Army medics and Winnipeg Police moving patients to Deer Lodge Hospital during the 1950 flood. (Courtesy of WCPI)*

The following day, Sunday, May 7, 1950, the dikes around the St. Boniface sanitorium (now the St. Amant Centre) became unstable, necessitating the evacuation of eighty patients, followed by eighty five the following day. This

116 "Another Four Institutions Still Battle To Halt Water." *Winnipeg Free Press.* May 6, 1950.

time, a team from Fort Osborne Barracks with six army ambulances, one army bus, and two three-ton army trucks moved the patients to WGH, Misericordia, and Deer Lodge Hospitals. Only ten patients remained: either too seriously ill to move or babies in incubators.[117]

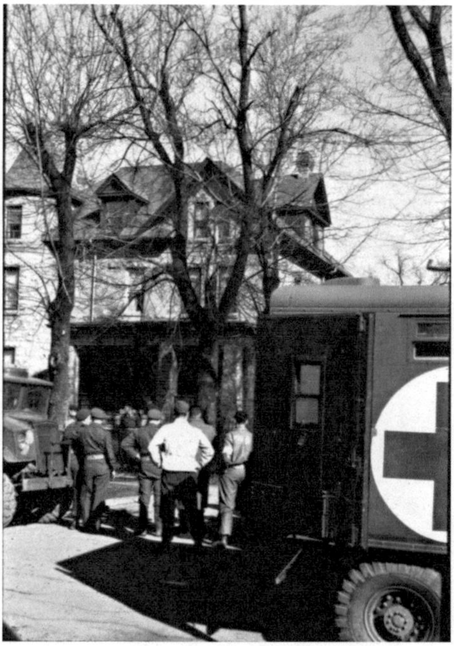

*Canadian Army ambulances evacuating residents from seniors' homes during the 1950 flood. (Courtesy of WCPI).*

By May 12, there was insufficient room to house all of the 450 St. Boniface Sanitorium patients in Winnipeg, so two planes of the Saskatchewan Air Ambulance Service began flying patients to Regina. A temporary staging hospital for 150 people was set up at the RCAF barracks at Winnipeg's Stevenson field.[118] To speed up the process, RCAF also used two aircraft and five army ambulances to transfer 36 patients from the Sanitorium and Deer Lodge Hospital to Yorkton, Saskatchewan. Two days later, on May 14, using eleven Dakota aircraft, 164 patients were flown by RCAF to Regina, Prince Albert, Saskatchewan, and Fort William, Ontario. To accomplish this feat, the army ambulances shuttled patients from Winnipeg-area hospitals to Stevenson Field all day.[119] To understand the process, it's useful to know that the World War II vintage ambulances used by the army during the flood could transport four patients at a time. Private ambulance services in Winnipeg at that time had nothing that could match that capacity.

Fortunately, all patients in Winnipeg's municipal hospitals were safely evacuated, but it was painfully evident that Winnipeg didn't have the capacity for major emergency medical transport without using significant outside resources.

117 "Army Evacuates 659 Patients in 4 Institutions As Precaution." *Winnipeg Free Press.* May 8, 1950.

118 "Airlift Takes First Patients to Regina Refuge." *Winnipeg Free Press.* May 12, 1950.

119 "Aged Patients Leave City in RCAF Planes." *Winnipeg Free Press.* May 15, 1950.

With the disappearance of funeral-home and hospital-based ambulance services, the start of private, ambulance-specific services, an ineffective police ambulance service, the fire department's ambulance service, and the inadequacies demonstrated during the 1950 flood, combined with knowledge about emergency care garnered during the upcoming Korean and Vietnam Wars and the lessons learned from the creation of North America's highway system, the next quarter century would create profound change in Winnipeg's ambulance services.

Whether it will be an improvement is anyone's guess.

## 1950-1975

# The Birth of EMS

The two decades between 1950 and 1970 saw the birth of modern emergency medicine. As an indirect result, the roots of paramedic programs began evolving during this period.

Until the 1950s, with exceptions, the objective of prehospital care was to get the sick and injured to a hospital (or doctor's office). The ambulance, for the most part, was just a form of conveyance. It could have been easily replaced by a taxi, a bread truck, or a donkey.

Unfortunately, getting a casualty to medical care didn't necessarily improve the chances of survival. Whether it was a physician's office or the hospital "accident ward," tended by whichever doctor or intern wasn't otherwise busy, often little could be done for the casualty. If they were still breathing and had a pulse, their injuries were bandaged by whatever staff was available. Without breathing or a pulse, it was the end of the story.

By 1970, it was accepted, at least in theory, that the absence of a pulse/heartbeat did not necessarily mean the casualty was dead, and the absence of breathing was frequently another fixable problem. With trauma—significant damage to the body—it was discovered that treating the body as a series of interconnected systems (as opposed to viewing the most obvious injury as *the* problem), leads to significantly increased rates of survival and successful recovery. Connected to this was the new understanding that the speed in beginning medical treatment—that is, care starting within the first five minutes, ideally at the scene—greatly increases the potential for a positive outcome.

As discussed, the 1930s and 1940s laid the groundwork for Winnipeg's prehospital emergency care metamorphosis. Thanks to experiences garnered during the First and Second World Wars, and the ongoing promotion of first aid by St. John Ambulance, there was a growing insight that immediate care meant many seriously injured or sick people had a greater chance of being kept alive.

Unfortunately, due to Winnipeg's poor economic health, that metamorphosis started a trend of haphazard, patchwork emergency response that would plague the city for the next quarter century. As noted, by 1950, the Winnipeg General Hospital's ambulance service had folded and Bardal Funeral Home had discontinued its railway-focused quasi-emergency ambulance. Some funeral homes were providing non-emergency ambulance transport. For emergencies, the options were either the Winnipeg Police's ambulance, which arrived *sometimes*, as availability and personnel allowed, or the Winnipeg Fire Department's rescue squads, a new one with patient-transport capability, and an older one, without patient-transport capability but with the latest first aid and oxygen-delivery equipment.

While there were some resources, there was much room for improvement!

The 1950s and 1960s provided the inventions and concepts needed to create our modern EMS. These set the parameters for evolving EMS in both Winnipeg and virtually every other North American city. The next six decades have been spent refining the advances made during this period.

Understanding the bigger picture makes it easier to grasp both the milestones and deficits of Winnipeg's EMS evolution. The next sections will discuss some of these developments.

## AED/CPR

Arguably, one of the biggest game changers in emergency care came with the invention of the Automated External Defibrillator (AED) and the development of "heart massage" or cardiopulmonary resuscitation (CPR).[120] Until the 1970s, when a person's heart stopped, it meant that they were dead; no ifs, ands, or buts. With about half of deaths in North America being related directly to heart or stroke, and with virtually every

120 Like most of the history of emergency medicine, the recording of the evolution of defibrillation and resuscitation is at best, "hit and miss". With so many different groups working at finding solutions, often in vacuums, there are many versions of history. This section is based on research by Hazzard (2022), Bell (2009), and Rapport (2019).

death being related to no heart beat or breathing, keeping the heart going and the lungs processing air is crucial to survival.

When electricity became a part of modern living in the 1920s, electrocution immediately became a collateral problem, affecting both customers and employees of electric power companies. With life and death becoming a work-place issue for their employees, New York's Con Edison company began supporting research on how delivering electric shocks could be used to restart human hearts. Relying on research from 1899, when Swiss doctors discovered that small electrical shocks could cause ventricular fibrillation in dogs, and larger shocks could reverse the effect, the search was on!

Several American, European, and Russian medical research teams were working on creating ways to restart a heart with electrical shocks. While many defibrillator prototypes were being developed, the challenge was that none of the teams could do it without cutting open the patient's chest, exposing the heart, and applying electrical charges directly to the heart muscle. Besides not being overly practical outside of a hospital setting, this technique was also messy. In a nutshell, the treatment was useless when the goal was to revive an electrocuted hydro lineman, lying at the side of the road with no heartbeat after touching a high-voltage powerline.

A breakthrough occurred in 1950, when William Kouwenhoven, an electrical engineer/medical researcher at Johns Hopkins University in Baltimore, Maryland, discovered that he could revive paralyzed dogs by placing electric charges on their hearts from outside of their chests—external defibrillation. With this discovery, Edison Electric offered Kouwenhoven research funds to develop a portable defibrillator. The results seemed promising.

Over the next few years, Kouwenhoven worked on developing a defibrillator that was more portable than his original 280-pound prototype. Everything about the device was heavy, including the 10-pound paddles that were placed on the patient's chest. The heavy paddles led to another discovery in 1956. When the paddles were placed on the dogs' chests, even without electricity, the weight caused the otherwise motionless heart to move and the blood to start circulating. With this new discovery, Kouwenhoven and his team started pushing and prodding and eventually discovered that by pressing repeatedly on the anesthetized dog's sternum, indirectly compressing the dog's heart, they could keep the heart alive for up to twenty one minutes.

This newest discovery reduced the need for a portable defibrillator. By pushing on a person's chest repeatedly for twenty one minutes, providing there was an efficient ambulance service, there was enough time to get the casualty to a hospital and use the 280-pound defibrillator.

Progressing, in 1954, James Elan, a physician from Austin, Texas, discovered that the air we excel from our mouths contains more oxygen than what we need to breathe. While ignored by most people, in 1956, Peter Safar, the chief of anesthesiology at Baltimore City Hospital and artificial respiration fanatic, spotted the benefit of Elan's research immediately.

Safar had already figured out that the current methods of artificial respiration all had a small but common problem; they didn't work. By taking Elan's research, he re-introduced a method of artificial respiration that both worked and had been ignored for almost 200 years—mouth-to-mouth resuscitation. (In 1740, the Paris Academy of Sciences was recommending that mouth-to-mouth resuscitation was the best way to revive drowning victims.[121] However, it was eventually ignored as manual resuscitation techniques came into vogue. My theory is that as people during the Victorian-era became more prudish, kissing in public, and anything that looked like kissing, was rejected. Hence, mouth-to-mouth resuscitation was punted in favour of techniques that didn't seem remotely sexual.)

One of the benefits of mouth-to-mouth is that it's not complicated. Safar believed that resuscitation had to be doable by non-doctors. In his experiments, Safar typically recruited young Boy Scouts to help demonstrate. His rationale was simple: *If a child can do it, anyone can.*

Things came together, and in February 1959, the researchers at Johns Hopkins University used a combination of external heart compressions and their defibrillator to successfully revive a surgical patient. Eleven months later, Baltimore firefighters had their first "save". Responding to a cardiac arrest, they immediately started chest compressions on the casualty, continuing in the fire department's ambulance until they reached Baltimore City Hospital. There, successful defibrillation enabled the casualty to walk out of the hospital six weeks later.

Dr Safar had a knack for connecting the dots. After forty eight different experiments proved that his mouth-to-mouth resuscitation worked,

---

121 Heart and Stroke Foundation. "The Amazing Story of CPR." at https://www.heartandstroke.ca/articles/the-amazing-story-of-cpr. Accessed August 30, 2024.

he noticed Kouwenhoven's discovery of using chest compressions for maintaining a stopped heart. In September 1960, Safar and his team joined forces with Kouwenhoven and his team at the Maryland Medical Society's annual convention. By combining chest compressions with mouth-to-mouth resuscitation, Safar and Kouwenhoven demonstrated that a technique they called cardiopulmonary resuscitation (CPR) worked better than either of their respective techniques did separately. The combination enabled a rescuer to technically keep a "dead" person alive indefinitely. In fact, anyone who has knelt beside a non-breathing casualty, doing CPR, and reciting the mantra:

"Airway,<br>
Breathing,<br>
Circulation,"

is taking the words out of Kouwenhoven's and Safar's mouths; they created the procedure.

While having a defibrillator in the hospital was a game changer, and having CPR as a tool to get the casualty to the hospital to be defibrillated was useful, the research team still hadn't accomplished their ultimate goal, to create a portable unit that could be taken to the casualty. Kouwenhoven's team at Johns Hopkins University kept hammering away; now with the financial support of both Edison Electric and the Mine Safety Appliance Company, both of which had vested financial interests in being able to restart hearts at remote locations.

By May 1959, using the additional technical skills that the Mine Safety Appliance Company brought, i.e. manufacturing portable rescue equipment, Kouwenhoven and his team had developed a forty five pound prototype, built into a fiberglass suitcase. The team built a number of units and between 1959 and 1962, ran multiple experiments; both in hospital settings and in the field. After ten successful defibrillations in 1962, the portable device was declared usable.

Over the next sixty years, portable defibrillators have continued to evolve. In 1978, the first fully Automated External Defibrillators (AEDs) were developed, and computer technology of the 1980s significantly advanced the design, while reducing the price.

AEDs have now reached the stage where any person with rudimentary training can use one to save a life.

## Defibrillation at the Scene

While the portable defibrillator's development was completed in 1962, somebody needed to actually make it work in the real world. This somebody came in the form of Frank Pantridge, a cardiologist at the Royal Victoria Hospital in Belfast. Through real-world observation, Dr. Pantridge noticed that despite having defibrillators in the hospital, many cardiac arrest patients, particularly those with myocardial infarction or ventricular fibrillation, simply didn't survive long enough to get to the hospital. At the same time, Pantridge noticed in the cardiac ward that thirty out of sixty three patients experiencing cardiac arrests were resuscitated successfully. When the arrest occurred in the general medical ward, thirty one percent survived. This is because 50 to 60 percent of all heart attack deaths occur within the first hour after onset; before ever reaching the hospital.[122] This gave Pantridge the idea of a Mobile Cardiac Unit.

As a result, in 1966 (January 1, to be precise), Dr. Pantridge and his colleagues put the Belfast Royal Victoria Hospital Mobile Cardiac Care Unit, or the "MCCU" or "Heartmobile" into service. Equipping a battered old ambulance with a portable defibrillator, the unit rolled with a physician and nurse whenever the hospital received a report of a possible heart attack. Arriving as quickly as possible, they went to work at the scene, trying to revive the casualty.

After reviving more than 300 people, Dr. Pantridge and his team published their results in two 1967 articles in *The Lancet*, an England-based publication and one of the premier medical journals at the time. While there was little interest from Pantridge's colleagues in Europe, first responders in North America were a different story.

Almost immediately after reading of Pantridge's successes, cities across North America began setting up their own versions of the Heartmobile. The key difference was that in North America, the units were often staffed by non-physicians. In 1967, Miami, Florida began their fire-based paramedic service, focusing primarily on cardiac arrests. Using electrocardiogram (EKG) telemetry equipment to transmit heart rhythms to the city's Jackson Memorial Hospital, firefighters were instructed, via radio, how to medicate, intubate, and defibrillate the patient.

122 Barkley (1978): 135

A year later, in 1968, St. Vincent's Hospital in Manhattan, New York, initiated their physician-staffed Mobile Cardiac Care unit. Following closely behind was Columbus, Ohio, which introduced their fire department's "Mobile Intensive Care Unit," utilizing a combination of physicians and emergency medical technicians. In 1969, Seattle firefighters using a converted, oversized, and impossible-to-handle motorhome nicknamed "Moby Pig," started their Medic One program. At the end of 1969, Los Angeles County Fire Department introduced their Rescue Heart Unit staffed by newly trained firefighter/paramedics. This program quickly evolved into the paramedic program made famous by the 1970s television series *Emergency!*

The first appearance of a mobile cardiac unit in Canada appears to be the Ontario Hospital Services Commission's 1969 *Cardiac One* experiment. Using a Toronto Department of Emergency Services ambulance, telemetry equipment, a portable defibrillator, and an intern from Toronto General Hospital, for July and August of 1969, the unit responded to cardiac calls throughout Toronto.[123] Little appears to have been written on this program. With the portable defibrillator and heart monitor powered by lead-acid car batteries and weighing around 45 kilograms (99 lbs.), it seems that the technology used was not sufficient. After the pilot program ended, emergency cardiac care does not appear to have gained further traction in Toronto until advanced life support-level paramedicine was introduced in 1981.

The following year, in 1970, Dr. Peter Cohen, head of Calgary Hospital's emergency department and a co-owner of Aaron's Ambulance Service in Calgary, created his "Resuscicar". Based on a Ford Econoline van, it was designed as a mobile treatment center with a large, operating room-sized hydraulic examination table in the back, along with the usual equipment found in a Heartmobile of that time period. While not entirely practical, it again showed how on-scene defibrillation was crucial in keeping cardiac arrest patients alive. The challenge was that Cohen had wanted it to be physician-staffed, but few doctors were willing to work in it. A year after Aaron's Ambulance started its Resuscicar, Calgary started its paramedic program, and Dr. Cohen moved to Montreal. There, he started another

123 Ontario Paramedic Association. "History of Paramedics in Ontario." at: https://www.ontarioparamedic.ca/before-911/history-of-paramedics-in-ontario, accessed July 1, 2024, and Newton (2015): 160.

Resuscicar program, a mobile intensive care unit operating out of the Royal Victoria Hospital.

At the same time as Cohen was creating his version of the Heartmobile in Calgary, the Saanich fire department on Vancouver Island, British Columbia started its Coronary Care ambulance. After setting up coronary care units in Victoria's St. Joseph's Hospital and Royal Jubilee Hospital, Victoria cardiologist George Woodwark realized that Pantridge was correct; a key component of cardiac arrest survival required proper prehospital care. Under Woodwark's tutelage, Saanich firefighters, who were already running the city's ambulance service, received six months of specialized cardiac training. Using a Physio Control Lifepak 33 defibrillator, a telemetry transmitter with heavy-duty radios mounted in the ambulance, and standard cardiac drugs at the time—lidocaine and atropine—the firefighters were able to treat cardiac arrests all over the Saanich peninsula.

Almost immediately it became apparent that the fire department's stretched Cadillac ambulance did not have the interior space to work/carry the needed cardiac equipment. The department quickly acquired one of the new GMC vans to serve as its Heartmobile. Saanich's unit continued saving lives until the creation of the British Columbia Ambulance Service in 1974.[124]

Most Heartmobiles or Mobile Cardiac Care Units proved their worth (and necessity), and then were merged with, absorbed into, or created the basis for their local paramedic ambulance services in the early to mid-1970s.

## Ambulance Design

Prior to the 1960s, most civilian ambulances were passenger cars modified to carry prone casualties. More often than not, they were custom-built, stretched vehicles; the same stretched custom chassis was used for both Hearses and ambulances. Where budgets didn't allow, conventional station wagons were often used.

There were exceptions, some fire departments, including Winnipeg's, used large commercial van-type vehicles, and other service providers, such as the municipal hospital, used panel trucks. In reality, all that was needed at that time was a vehicle long enough to transport a body in

124 Klein (2018): 46-50.

horizontal position. Whether the body was dead or alive really didn't matter. For the most part, until the 1960s, ambulances were more or less elongated taxis.

This common use is best illustrated by the production of *combination cars*. In the early 1940s, professional car manufacturers started offering combination cars for budget-minded funeral homes: stretched station wagons that could be converted from a Hearse to an ambulance, or vice-versa in a matter of minutes. Pondering that concept for a moment, it becomes readily apparent that the equipment carried by ambulances was minimal—flashing lights, a gurney (a stretcher on wheels), a folding seat for the attendant, and *maybe* a box with first aid supplies and/or oxygen. Everything needed for a full-out "you call, we haul, that's all" response.

A related problem during this era was that most car-based ambulances didn't have room for more than the casualty and a seated attendant. As shown with the Saanich Fire Department's Cadillac ambulance, once firefighters were taught how to manage cardiac arrests, it became apparent that there was no room for the equipment.

One of the first published analyses highlighting the problems with traditional civilian ambulance design occurred after a serious train accident in London, England. In October 1952, at the Harrow and Wealdstone Rail Station, just outside of London, three trains crashed into the train station during the morning rush-hour commute. The end result was 112 dead and 340 injured passengers (of the 157 taken to hospital, 88 had serious injuries). Using existing emergency services, it took over four hours to evacuate the seriously injured, and almost twenty hours to remove all of the casualties.[125] Many of the deaths occurred because the casualties did not receive medical care quickly enough. The accident resulted in an acknowledgement of the need for ambulances to be able to carry multiple casualties, have medical supplies, and have sufficient interior space to treat casualties enroute to the hospital.

While the Harrow and Wealdstone crash got the ambulance industry thinking about increased capacity and size for ambulances, it was not an entirely new concept. In 1934, the Miller-Meteor ambulance company pioneered the "high headroom" ambulance, by taking a Ford 40 sedan chassis and increasing its height to fifty two inches of headroom

125 https://en.wikipedia.org/wiki/Harrow_and_Wealdstone_rail_crash, accessed October 14, 2023.

by adding several inches just below the windows. This enabled the unit to carry four patients—two on stretchers and two on ceiling-suspended cots. These units were rare, custom-built, and typically bought by fire department rescue squads as opposed to funeral homes or ambulance services[126]. Miller-Meteor subsequently made the fifty two inch headroom into a production model in 1950, called the "First Aider High Headroom Ambulance." To capture the demand for these types of vehicles, in 1942, the Henney-Packard Motor Company introduced their "Civil Defense Ambulance." It was a modular ambulance with headroom of fifty six inches, and could carry twelve adults, twenty children, or four stretchers and four attendants. Only ten were built.[127]

While the need for carrying capacity and a large working area is a necessity today, it is important to remember that before the transitional period of the 1950s and 1960s, ambulances were glorified taxis. Other than the fire departments, rescue squads, and hospital-based ambulance services around North America that provided advanced first aid enroute to the hospital, not many ambulance operators had a need for a large working area in their vehicles' passenger compartments.

It is one of these exceptions that resulted in the invention of the "modular ambulance"; the ambulance design that is currently used for all of Winnipeg's ambulances, and most ambulances in western and central Canada. The Baltimore Fire Department, which, as noted above, was instrumental in using CPR to keep cardiac patients alive, in 1960 started converting heavy, one-ton Chevrolet panel trucks for use as their ambulances. They worked well and gave firefighters sufficient space to do first aid/CPR on patients as they raced to the hospital.

A problem arose in 1963 when Chevrolet discontinued the one-ton panel truck. Baltimore's fire chief, Mike McMahon, discovered that the new ¾ ton panel trucks didn't give firefighters enough room to properly give CPR. As a result, McMahon contacted the Swab Wagon Company, an Elizabethville, Pennsylvania-based company that had been building ambulance and rescue vehicles since 1868 and asked them to invent *something* on a one-ton truck chassis. The result was essentially a light truck chassis with a box mounted behind the cab that was slightly higher and wider than a panel truck. The result revolutionized ambulance design,

126 McPherson (2010): 143
127 McPherson (2009): 165-166

as it created an appropriate-sized working-space for casualty-care. With fifty four inches of headroom and much wider than an automobile, Baltimore's modular ambulances were large for the day (see image below). Being truck-based, it didn't have the smooth ride of a Cadillac or Pontiac-chassised stretched automobile ambulance, but the extra space it provided for giving life-saving care enroute to the hospital significantly over rode this disadvantage.

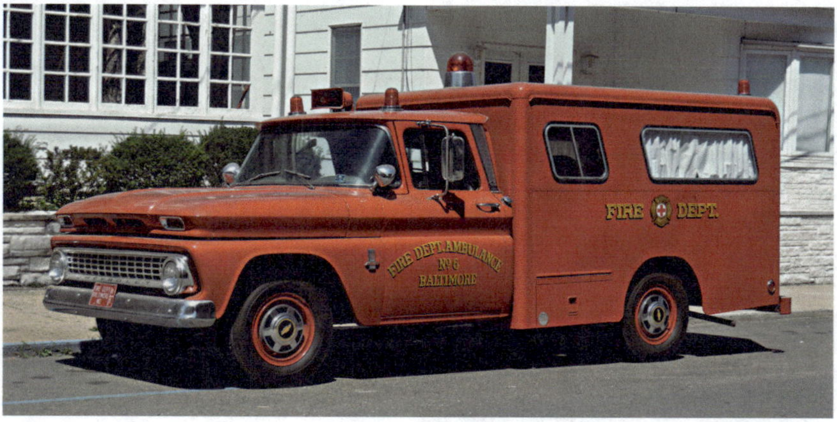


*Baltimore (Maryland)'s 1963 Swab modular ambulance – the unit that started the modern ambulance trend. (Courtesy of Michael Martinelli).*

After Baltimore bought a fleet of these modular ambulances, Chief McMahon began promoting them as *the answer* to emergency care.[128] While the modular ambulances revolutionized prehospital emergency transportation, they also have the benefit of reducing the long-term cost. As the "box" is bolted on to a truck chassis, when the chassis wears out, the box is simply transferred onto a new chassis, reducing the frequency of purchasing new ambulances. According to Crestline Coach, an ambulance manufacturer in Saskatoon, Saskatchewan, most chassis only last a maximum of four to five years, but the ambulance body can last ten to fifteen years.[129]

There was now a solution for ambulance providers who wanted more space in their vehicles than a stretched station wagon or Hearse could provide. Unfortunately, there was still a problem: Both modular truck-based units and high-headroom passenger car ambulances were custom

128 Bell (2007): 220-223.
129 Online interview with Scott Sawatsky, Crestline Coach, September 10, 2024.

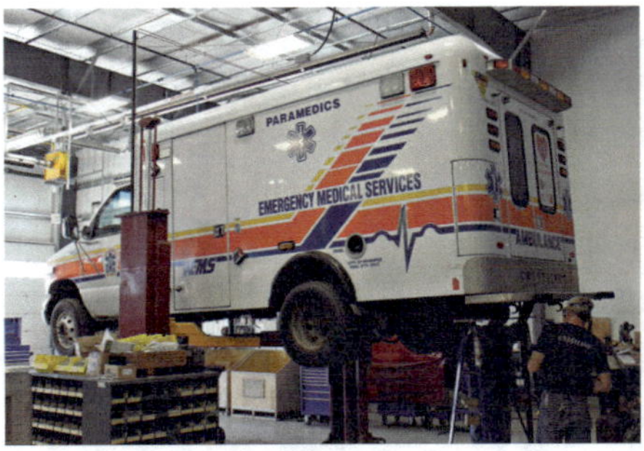


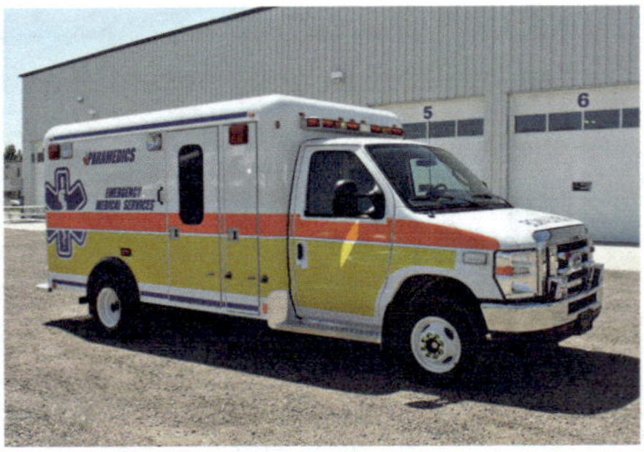

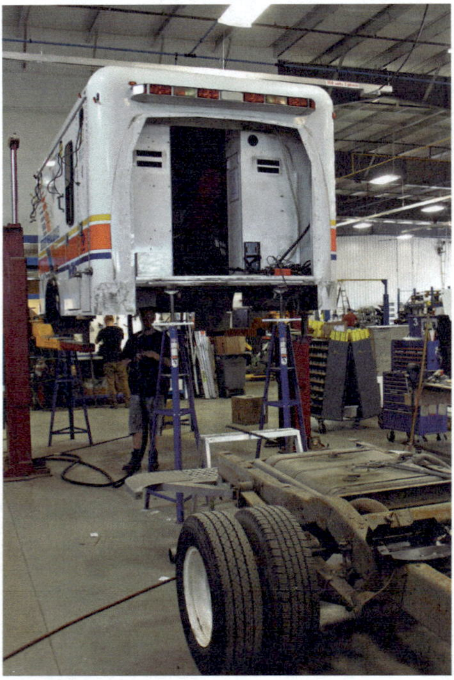

*One of Winnipeg's older modular ambulances receiving a new chassis in 2014. (Courtesy of Crestline Coach).*

built. For many services with a limited budget, such as Winnipeg Police's ambulance service, the trusty station wagon, with no extra space, was all that many ambulance services could afford.

However, this changed in 1968.

Whether in response to the growing need for improved vehicles for ambulance work, or a response to a consumer demand for larger commercial vehicles, in 1968 (as a 1969 model), Ford introduced its second generation Econoline van. It was bigger, taller, and wider than any van or panel truck previously produced. While seriously underpowered, for the first time, the Ford Econoline provided a reasonably priced, commercially built vehicle which easily could be converted for ambulance work. It provided a patient working area that was more expansive than even the largest high headroom passenger car ambulance could provide.

Quickly spotting the opportunity, in 1968, the Superior ambulance company introduced a Ford Econoline van-based ambulance, the first major coach builder to introduce a standard product that was not based on a passenger car. In 1969, the Miller-Meteor Motor Car Division followed suit with the Wayne Sentinel Ambulance, based on a Chevrolet

Suburban chassis. It had fifty inches of headroom, could carry four patients, had medicine cabinets with roll-up doors, and 129 square feet of working space (103" long and 50" wide). Interestingly, both vehicles were advertised as "budget stretchers" as opposed to having a larger working space for providing care. It was apparent that ambulances were still deemed by many ambulance services to be transport vehicles as opposed to a platform for providing enroute medical care.

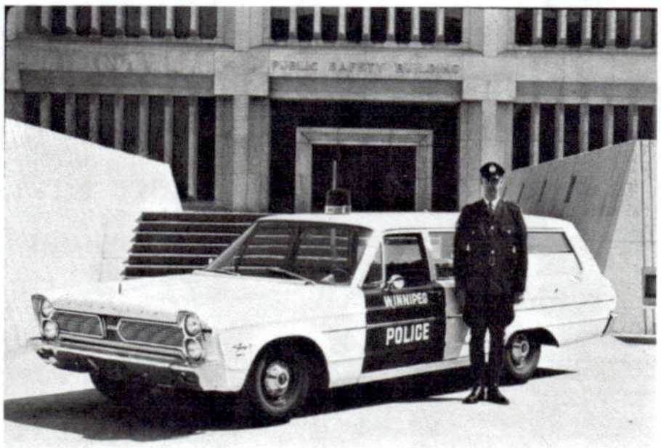


*Winnipeg Police Department's 1966 Plymouth station wagon ambulances were an example of the more common vehicles used by budget-conscious EMS providers. (Courtesy of WPS Archives)*

Two years later, in 1970 (for the 1971 model year) Dodge jumped into the full-sized van/ambulance market by introducing the Tradesman van. The role as an EMS vehicle was solidified in 1973 with the introduction of Dodge's Maxivan/Maxiwagon (depending on whether the rear area had windows or not); a Tradesman or Sportsman van with an eighteen-inch body extension. Designed by the same company that produced the Plymouth Roadrunner, the Charger Daytona (the world's fastest production car at the time), and the Dodge Super Bee, the extended Maxivan was both roomier and more powerful/faster than the Ford Econoline van. This made it ideal for EMS work. If believed, Calgary paramedics claim that in the early 1970s, the RCMP clocked them doing 188 km/h (117 mph) both ways during one response in their Dodge van-type ambulance.[130] While perhaps not the safest way to run emergency calls, it does highlight the Dodge van's capacity.

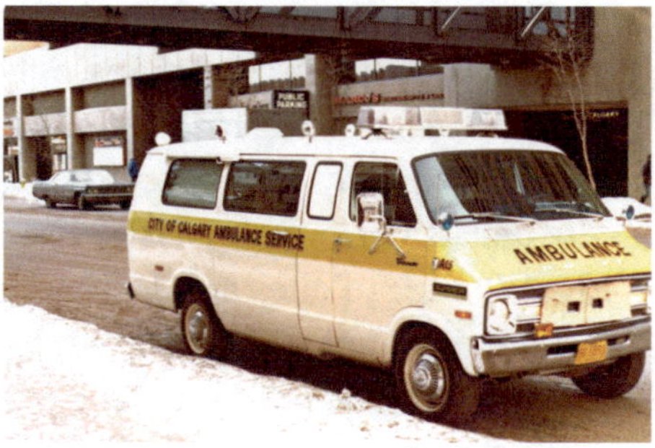


*One of Calgary Ambulance Service's allegedly 180 km/h-capable Dodge-van based ambulances. (Courtesy of Stan Stone)*

As an example of the size of these units, when Wayne Ambulance Corporation introduced

130 Duncan (2019): 39.

the Medicruiser in 1973, a stretched Dodge Maxivan, it had sixty one inches of headroom, and 310 cubic feet of space in the patient's compartment. In Winnipeg, by the early 1970s, both Seven Oaks and Veterans-Prince Ambulance services, as well as the Winnipeg Police, were running Dodge Tradesman-based ambulances, mainly of the Maxivan variety.

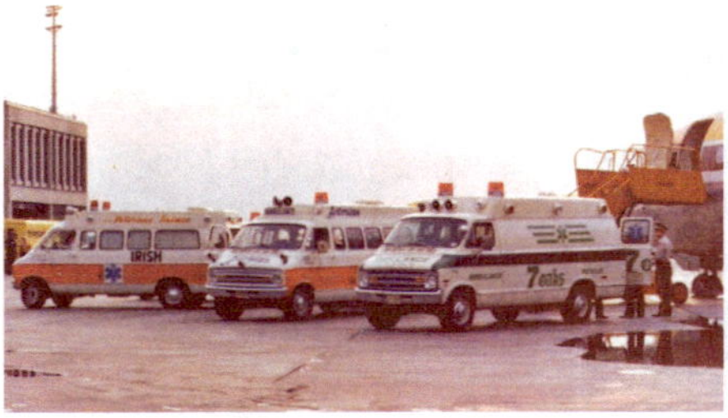

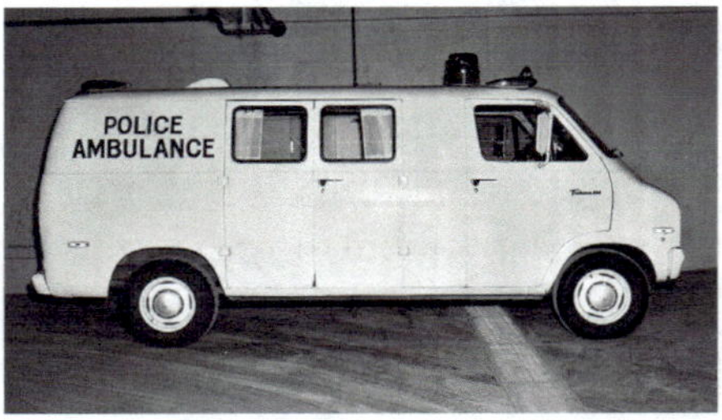


*Some of the early Dodge ambulances in Winnipeg. Private ambulances at a 1974 mock airport disaster (Courtesy of Peter Adsten @ EMS Classics) and Winnipeg Police's last ambulance—acquired in January 1972. (Courtesy of WPS Archives)*

While the 1966 US "White Paper" (discussed in more detail in the next section) recommended that there be an "implementation of recent traffic safety legislation to ensure completely adequate standards for ambulance design and construction...," nothing formally happened in either Canada or the US for another eight years to clarify appropriate ambulance design. Surprisingly, any vehicle could be called an "ambulance."

Finally, in 1974, the US Department of Transport introduced "KKK-A-1822," the standards for purchasing ambulances using US Federal funds. Under these regulations, only three types of ambulances could be acquired when using federal funding: "Type I"—a transferable modular ambulance body on a truck chassis (similar to the original Baltimore fire department's unit); "Type II"—a customized van (such as used by the Winnipeg Police and Winnipeg's private ambulance providers the early 1970s); and a "Type III"—a hybrid of types I and II: a transferable modular ambulance body on a cut-away van chassis (used on Winnipeg's current ambulances).

While there were no legal restrictions as to what could be used as an ambulance, manufacturers had little financial incentive to build models that would not qualify for US federal funding. This also affected Canada, in that for the most part, the US manufacturers were only building

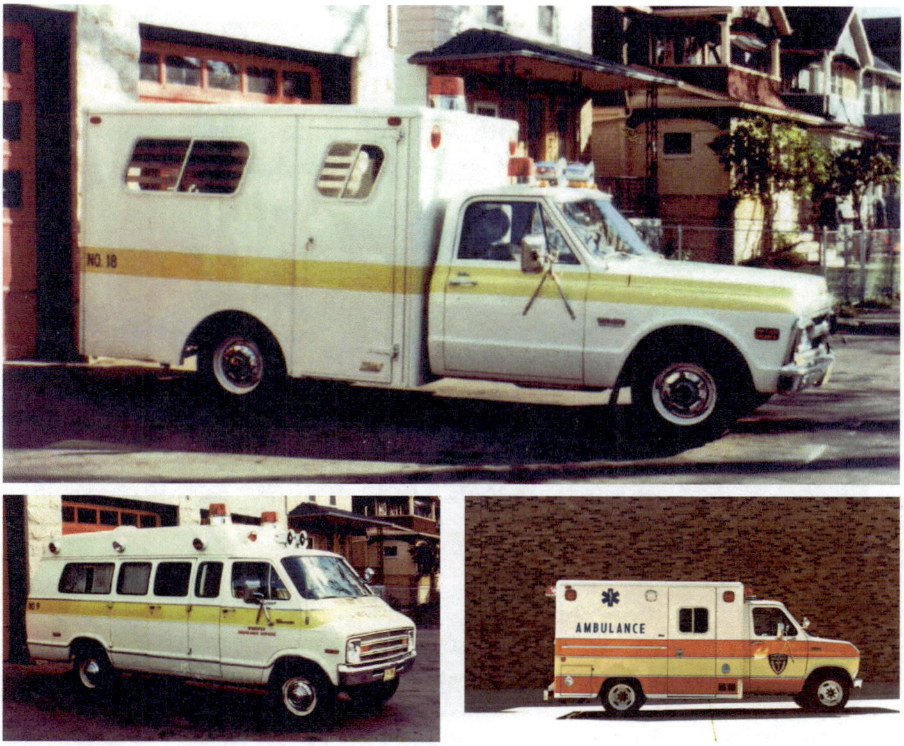


*Early Winnipeg Types I, II, and III ambulances. The Type I was Winnipeg's first modular, built by the Lawrie Wagon and Carriage Company, on a 1972 GMC chassis for Wylie Rescue Ambulance. (Courtesy of Stan Stone)*

Type I, Type II, or Type III units, and Canadian manufacturers, wanting to attract American customers, had to stick to US requirements.

There were still some ambulance services that purchased stretched station wagon/Hearse- type ambulances. Given that the KKK-A-1822 standards only applied to ambulances being purchased using US federal funds, there was nothing illegal about doing so. However, as more ambulance services were providing prehospital emergency medical care, the need for increased interior space made stretched passenger cars less and less practical. As a result, they were typically only bought as non-emergency, transfer ambulances.

The production of passenger car-based ambulances finally ended in 1977. With the North American fuel crisis in full swing, American car manufacturers began "downsizing." Former full-sized car manufacturers, such as Cadillac, Pontiac, Oldsmobile, and Dodge began building smaller vehicles. It became impossible, using passenger cars, to custom-build vehicles with enough room to transport a patient and attendants, not to mention carry the now standard medical equipment. While the Hearse industry continued, their primary passengers never complained about the cramped space: Death tends to make you quiet. Passenger car-based ambulances disappeared forever.

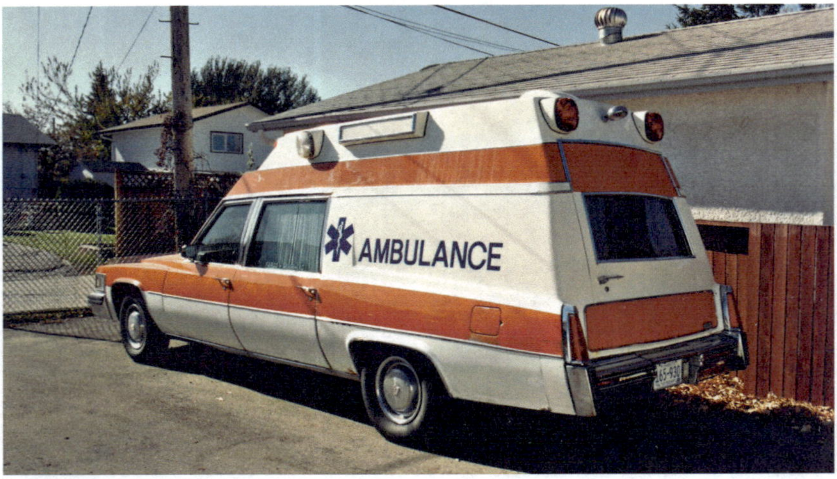


*One of the last passenger car-based ambulances built; a 1977 Superior-Cadillac. (Courtesy of Brian Schuff)*

## The White Paper

A huge influencer on the evolution of modern EMS was the 1966 US National Academy of Sciences' Committee on Trauma and Committee on Shock's paper: *Accidental Death and Disability: The Neglected Disease of Modern Society*, often referred to as: "the White Paper."

Several factors including the increased carnage on American highways, the increasing skills/success rates of medics in the Korean and Vietnam wars, the Harrow and Wealdstone Rail Accident, and the newly evolving specialty of "emergency medicine" resulted in the American National Research Council putting together a project in 1963 to investigate accidental death and injury in the context of it being a national health issue. The researchers were directed to not only pay attention to accidental injury and death, but to study the initial treatment of injuries, and how such might affect the overall outcome.

The result of the three years of research was the forty four-page report which provided a blueprint for improving emergency medical services. Using the head-turning statistic:

> "... that a soldier shot in the Viet Nam jungle has a better chance of surviving than a housewife seriously injured in an accident on an American highway..." [131]

The White Paper captured the continent's attention.

The paper provided a series of recommendations that led to significant reforms in both the US and Canada. These included:

1. Accept that accident prevention, through both education and legislation, is crucial for reducing a significant number of deaths and injuries;
2. Emergency responders, including ambulance attendants, firefighters, police officers, and rescue squad personnel must have proper training in cardiopulmonary resuscitation and other life saving techniques. The public also needs to be trained in CPR and advanced first aid.
3. Legislation must be implemented to clarify adequate standards for ambulance design, equipment, and supplies, as well as the qualifications of ambulance personnel.
4. Determination of proper standards for radio equipment to be used between ambulances, emergency departments, and other health-related agencies.
5. Develop proper hospital emergency departments throughout the nation and develop seamless connections between emergency departments and hospital intensive care departments.
6. Create trauma departments in selective hospitals and significantly increase the research in trauma medicine.

The White Paper's recommendations had a profound impact on emergency care in North America. As it came out, the US *National Highway*

---

131 National Academy of Sciences and National Research Council. *Accidental Death and Disability: The Neglected Disease of Modern Society.* The National Academies Press, 1966,

*Safety Act* established the US Department of Transportation (DOT). The DOT, in turn, in 1967 unveiled its new EMS standards, which made federal funding for highway projects contingent on states creating a program to ensure that victims of highway accidents receive "prompt emergency care." In a nutshell, states were expected to legislate training and licensing standards for ambulance and rescue personnel, equipment, and communications equipment. These requirements were followed with the threat of withholding federal funding for highway construction/maintenance for states which did not develop proper EMS regulations. In summary, it was the first time that a policymaker in North America had attempted to create EMS standards. While it did not address ambulance design and paramedic training, it was a start.

With EMS standards evolving in the US, given the close connection between the two countries' economies, the standards were quickly followed and adopted in Canada.

## Emergency Medicine

Another key factor in the development of modern EMS was the creation of the specialty of emergency medicine. Good prehospital emergency care works hand-in-glove with hospital-based emergency/trauma care. A good emergency department can't do much if it's only receiving corpses, and a great prehospital EMS is relatively useless if the sick or injured patients don't receive proper care upon arrival at the hospital.

It's important to not confuse modern emergency medicine and hospital emergency rooms and trauma centers with the "casualty wards" and "emergency hospitals" that emerged in the late 1800s. Casualty or accident wards, such as the one within the early Winnipeg General Hospital, were often staffed by interns or physicians with little experience in emergency medicine. They were created more often as an afterthought, for treating those patients coming in the door with whom no one quite knew what to do.

Emergency hospitals, as found in larger American cities, were a bit different. While they typically had minimal equipment or staff with formal training, they were often staffed by police surgeons (physicians employed by the local police department). Through extensive practice, the police surgeons became skilled at treating stab and gunshot wounds. While Winnipeg Police had a surgeon on staff in the early 1900s, records are sparse as to how much he was involved in assisting with the injuries that Winnipeg's sixty-odd bars regularly created.

Nevertheless, without equipment such as defibrillators, resuscitators, trauma dressings, and anti-shock equipment, there was little that even the most competent and dedicated police surgeons or casualty ward interns could do.

The Korean and Vietnam wars did wonders for creating knowledge that proper, immediate treatment of life-threatening injuries could result in preservation of life. In particular, it became readily apparent during the Vietnam War, "… many factors contributed to the low mortality rate of casualties, such as rapid evacuation, the availability of whole blood, well established forward hospitals, advanced surgical techniques, and improved medical management…"[132] Perhaps most crucial: "The average time lapse between being wounded and reaching a hospital was usually less than one hour and, as a result, less than 1 percent of the casualties died of their wounds within the first 24 hours."[133] This new learning about casualty care provided the base for modern EMS and emergency medicine. In a nutshell, it became clear that emergency medical interventions needed to start immediately, followed by properly trained emergency physicians and surgeons providing advanced medical care within the hour.

This knowledge expanded to North America and resulted in a rapid change in civilian casualty care, creating a new, unconventional, but effective approach to treating injuries. As explained by the Canadian Medical Association: "Emergency medicine focuses on the recognition, evaluation and care of patients who are acutely ill or injured. It is a high-pressure, fast-paced specialty that, because of its diversity, requires a broad base of medical knowledge and a variety of well-honed clinical and technical skills. Emergency physicians must be prepared to treat patients of all ages and a nearly infinite variety of conditions and degrees of illness—often before a definite diagnosis is made and within time-restricted circumstances."[134]

As returning army physicians and surgeons began incorporating the lessons from the Korean and Vietnam Wars into their care regimes,

132 King (2021): 214.
133 King (2021): 215.
134 Canadian Medical Association. "Emergency Medicine Profile". December 2019: 4.

the understanding and acceptance of these techniques quickly spread. The Emergency College of American Physicians was created in 1968 in response to the need for physicians skilled in managing emergency patients. In 1970 the University of Cincinnati created the first emergency medicine residency program. Recognizing a good idea, the following year, the Royal College of Physicians and Surgeons of Canada (RCPSC) took notice, and proposed that educational programs be developed in the discipline of emergency medicine (EM). By 1972, the proposal for an EM specialty was accepted and Montreal's McGill University created the third North American (and first Canadian) emergency residency program. By 1975 there were thirty-two university level emergency residency programs, including three in Canada at: McGill, the University of Western Ontario, and Queen's University at Kingston.

The interest in EM was infectious. In 1976, the American Board of Emergency Medicine (ABEM) and the Society for Academic Emergency Medicine were born. After the American Board of Medical Specialties (ABMS) first voted one hundred to five *against* the application for specialty status (1977), the application was reconsidered, and emergency medicine was subsequently approved as a specialty in 1979.

Canada was not far behind. In 1978, the Canadian Association of Emergency Physicians was formed and by 1981 emergency medicine had been approved by the Royal College of Physicians and Surgeons of Canada as a recognized specialty. The first fellowship certificates were granted by the Royal College of Physicians and Surgeons of Canada in 1983.

Today, despite emergency medicine having been formally recognized in Canada for almost fifty five years, many emergency room physicians are not emergency or trauma-certified specialists, but doctors who have completed their family medicine residencies. As with paramedicine, it is a profession that is still evolving.

## *Emergency!*

It may seem unbelievable that a television show could stimulate an international evolution in prehospital emergency care, but in the early 1970s, Universal's television show *Emergency!* did just that. As television viewers watched firefighter-paramedics John Gage and Roy DeSoto keep casualties alive by using the latest emergency care techniques, the demand for (and acceptance of) emergency paramedics spread across the continent. While not directly responsible for creating paramedic services, the show created a public understanding, and more importantly, a taxpayer demand for municipal EMS programs. During the 1973-74 period, a year after *Emergency!* premiered, paramedic-level EMS programs were initiated in at least 24 American states.[135]

The *Emergency!* story began in 1969, when the Los Angeles County Fire Department (LACFD) started its emergency cardiac care program, with six firefighter/paramedics. Over the next year and a half, it morphed into a full prehospital emergency paramedic program, with seven squads. In the Los Angeles County program, two firefighter/paramedics respond in pick-up truck sized rescue squads to serious emergency medical calls. The patients, once stabilized, were transported to hospital by private ambulances (accompanied by one or both paramedics).

In late 1970/early 1971, television producers Jack Webb and Robert Cinader, after watching the success of police drama *Adam* 12, got the idea to produce a firefighter rescue show. After being rejected by the Los Angeles Fire Department, their discussions with the LACFD's public information officer got a more positive reception. After hearing about LACFD's new paramedic program, and Cinader doing several ride-alongs with real paramedics, the Webb-Cinader duo became captivated with the idea of a television series on paramedics.

Not wasting time, Cinader reached an agreement with LACFD to use their equipment and expertise and began filming in November 1971. Almost immediately, the show was bought by the NBC television network. From the airing of the premiere on January 15, 1972, it ran for five and a half years. During this period, Cinader produced 122 one-hour episodes as well as the two-hour premiere and six two-hour movies.

What made the show particularly effective was that, in light of his personal slogan: "Educate Through Entertainment,"[136] Cinader made more than 500 trips with squads during the five years of filming to verify the accuracy of the techniques used in the show. As well, to ensure the rescues and medical emergencies were believable, all incidents were based on either documented emergency medical calls or LACFD practice scenarios.

135 Page (1979): 137.
136 Yardley, et al (2008): 48.

The show was extremely effective in introducing the North American public to paramedics, following the paramedic actors as they responded to medical calls. It also highlighted the emerging area of emergency medicine; watching Drs. Joe Early and Kelly Brackett and their hospital emergency department team keep patients alive.

Besides immersing the viewing public in prehospital emergency care and modern emergency medicine, it also created an acceptance of devices critical to the work of paramedics. For example, the paramedics used a Datascope Model 850 Dual Trace Physiological Monitor, an EKG/defibrillator. Through watching its use each week, the viewing audience learned that out-of-hospital cardiac arrests could be reversed, providing there's a quick initial response.

In a brilliant marketing strategy, the Modular Ambulance Corporation, a large Dallas, Texas-based custom ambulance manufacturer, contributed both Type I and Type III modular ambulances to the show. By seeing these units being regularly used, the viewing public began viewing modular units as being *proper* ambulances.

Similarly, two rescue tools that are often seen in action at motor vehicle accidents got their first wide-spread exposure during *Emergency!*. For starters, the Partner K-12 power saw gained a reputation as being the "problem solver." Invented in 1958, the Partner box saw, or open-ended circular saw, was originally designed for quick rescues of airline passengers. It enabled rescuers to cut through the fuselages of downed aircraft.[137] By adding different blades, it could cut through concrete, rebar, steel, and almost any other obstacle entrapping people. As highlighted in *Emergency!*, it quickly gained acceptance as the "go-to" heavy rescue gadget.

Like the K-12 saw, the Hurst "Jaws of Life" system (and various imitations) has become the quintessential tool for motor vehicle extrication. Hurst's hydraulic rescue system was originally invented in 1961 for the automotive racing industry. Unlike the K-12 saw, which sent off sparks, the Hurst tools use phosphate ester fluid, which is both nonflammable and doesn't conduct electricity. This makes them ideal for situations where there is spilled gasoline and the potential for fire. Unlike the K-12 saw that was already in wide use, the Hurst tools were fairly new. Seeing the benefit of *Emergency!* for marketing their rescue tools, Hurst offered

137 Yardley, et al (2008): 114.

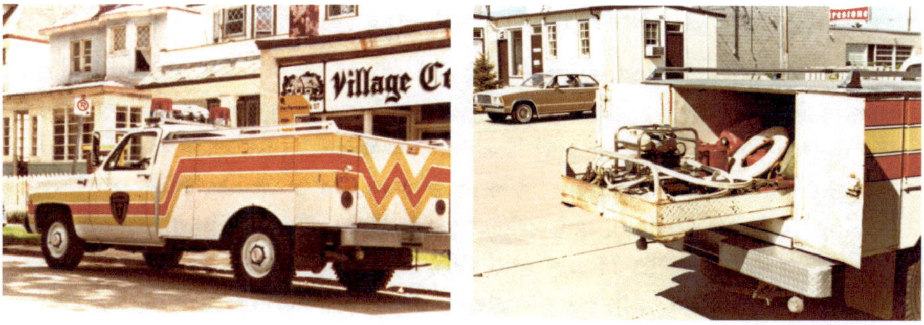


*Winnipeg's early Extrication Unit and Hurst Jaws of Life cutting tools in 1976. Note the "W" in early Winnipeg Ambulance vehicle graphics. (Courtesy of Stan Stone)*

a set to the show's production company. While Cinader was active in promoting modern emergency equipment, he initially rejected Hurst's offer, because the Jaws of Life weren't used by the LACFD. Hurst rectified the situation by donating a set to the LACFD and providing training to their firefighters. Cinader then accepted the donation of Hurst tools for the show and featured them as a common rescue tool. Soon, Hurst tools were being noticed and acquired by rescue services across North America; including those in Winnipeg.[138]

## The EMS Evolution's Effect on Winnipeg

In a nutshell, a number of major changes in North America in the decades preceding 1975 affected the overall emergency medical industry. But how did these changes affect Winnipeg?

After incorporation in 1873, Winnipeg had a significant lack of emergency ambulances for the first seventy five years. This changed in the late 1950s/early 1960s, as private enterprise saw a business opportunity and latched on. With insufficient emergency ambulance coverage in the city, and current non-emergency ambulance providers not seemingly interested in filling the gap, a new group of commercial ambulance companies began to breed in the city.[139]

138 Yardley, et al (2008): 113.

139 As there has never been a concerted effort to trace the history of Winnipeg's EMS history, the dates provided are approximate, based on the best information available as per Winnipeg Directories, Provincial incorporation records, and local newspaper articles.

## The Growth of Private Ambulance Services

While Winnipeg's first private ambulance companies—businesses that made their income exclusively from providing ambulance services (not including funeral homes and hospitals)—started just after the Second World War, they ultimately weren't economically viable. Nevertheless, seeing the business potential, either by purchase or amalgamation, in 1954, the Leiman Brothers; Henry and Bill, and their brother-in-law, Norm Warren purchased both the Greater Winnipeg Veterans Ambulance and Prince Ambulance, creating the Veterans-Prince Ambulance Service.

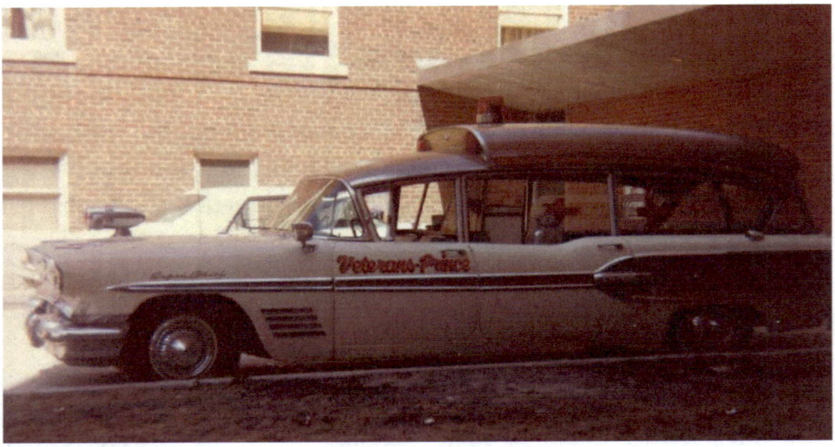


*Veterans-Prince's 1958 Superior(?) Pontiac Ambulance. (Courtesy of the Ken Burdyny Collection)*

Seeing the success of Veterans-Prince Ambulance Service, in 1955, William Charles Saunders started Astorian Ambulance, providing another private emergency ambulance service. Shortly after its creation, the Leimans also acquired Astorian Ambulance. While it was a reasonable business opportunity, it soon became evident that in order to be profitable, there needed to be minimal competition and a high volume of calls. As shown by Arinbjorn Bardel thirty-five years before, a high volume of emergency calls from the railway companies was great for business, but when the calls started drying up, the private ambulance business was no longer profitable.

Inspired by the Leimans and Saunders, in 1957, Don Irish bought a 1944 Packard, a 1949 Dodge, and a 1952 Chrysler, all sedan-based, side-loading ambulances (ambulances that are loaded by opening the curbside, passenger door; you can't get much closer to a taxi cab than that!) and formed Irish Ambulance Service. Following the multiple name approach, in 1963 Irish also began advertising as "Transcona Ambulance and Invalid Car Service". As we'll see, he eventually sold the company to Bill Leiman in 1965 and then started another, competing ambulance service.

To give the Leimans a run for their money, in 1959, Gerald Maeren started Metropolitan Ambulance. Following Irish's style, he acquired a 1949 Flxible Buick and a 1949 Packard; both side-loading ambulances

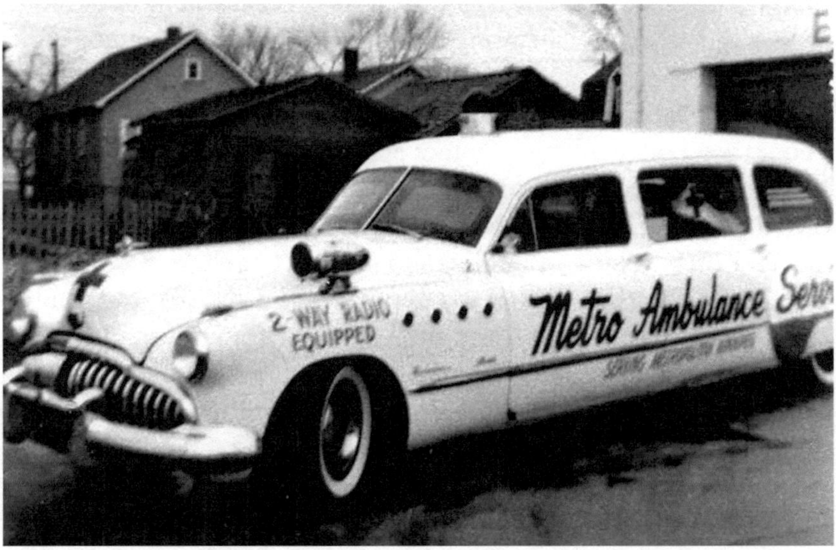


*Metropolitan Ambulance's 1949 Flxble Buick side-loading unit. (Courtesy of Peter Adsten @ EMS Classics)*

To ensure he was easy to find, given the need for a high volume of calls in order be financially viable, in addition to Metropolitan Ambulance, between 1963 and 1967 Maeren registered a number of other trade names including: "AAA," "Amalgamated," "Metro-Assiniboia," "Metro-Fort Garry," "Metro-West Kildonan," "Metro-North Winnipeg," and "St. Boniface." It appears that his marketing worked well, in that he quickly began acquiring more ambulances for his fleet, including: two National Chevrolet station wagons (a 1961 and a 1962 model), a 1963 Cotner-Bevington Oldsmobile, a 1965 Miller-Meteor Cadillac, a 1969 Superior Pontiac, a 1973 Superior Pontiac, and a 1975 GMC van.

Not to suggest that the Leimans were into creating monopolies, but it appears that they were worried about Maeren's success. After Don Irish bought his first new ambulance, a 1964 Ford station wagon, they bought Irish Ambulance Service as well. Then in 1970, Doug James started up Seven Oaks Ambulance and Rescue, with a 1967 Superior Pontiac ambulance bought from United Rescue Services. Within a couple of years, Seven Oaks merged with the Leimans' growing enterprise. To keep up with Maeren's marketing style. Leimans also used the names: "Astorian," "Crestview," "Professional," "St. James," "Irish," and "7-Oaks" for Astorian-Veterans-Prince advertising and promotion.

As a quick aside, while using multiple names was a common strategy in the private ambulance industry, an equally important strategy was to acquire one or more "fast" phone numbers. Before touch-tone phones were invented, most homes and businesses had rotary phones. Each number dialed had to *click* the respective number of points for each digit in the phone number. For example, "9" had nine *clicks* and "4" had four *clicks*. It took an extra second for each two clicks. So, for example, Gerald Maeren acquired the number "233-4467" for AAA Ambulance. It had twenty nine clicks, or took about fifteen seconds to dial. Irish Ambulance acquired the numbers "338-1717"—thirty clicks, and "943-3053"—a mind numbing thirty seven clicks or nineteen seconds to dial. John Wylie got one of the fastest numbers: "284-4225," which took twenty seven clicks, or twelve seconds to dial.

This is one of the reasons why, in 1975, Winnipeg switched its emergency number from 999 to 911. The switch removed sixteen clicks, or eight seconds, from the dialing time needed in an emergency. While "1" would seem like the quickest first number to use, because it was already reserved for long distance calls and it was the easiest number to accidently dial on a rotary phone, it was not a viable option.

It appears that in the Wild West of ambulance trading, the Leimans didn't ask Don Irish to sign a non-competition agreement as a condition of selling his company. As a result, in 1970, after selling to the Leimans, Irish started Reliable Ambulance, and subsequently bought out St. Francis-McGee Ambulance Service; a small ambulance company started in about1960 by Charles Berard. Irish then began operating his new ambulance service under the names "Reliable Ambulance Service" and "St. Francis-Norwood Ambulance," running two 1959 Superior Pontiacs.

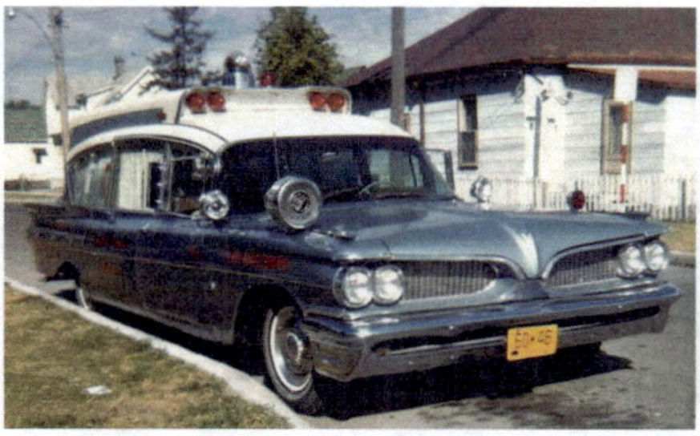 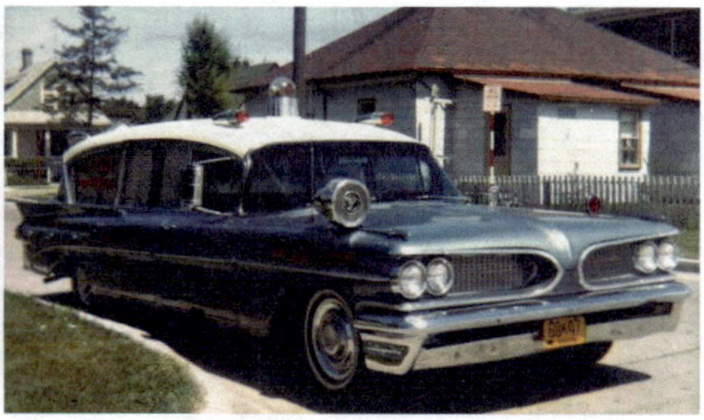

*While St. Francis Ambulance had two 1959 Superior-Pontiac ambulances, interestingly they were different models. Left is a forty eight-inch high top model (possibly capable of carrying four very cramped patients) while right is the standard forty two-inch model. (Courtesy of Peter Adsten @ EMS Classics)*

Irish also acquired a 1966 Superior Pontiac, a 1973 GMC Wayne van-type, and a home-built 1974 GM Suburban.

There was a visible change in the new entries to Winnipeg's ambulance market beginning in 1966. In that year, the US National Research Council published the previously discussed "White Paper." It emphasized how there were too many people dying in motor vehicle accidents because of too few trained responders/too many underequipped ambulances. As a result, Washington assigned the Department of Transportation to develop emergency medicine standards for ambulances. Interestingly, the White Paper noted that the US national average response time for an ambulance was forty minutes.[140]

In apparent response to the White Paper and the related emerging trends in the US, in 1966 former Irish Ambulance employee John Wylie created "Wylie's Rescue Ambulance". Starting with a 1957 Superior Cadillac, he moved to a 1967 Superior Pontiac (high headroom, four-stretcher), a 1972 Laurie Carriage Works/GMC modular, a 1973 Superior Pontiac, and a 1974 Superior Pontiac. Wylie was a unique guy himself, and his service reflected his attributes. In a period when many Winnipeg ambulances carried minimal equipment, Wylie's rigs, besides carrying oxygen and an array of medical supplies, also carried fire extinguishers and the basic extrication tools needed for assisting at motor vehicle accidents. As well, when most of the city's ambulances, except for the fire department, barely had room for one patient, Wylie acquired a custom-built, high-headroom. four-patient ambulance, and in 1972, bought the city's first modular, truck-chassised ambulance (see image on page 85). Perhaps equally unique was the training

140 Barkley (1978): 148.

of Wylie's staff. While staff had the required first aid certificates, Wylie also required all staff to attend autopsies at the Health Sciences Centre, enabling them to better understand the human body. The superior equipment and staff training made Wylie's Rescue one of the city's premier private services, giving him clients who often had more political influence.

Also jumping into the fray in 1966 was tow truck operator Ken Burdyny. Making the connection between car accidents, tow trucks, and ambulances, he started a "one stop" enterprise called Riverview and Kildonan Ambulance. Being a mouthful, the name was quickly changed to simply Riverview Ambulance. In his fleet, Burdyny ran a 1957 Superior Cadillac, a 1959 Memphis Chrysler, a 1966 Gateway Autobody Chrysler, a 1972 GMC van—home built, and a 1974 Oldsmobile Cotner-Bevington. The 1966 Gateway Chrysler was particularly unique in that its front and rear roof top tunnel lights were taillights from a 1962 Mercury Monterey, the taillights from a 1959 Buick, and the rear door from a 1954 Ford Sedan Delivery. While I'm not sure how well it worked, it certainly was an interesting vehicle!

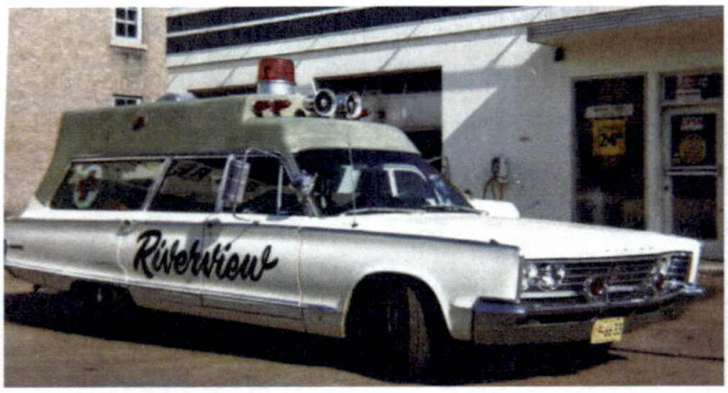


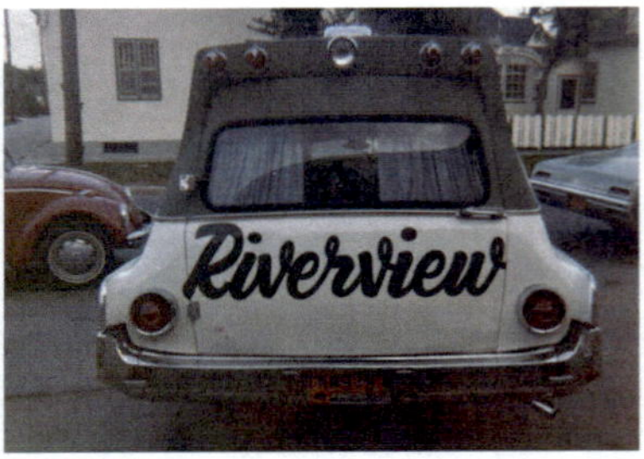


*Riverview's 1966 Gateway-Chrysler ambulance. (Courtesy of the Ken Burdyny Collection)*

Seeing Burdyny's success in using his towing business to acquire corollary ambulance business from car accidents, in 1968 the Leach Brothers, Gerald and Gary, owners of United Towing followed suit. Utilizing a 1967 Superior Pontiac, a 1970 Wayne Chevrolet Suburban, a 1972 Superior Pontiac (destroyed a year later), and a 1974 Cotner-Bevington Oldsmobile, they used their towing services as a stepping stone to enter the ambulance business; rebranding it as United Ambulance and Rescue Services.

The problem with ambulance services prior to the mid-1970s was that with notable exceptions, they were often glorified taxi services using station wagons. Whether the person was dead or alive really did not matter, as both got similar treatment; a quick ride to the nearest hospital. At the time of expansion of private emergency ambulances, there were minimal requirements to run an ambulance service. As of 1962, all a person needed was a chauffeur's license. A first aid certificate was required, but the requirement was often ignored or not enforced. More often than not, especially before the 1966-era, an ambulance would arrive with a driver and stretcher, but no attendant or first aid supplies.

## Winnipeg Gets Closer to a Public Ambulance Service

The 1957 election of Mayor Stephen Juba provided stimulus for policy changes that would impact Winnipeg's EMS for the next sixty years. His policies would also lead to the creation of the Winnipeg Ambulance Service. Juba was a huge fan of big American cities, and from his first day in office, for good or bad, over the next twenty years he worked tirelessly to grow Winnipeg into the equivalent.

In November 1960, Juba facilitated the creation of the Metropolitan Corporation of Greater Winnipeg, or "Metro Winnipeg," a governing body that provided partial joint leadership for the municipalities surrounding the City of Winnipeg. Its membership included Brooklands, Tuxedo, Charleswood, Transcona, West Kildonan, North Kildonan, East Kildonan, Old Kildonan, St. Boniface, St. Vital, and Fort Garry. Until the creation of Unicity in 1972, it managed joint services such as transit,

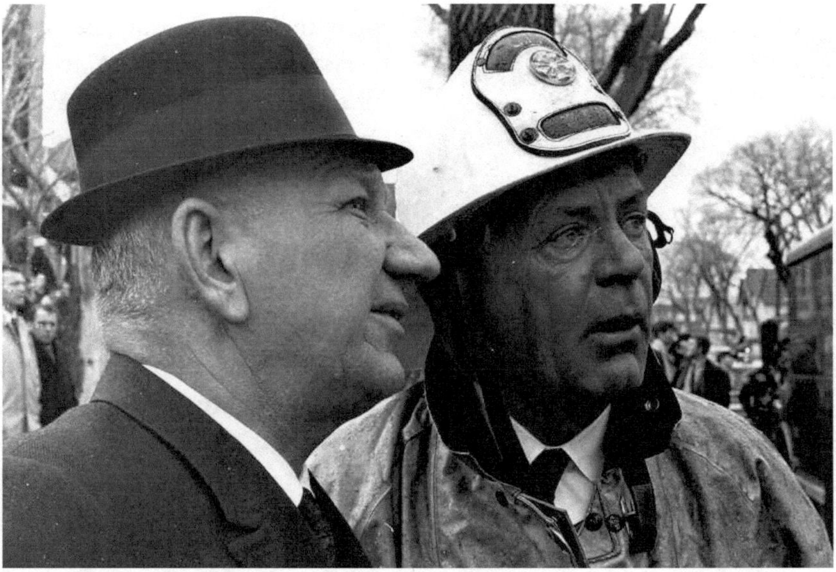

*Mayor Stephen Juba in one of his favourite roles, supervising the Winnipeg Fire Department (with Chief Cam Shewan). (Courtesy of FFHSW)*

waterworks, and parks. As Juba's ultimate goal was to create one unified city, from the beginning of his first term he worked at ensuring that municipal services could be Metro Winnipeg wide.

Even before the creation of Metro Winnipeg, Juba facilitated the creation of a single, three-digit emergency number for all of the member municipalities. While traveling through Europe in the mid-1950s, Juba noticed that many areas had a three-digit telephone number that would connect the caller to all emergency services. Always looking for practical ways to improve Winnipeg, not to mention help in creating his unified city, he gleefully brought the idea back. With the help of the Manitoba Telephone System, a system similar to that used in England was developed. With the new system, a person could dial 999 on their phone and an operator would immediately direct their call to the most appropriate service. This replaced the then-existing thirty two separate, seven-digit emergency numbers found in Metro Winnipeg with the one three-digit number. Winnipeg was the first North American city to implement the three-digit emergency phone number.

The proposal combined emergency service phone numbers for sixteen different municipalities. Some municipal leaders were upset with the cost, which was a proposed annual fee of 10.77 cents per person in their municipality; believing this was too extravagant. Alderman Albert Bennett (Winnipeg Police Commission's chair) proposed a way to cut costs by hiring women as operators, at a cost of $200/month, instead of $345/month for male personnel. This cut one quarter of the cost to the municipalities and was accepted by city council. Councillors were reassured by Mr. Bennett that "this arrangement will not affect the efficient operation of the proposed system." [141] For con-

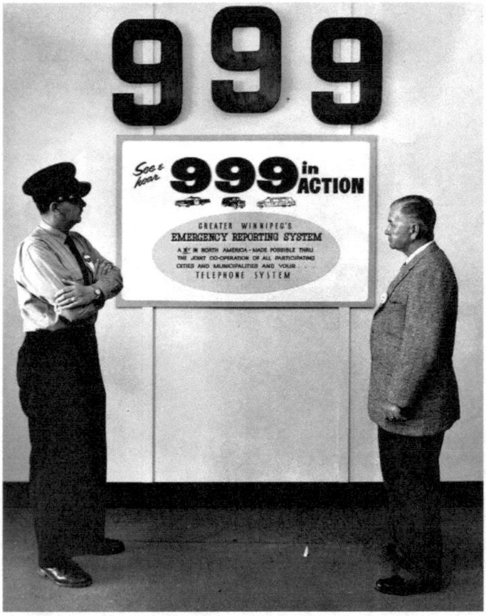


*Display at Winnipeg's 1959 Red River Exhibition demonstrating the new 999 emergency number. (Courtesy of FFHSW)*

141 "Three Digit Emergency Dialing in Winnipeg." 2019 *Winnipeg Police Museum Annual Report*: 28.

text, $200 in 1959 equates to roughly $1,780 in today's market. The reference to hiring of female employees as a way to "cut costs without affecting efficiency" is such an odd and embarrassing contrast to today, where Winnipeg has several dozen female firefighters and almost half of its paramedics are women.

On June 21, 1959, Winnipeg commenced operation of the first three-digit emergency phone number in North America[142]. By dialing "999", Winnipeggers had instant access to police, fire, ambulance, a doctors' directory, and the poison control centre. A team of nine women—eight operators and a supervisor—working in shifts of two, directed the 300 calls per day to the appropriate emergency service within the applicable municipality.[143] By contrast, New York City, the first city in the United States to get a three-digit emergency number, didn't acquire their system until 1968.

Today the system handles 1,300 calls per day and employs more than 100 staff.[144] Considering that the city's population has grown significantly since 1959, this may not seem like a large increase. However, since the system's introduction, Winnipeggers are now better educated as to what constitutes an "emergency". There are now fewer calls reporting overflowing toilets and cars running out of gas than when the emergency number was first introduced.

Throughout North America, there was a growing recognition that a three-digit, "one stop" emergency telephone number was an asset. In 1957, the International Association of Fire Chiefs recommended the use of a single number for reporting fires. Little happened for ten years until the President's Commission on Law Enforcement and Administration of Justice recommended that a nationwide, single number be established for reporting emergencies. Apparently, recommendations from the White House have a greater impact than those from the national fire chiefs' association.

Within a year, the American Telephone and Telegraph Company (AT&T) announced that it had researched and developed the 911 number and would introduce it as the emergency code throughout the United States. AT&T's research found that the digits 911 are quick

142 "City's 999 Only One On This Continent." *Winnipeg Free Press.* June 20, 1959.

143 Scott Billeck. "Three-digit emergency line in Winnipeg turns 60." *Winnipeg Sun.* June 21, 2019.

144 Ibid.

to dial (sixteen fewer *clicks* on a rotary phone than 999), easy to find in the dark, and had never been authorized as an office code, area code, or service code. The U.S. congress quickly passed legislation making 911 the standard nationwide emergency number. With 911 being standardized in the United States, Canadian cities quickly followed suit. On June 22, 1975, the Manitoba Telephone System switched Winnipeg's emergency number to 911.

The 911 dispatch system has continued to evolve with new technology. For example, in 1980, it became possible to instantly trace a call to 911. While this may seem simple today with caller ID, in 1980, before this breakthrough, it would take 911 operators up to two hours to trace a call when the caller disconnected (or passed out) before they could identify themselves.[145] Today, the technology has evolved further to enable a 911 operator to identify a cell phone caller's precise location the instant a call for help is received.

In Winnipeg, tied to the use of the new emergency number came a heated City Council debate as to whether fire department rescue squads should be used for emergency patient transport in non-fire situations. With the ultimate goal of combining the sixteen municipalities that formed Metro Winnipeg, an underlying problem was that the cost of using fire rescues as ambulances would be cost prohibitive. Winnipeg's fire department was already running two rescue squads as ambulances and added a third in 1961.

At the time, the city's protection committee ordered that the rescues not be used in situations where an ambulance was more appropriate. The committee's rationale was that as the rescue squad was a firefighting vehicle, it should not be used for transporting injured people, particularly when the injury was not fire related. Given the state of ambulance services in Winnipeg, such an order was ignored as being impractical. At the time, fire rescue squads were the only vehicles in Winnipeg that were carrying resuscitators and had staff consistently trained in first aid. Failure to have firefighters respond would have meant a significant increase in deaths from chokings, drownings, electrocutions, and cardiac arrests.

However, in an effort to reduce the number of medical calls which would be directed to the fire department, an obvious need for the future

145 "New system would trace all 911 calls." *Winnipeg Free Press*. April 17, 1980.

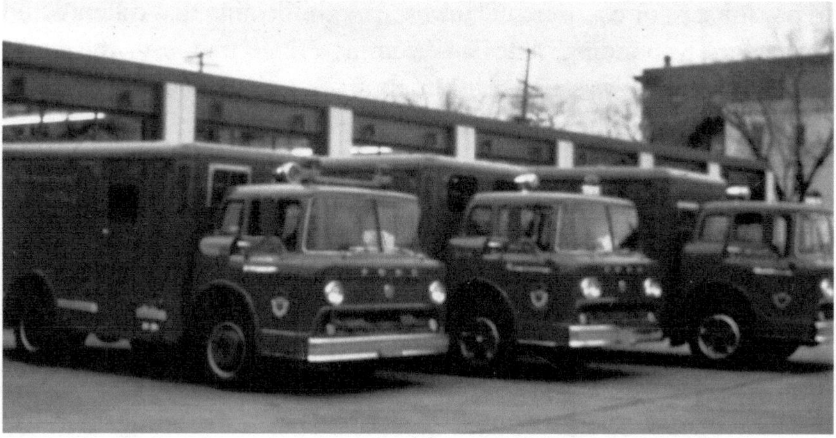

*Winnipeg Fire Department's 1961 fleet of rescue squads. WFD's contribution to the city's 1960's ambulance debacle. (Courtesy of FFHSW)*

Unicity, in July 1959 the city's finance committee awarded a municipal contract for all emergency medical calls to a private ambulance provider. After taking bids from both Astorian-Veterans-Prince Service and Irish Ambulance Service, the finance committee awarded the contract to Astorian-Veterans-Prince.[146]

This was more of a knee-jerk reaction by the city, aimed at reducing costs. There was no effort, whatsoever, to create a proper ambulance service for Winnipeg. City Council did not provide any type of subsidy to Astorian-Veterans-Prince for responding to 999 calls, did not assist in collecting ambulance fees, continued to provided free ambulance services through both the police and fire departments, and continued to allow other private ambulance companies to compete with Astorian-Veterans-Prince for the same small piece of the pie.

The results can best be described as *wacky*.

As was quickly shown, Astorian-Veterans-Prince was placed in the awkward position of needing to screen referrals from the 999 dispatch centre to first determine whether the callers had the ability to pay. The city had created a situation where Astorian-Veterans-Prince was contractually required to respond to ambulance calls throughout Metro Winnipeg, and yet if the callers couldn't (or wouldn't pay), that was Astorian-Veterans-Prince's problem. If Astorian-Veterans-Prince didn't confirm payment, they were stuck with the potential of having no funds

146 "Vets Ambulance for City Work." *Winnipeg Tribune.* July 10, 1959.

to pay for staff or equipment. However, by confirming that callers could pay before responding, Astorian-Veterans-Prince met with the ire of city councillors. It was a no-win situation.

The silliness of the situation was best captured in a December 1959 *Winnipeg Tribune* article, where Henry Leiman, president of Astorian-Veterans-Prince, explained that they couldn't compete with the city's free ambulance services. Alderman Bennett retorted that: "either the City should operate a regular ambulance service and charge for routine trips or we should require the private companies to answer every call they are given under threat of losing their city license."[147] Despite having been an alderman for four years at the time, Bennett appears to have been out of touch; various public groups had been advocating for a city-run ambulance service for the previous fifty years!

Mr. Leiman's concerns were further exemplified when Astorian-Veterans-Prince was dispatched by Winnipeg's emergency call center to medical calls at both a private residence and the arena. In both cases, Astorian-Veterans-Prince units arrived to find a police ambulance already dealing with the call—despite the fact that the mandate of the police ambulance service was to respond to medical calls involving: " … street accidents, accidents, persons collapsing, etc, in places in which the public has access or public places, industrial accidents, fires…" In response to criticism, the the police chief replied: "This is the intended use of police ambulances, but there will be occasions when the police arrive at a place that does not come under the intended use, and then humanity and common sense must dictate."[148] On the surface, a perfectly reasonable explanation. Unfortunately, it also suggested that the private ambulance services were expected to operate at a loss in order to accommodate the city's failure to follow both their own policies and create a proper public service.

The civic debate in 1959, combined with concerns about ambulance services in general, helped to stimulate a 1961 review of ambulance services by Metro Winnipeg's Civil Defence Department. The review resulted in a scathing report, severely criticizing ambulance services in Greater Winnipeg. It found that of the five private ambulance companies: Astorian-Veterans-Prince Service (five units), Irish Ambulance Service (three units), Metropolitan Ambulance Service (two units),

---

147 "Ambulance Payments Criticized, Defended." *Winnipeg Tribune.* December 10, 1959.
148 "Say Police Ambulance Doing Private Work." *Winnipeg Free Press.* January 22, 1959.

St. Frances/McGee Ambulance Service (two units), and St. Boniface Ambulance Service (one unit), as well as the City Police ambulance and a prisoner transport wagon (listed as an alternate ambulance) and the Department of Veterans Affairs ambulance, none provided a quality level of care. There were only a handful of full-time employees operating the sixteen units. The remainder of staff were either part-time or on-call. The report noted that only 29 percent of ambulances carried an assistant; most units arrived at an emergency with only a driver.

With notable exceptions, the service provided by the private companies ranged from moderately poor to awful. Other problems with ambulance services in Winnipeg included: inefficiency in handling casualties; lack of attention in ambulances; refusal of operators to accept patients unless the charges for that trip were paid in advance in cash; lack of cleanliness of the ambulance; aggravation of a patient's condition through a lack of knowledge of elementary first aid; inability to obtain an ambulance as the operator only runs the ambulance as a sideline to some other business; and a lack of equipment in the ambulance, or if the equipment is present, lack of knowledge of how to use it.[149]

The report went on to note that in a survey of Winnipeg ambulance operators, 66 percent could only carry one patient, 29 percent carried an assistant - the rest only had a driver, and only 49 percent had received *some* first aid training.[150] Perhaps the most quirky part of the ambulance situation was that of the sixteen units operating in the city, almost a quarter were operated by funeral homes.[151] This created a potential conflict of interest, in that if the seriously injured casualty being transported did not arrive at the hospital fast enough, the funeral home would likely get additional business. A bizarre problem, with disturbing ramifications.

While this picture seems horrific, context is important. It is worth remembering that prior to January 1, 1962, a few months *after* the report came out, neither Winnipeg nor Manitoba had any laws respecting ambulances. The Civil Defence Report seems to have been the stimulus for the first City of Winnipeg ambulance bylaw. Further, as both the police and fire departments were providing free ambulance

149 Civil Defence Department. *Extracts from a brief submitted to the Manitoba Medical Association on ambulance services in Metropolitan Winnipeg.* Metropolitan Corporation of Greater Winnipeg, 1961: 1.

150 Civil Defence Department: 2.

151 Civil Defence Department: 14.

services, it was extremely difficult for private ambulance companies to be able to charge enough to acquire either proper staff or adequate equipment. Finally, the report mentioned that "a quarter" of the city's private ambulances were operated by funeral homes. This statement is misleading, given that Winnipeg's funeral homes had ceased providing emergency ambulance services in the 1930s. Despite this allegation, *none* of the sixteen ambulances listed in the Civil Defence Department's report were operated by funeral homes. At the time, funeral homes in Winnipeg were only providing *invalid* or transfer ambulance services. Given the data utilized and the timing of the report, it seemed unrealistic to expect any other level of quality for Winnipeg's ambulance services.

The Civil Defence Department's report recommended that a centralized Winnipeg agency be set up to manage the ambulance service. It cited Vancouver, British Columbia as having a model to follow, with both privately and publicly owned ambulances being used to provide needed emergency medical services. The privately-owned ambulances were assigned districts and responded to all calls in their area.

At page 5 of their 1961 report, the Civil Defence Department noted:

> . . . The cycle of an ambulance service as evidenced in Winnipeg is for one or two men to purchase the cheapest possible unit, plastering it with their name or the name of their service, attracting attention by racing all over town with screaming sirens as a form of self-advertisement, accepting all and every call, even when they know rival units have already been notified, making their service pay by dint of hard work and long hours, and eventually taking on an extra employee to relieve them to a certain extent. They develop a credit rating, improving all the time, enabling them to invest in a bigger, somewhat more modern and more gawdy unit, which is probably a unit previously accepted in part exchange when some other ambulance service has bought a new unit. They operate these two units for a time, trying to undercut all competitors and thus forcing some of the more efficient services who cannot match these charges to bankruptcy whereby they, the less efficient and newer service, are able to obtain more work and thereby expand their service, possibly by the purchase of some bankrupt units, until finally, they too, having to employ more personnel, and because they are

> running more expensive units, have to make higher charges which cannot be reconciled with the running of their old decrepit original unis, which they therefore sell. The whole cycle is then repeated by some other man buying up the cheap unit they have just sold and starting a service until he too drives the now expanded service in its turn. This has happened not only in Winnipeg, but in all major cities, both in Canada and in the United States where haphazard ambulance services have been allowed to develop.[152]

Again, while the report's findings were alarming, the problems were ultimately a result of the City of Winnipeg's failure to take action. At the same time, the city did not have the financial resources to create a proper service. It was a no-win situation where there were dedicated ambulance personnel: firefighters, police officers, and private ambulance attendants, who wanted to provide services, the sick and injured who desperately needed aid, and a haphazard system that had hobbled along for eighty years, aggravated by the city's financial woes.

A further, often unmentioned aspect of having multiple for-profit ambulance services in a limited area was the nasty competitiveness. The conduct was similar to firefighters a century before, when there were multiple, independent volunteer fire companies operated in large American cities. Their fighting to be the "first in" to claim limited insurance company "rewards," in many cases led to thwarting their competitors while ignoring the fire.[153]

Winnipeg's private ambulance providers often obstructed each other's efforts to get paying patients. It wasn't unheard of for ambulance companies with one or two units to get mysterious out-of-town calls that would send their staff on "wild goose chases" for three or four hours, making them unavailable to respond to calls in the city.[154]

Similarly, it wasn't unusual for private ambulance providers to use police radio scanners and grab calls before a competitor could respond, or if arriving second, to park so that a competitor's rear door was blocked; preventing access to their stretcher.[155] While these tactics were

152 Civil Defence Department: 5.

153 Parker (2008): 34.

154 See for example, "Meanness." *Winnipeg Free Press.* April 29, 1961.

155 Interview with Wayne Farmer, former Astorian-Veterans-Prince attendant, October 18, 2023.

counterproductive, it appears that Winnipeg didn't have some of the more extreme competitive tactics, such as stealing keys to competitor's ambulances, stealing entire ambulances, and/or actually destroying competitors' vehicles by putting sugar in the gas tanks and ruining their engines, as seen in some other cities.[156] While pure speculation, the fact that key competitors in Winnipeg's ambulance industry were police officers and firefighters perhaps put a damper on some of the more destructive tactics.

While Winnipeg's private ambulance services often got bad reviews, both in the media and in official government reports, it's important to recognize that there was an equally positive and compassionate side to the industry. Unfortunately, this aspect was often unreported. Consider:

- In 1961, when the City introduced the new proposed ambulance bylaw, three of the four private ambulance company owners argued that the rules needed to go further, noting that better control and regulation would provide better service.[157]
- In a reported incident from December 1966, Veterans-Prince Ambulance Service received an emergency call. Not having resources close enough to respond, Veterans-Prince's dispatcher immediately contacted Irish Ambulance Service; the ambulance company that was closest to the reported address. Ambulance attendants from Irish responded immediately, and despite initially finding no heartbeat, using CPR resuscitated the patient twice enroute to St. Boniface Hospital.[158] It was only through this kind of inter-company cooperation that many patients survived.
- Particularly after 1966, as the insights of the *White Paper* began to spread, many of the city's private ambulance operators began investing in superior, modern equipment. There was a definite commitment on the part of many of the private operators to provide the best service possible. Unfortunately, the economics of competing with free services,

156 Duncan (2019): 6.

157 "Men Behind the Siren." The *Winnipeg Tribune*. August 22, 1961.

158 "Man Brings Woman Back To Life Twice." The *Winnipeg Free Press*. December 19, 1966.

> provided haphazardly by Winnipeg via the police and fire departments, made it difficult for the private owners to properly maintain these expensive vehicles.[159]

As Winnipeg rolled into the 1960s, in many ways, the city's ambulance problem was akin to Hans Christian Andersen's fable: "The Emperor's New Clothes." It seems that everyone involved, except for Winnipeg City Council, understood that Winnipeg's prehospital emergency medical services were a mess. Unfortunately, with no power or money to fix the problem, each involved agency and private business did what little they could to help rectify the situation.

As a result of the inane 1959 ban-fire-rescues-as-ambulances debate, the Winnipeg Fire Department added two extra rescue squads to its roster. Again, by building the squads in-house, and by transferring staff from seldom-used apparatus, such as the high-pressure units, the fire department was able to beef up their ability to provide efficient emergency medical care without hiring more staff.

Winnipeg Police, in response to the highly critical 1961 Civil Defence Department's report, added a second ambulance to its roster. In 1963, they acquired a new Cotner-Bevington Oldsmobile raised-roof *Seville* ambulance. As a standard wheelbase station wagon (as opposed to the stretched, Hearse-type vehicles used by the private service providers), it didn't have much room for providing care enroute to the hospital. Also, it was only staffed by a driver, with a second officer being picked-up enroute to act as an attendant. Nevertheless, it showed a commitment by Winnipeg's police to try and pull their weight, without adequate funding, in a messed-up system.

It appears that the 1966 White Paper had a significant impact on Winnipeg. Unlike the 1961 Civil Defense report which simply criticized Winnipeg's ambulance system, the White Paper, in linking the need for improved prehospital care with automobile accidents, provided concrete suggestions for improved emergency care. While city council's collective heads remained firmly buried in the proverbial sand, except when they came up for air and debated whether they should ban private ambulances from using their sirens, all of the other involved parties extracted lessons from the White Paper on how to improve services.

159 Miscellaneous interviews with John Wylie, Garry Leach, and Bryan Leach.

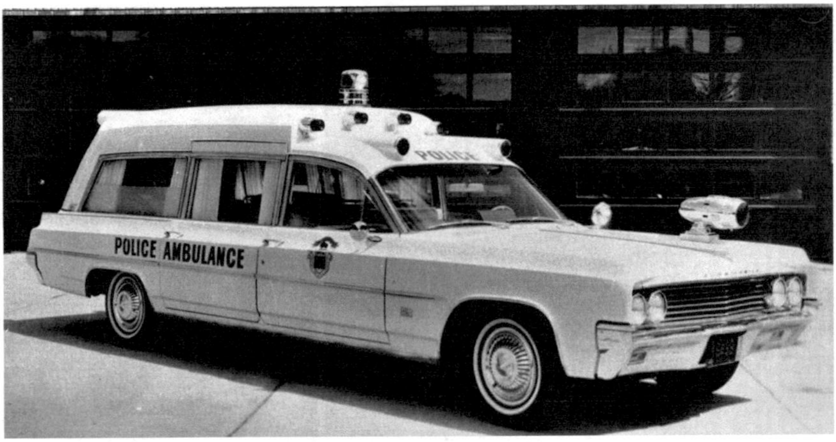


*In an effort to improve their ambulance service, in 1963, Winnipeg Police added a high headroom Cotner-Bevington Oldsmobile ambulance to their fleet. (Courtesy of Peter Adsten @ EMS Classics)*

The Winnipeg Fire Department had each of their rescues equipped with a direct radio link to Misericordia Hospital's newish emergency ward. As the rescues had been carrying emergency breathing equipment, including respirators and pulmotors since 1929, they were usually dispatched to the more serious medical emergencies such as cardiac arrests, choking, and electrocutions. With direct contact with an emergency room doctor or nurse, the rescue teams could get better patient care instructions enroute.

While firefighters didn't have extensive training in emergency care at the time beyond advanced first aid, emergency room doctors also did not have specialized training in emergency medicine or trauma care. This resulted in all involved, while trying their best, only providing a basic level of care to patients.

As mentioned, several private ambulance operators including John Wylie of Wylie Rescue Ambulance, Ken Burdyny of Riverview Ambulance, and Gerald and Garry Leach of United Rescue Services Limited, all created ambulance services which reflected principles outlined in the White Paper.

The Winnipeg Police also latched on to the White Paper's linkage between motor vehicle accidents and the need for ambulances. Purchasing two 1966 full-sized Plymouth station wagons, the WPD converted them into ambulances (albeit with extremely limited patient working space), and assigned them to its traffic division. Staffed by a single officer with a "senior" first aid certificate (roughly equivalent to today's sixteen-hour "Standard First Aid Certificate"), a second officer would be picked up enroute. While seriously underequipped and used primarily to transport accident victims to the hospital as opposed to providing any degree of on-scene emergency care, these two new ambulances were a definite improvement to the paddy wagons and even the older, single purpose-built ambulance previously used for medical calls. With the two new station wagon ambulances, WPD's ambulance fleet was up to four units.

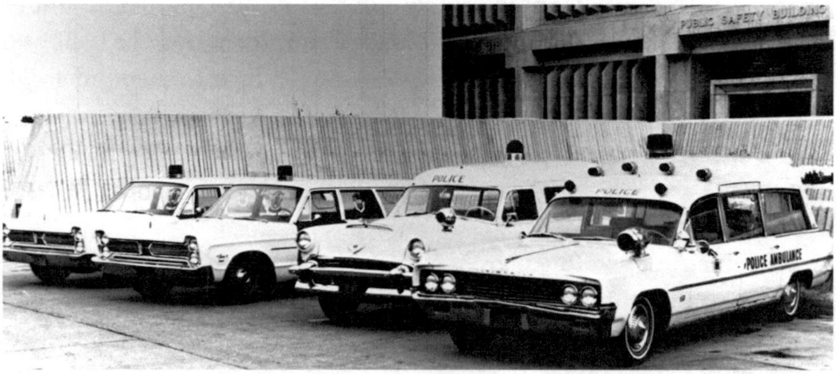


*Winnipeg Police's 1966 ambulance fleet, including the two new Plymouth station wagons on the left, proudly displayed in front of Winnipeg's newly opened Public Safety Building. (Courtesy of Peter Adsten @ EMS Classics)*

I can attest to the experience of riding in one of the WPD's Plymouth ambulances. After my dad, older sister, and I were involved in a motor vehicle accident in the late 1960s, one of WPD's traffic ambulances responded. My dad and sister were piled in the back; Dad on the gurney and Lise wrapped in a blanket on the floor beside him. Four-year-old me was plunked on the front bench seat, firmly squished between the two large officers with a rag pressed to my forehead, stopping the blood (after being hit by parts of the windshield) from splattering onto their uniforms. There was no room for an attendant to ride in the back. Perhaps not the most ideal way to transport three casualties to the Misericordia Hospital, but we got there quickly.

It's important to emphasize, again, that no criticism is being directed at the individual officers. They were relegated to doing a job they didn't want to do. They had signed up to be cops, not ambulance attendants, and to make matters worse, they were neither given the training nor equipment to properly accomplish the job they had been assigned. City

Council didn't want them to be providing ambulance services at accidents, and they were now stuck trying to figure out what to do with a four-year-old, uncoordinated due to cerebral palsy, who was bopping around spewing blood onto their uniforms. Kind hearted as they were, I can't blame them for tossing everyone into the cramped ambulance and trying to dump them off at the hospital as quickly as possible.

While the city's various ambulance providers were trying to improve their game, Winnipeg's City Hall did not follow. In October 1966, after being reminded that it would cost $365,000 to set up a municipal ambulance service,[160] the Winnipeg City Council simply shelved the issue and renewed its contract with Astorian-Veterans-Prince to respond to all 999 emergency medical calls. It further directed, apparently as a cost saving measure, that the police ambulances and fire department rescue squads were dispatched only when all of Astorian-Veterans-Prince's ambulances were busy.

Winnipeg's convoluted ambulance system became even less efficient when the Winnipeg Police Commission, which managed the 999 emergency call centre, determined that the contract with Astoria-Veterans-Prince also applied to all 999 calls coming from the surrounding municipalities;[161] an area almost double the City of Winnipeg's population and covering three times the land area.

Despite requests from the outlying municipalities to direct calls to locally based ambulance services, every call was handled by the one ambulance service based in Winnipeg. There were now six ambulances; three operating from a station in Winnipeg's West End and three others at satellite locations, responding to all calls in Metro Winnipeg. This often resulted in response times of fifteen to twenty minutes, with at least one call taking forty seven minutes for the ambulance to arrive.

Given that heart attack victims need help within a couple of minutes, results for medical emergencies were often negative. As with previous directions from city hall, the directive to not respond to medical emergencies was routinely ignored by both the police and fire departments. In 1959, the fire department responded to 450 resuscitation calls, in 1968, this was up to 1,973 calls, and by 1974, after the creation of Unicity, this

---

160 "Province Now In On Study." *Winnipeg Free Press.* June 27, 1969.
161 "Illegality Argument In Vain." *Winnipeg Free Press.* September 28, 1967.

had increased to 3,396.[162] Not only did the WPD ignore the City Council's directive, but in 1969, medical staff at the Winnipeg General Hospital were recruited to teach police ambulance officers how to use resuscitators, oxygen equipment, airways, and suction equipment.[163]

After recognizing that their plan for directing all 999 ambulance emergency calls to Astoria-Veterans-Prince didn't work, the police commission revised its directive in 1969. For the next three years, ambulance calls for the surrounding municipalities, directed through the 999 call centre, were redirected to those municipalities' police departments for response by an ambulance provider of their choice. However, when the suburban police departments subsequently merged with Winnipeg Police in 1972, the chaos started all over again.

To show the total confusion that reigned at city hall, in the midst of private ambulances improving their services and being directed by city council to handle all emergency medical calls, Winnipeg City Council began debating, yet again, whether to ban private ambulances from using their sirens.

In the spring of 1966, the Canadian Medical Association passed a recommendation that private ambulances be banned from using sirens. It seems that there were underlying beliefs that private ambulance operators were using their sirens as a means of advertising, and the extra couple of minutes saved getting to the hospital did not significantly affect patient outcome. (Unfortunately, probably true, given the hospital staff's lack of training in trauma and/or emergency medicine.)

As a result, both Winnipeg and St. James City Councils began debating bylaws which would prohibit the use of sirens by private ambulances.[164]

The debate continued for several years, with Astorian-Veterans-Prince Ambulance Service, which had the 999 ambulance contract, voluntarily not using sirens in 1968. By 1970, the debate seems to have died, and the proposed bylaws never actually passed. Regardless, the fact that the issue was given serious debate shows how little the city actually thought about the need for emergency care in Metro Winnipeg. Interestingly, Edmonton, Alberta followed Winnipeg's lead, banning sirens on private ambulances until 1971.[165]

---

162 Richardson Report: 7.

163 "Resuscitation Help Earns Chief's Praise." *Winnipeg Free Press.* January 9, 1969.

164 "Silent Sirens." *Winnipeg Free Press.* May 13, 1966.

165 Plumbtree (2011): 258.

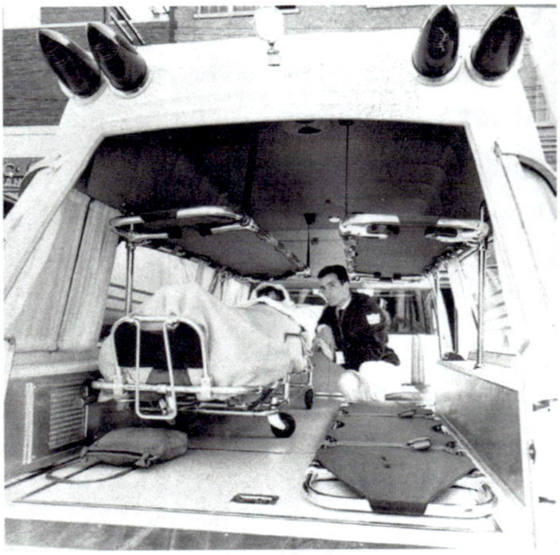

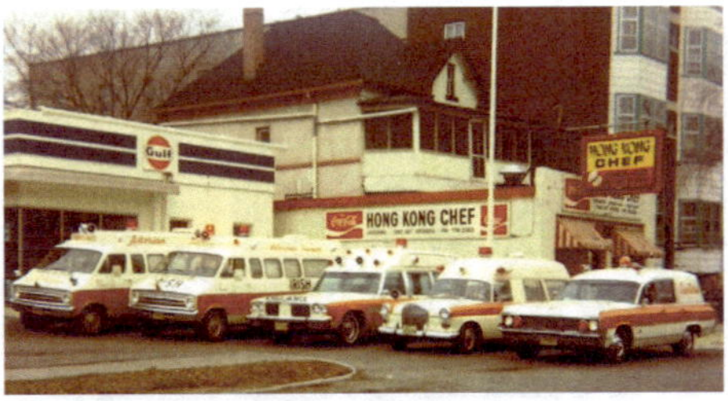


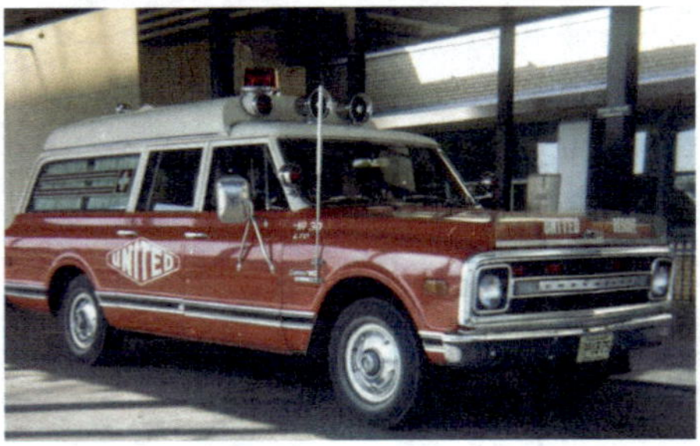


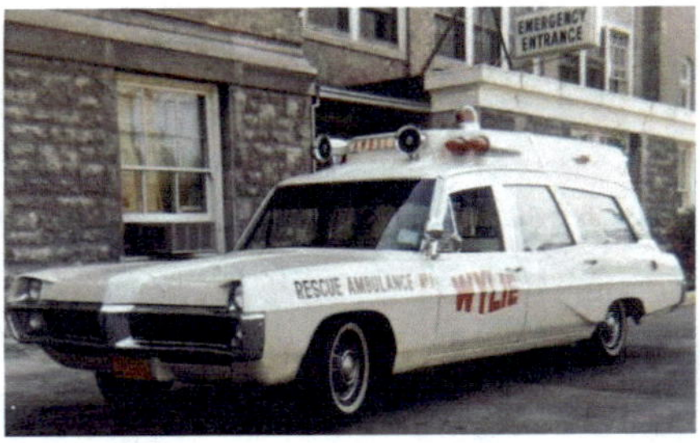


*An array of private ambulances used in Winnipeg in the late 1960s/early 1970s including John Wylie and his four-stretcher high top 1967 Superior-Pontiac (two stretchers are suspended from the ceiling), the Veterans-Prince-Astorian-Irish fleet, and the use of heavier Suburban-chassied ambulances such as United Rescue's 1970 Chevrolet. (Courtesy of Peter Adsten @ EMS Classics)*

In an effort to rectify the overall abysmal ambulance situation, in 1967, Astorian-Veterans-Prince's main competitors: Metropolitan Ambulance, Riverview-Kildonan, St. Francis, and Wylie ambulance services joined together to form the Winnipeg Ambulance Association. While they had an obvious underling financial motivation: each wanting a piece of the municipal pie, the end result of their cooperative effort would have provided an additional nine ambulances to respond to emergency calls in Winnipeg, resulting in faster response times.

The Winnipeg Ambulance Association, through its president, John Wylie, proposed that the city copy the ambulance dispatch model used (at the time) in Vancouver, British Columbia. The idea was that the city be divided into districts, with a private ambulance assigned to each district. When a call came in, the 999 dispatcher would simply cross reference the street address with the ambulance assigned to that district and alert the responsible ambulance company. The nearest police ambulance or fire rescue squad would be dispatched if the assigned ambulance was already on a call.

Unfortunately, there were two key problems with this proposal. First, Astorian-Veterans-Prince would not join the Association. Second, Winnipeg City Council had no interest in breaking its contract with Astorian-Veterans-Prince. Instead, ignoring the real issue, at a September 4, 1968 police commission meeting, the commission requested that the ambulance operators form a central dispatch operation with Astoria-Veterans-Prince and distribute the calls amongst themselves. At the risk of being repetitive, at this point Astoria-Veterans-Prince was refusing to work with the other private ambulance services, and the city was refusing to break their contract with Astoria-Veterans-Prince. Yet somehow, the police commission believed that their request would provide a workable solution.

After significant infighting, Astorian-Veterans-Prince finally joined the Winnipeg Ambulance Association. While owners Henry Leiman, Bill Leiman, and Norman Warren had initially demanded that Wylie's resignation as president and that they receive three votes on all decisions, the Leimans finally settled for just the resignation.

History indicates that Wylie had a profound ability to aggravate competitors and politicians alike. His "my way or the highway" approach irritated many people. However, there is little doubt that he had a commitment to improving emergency medical care for the citizens of Winnipeg. Throughout the late 1960s and early 1970s, Wylie took the recommendations of the White Paper to heart and spent countless hours lobbying for better prehospital care. During the period leading to the creation of Winnipeg's municipal ambulance service, Wylie was at the forefront of virtually every ambulance-related debate.

Despite Astorian-Veterans-Prince joining the Association, the members were never able to agree on a way to divide the city. Unlike the Vancouver model that was being suggested as a prototype, Winnipeg's private operators were not only competing against each other but were also facing free ambulance service from both police and fire, an issue which City Council was unwilling to seriously address.

For Astorian-Veterans-Prince to give up its lucrative contract and share with the other private service providers would have been financial suicide. As a result, the city council buried its collective head in the sand,

and once again, kept the status quo, referring routine ambulance calls to Astorian-Veterans-Prince.

After former city alderman and Winnipeg Blue Bombers business manager, Terry Hind, was recruited to try to mediate a compromise, the Winnipeg Ambulance Association collapsed in the spring of 1969. Ultimately, the real problem wasn't within the Association's power to fix. The solution wasn't in figuring out how to divide up the private ambulances' small piece of the pie; it was about overhauling the whole system.

## Changes in the 1970s

In February 1971, a second effort was made by the revived Winnipeg Ambulance Association to create a unified dispatch system with a government-subsidized zone system. As nothing had changed in the two years since originally proposed, Astoria-Veterans-Prince still had the city contract and city council didn't want to breach it, the proposal went nowhere.

While ultimately unsuccessful, the Winnipeg Ambulance Association's newest proposal did bring about publicized complaints from the Manitoba Professional Firefighters' Association and the Manitoba Safety Council about the continued use of fire department rescue squads as ambulances.[166] Although there seemed to be a general acceptance that a publicly operated, municipal ambulance service was the only way to ensure uniform, quality service, city council continued to refuse to accept responsibility for making change, and the status quo continued.

Many of Wylie's proposals in the last round of negotiations were based on equipping strategically placed fire department vehicles with medical supplies, using fire department personnel to provide paramedical-type services, and having ambulance personnel acting in a transport role.[167] It appears that these ideas were deemed too expensive or not practical at the time. However, as Winnipeg's EMS evolved, many of these early ideas became the norm.

On January 1, 1972, the unified city of Winnipeg, or "Unicity," was created—formally amalgamating all of the municipalities of Metro Winnipeg. While it took a couple of extra years to merge the respective police and fire departments, the writing was on the wall. It soon

166 Firefighters Seek Ambulance Service Standardization, *Winnipeg Free Press.* June 7, 1972.
167 Interview with John E.W. Wylie, April 4, 2004.

became apparent that the non-system of EMS that had evolved in Winnipeg would not work for a population twice the original size.

In June of 1972, the chiefs of the various fire departments comprising Unicity, city administrators, the provincial ambulance officer, and the Canadian Underwriters Association joined forces to try and find a solution. Besides the recurring, impractical recommendation that fire department rescue squads be used for firefighting and rescue work and not as ambulances, the committee didn't find a resolution.

The idea of not using the rescue squads as ambulances was punted almost immediately by Winnipeg City Council, and the chair of the city's finance committee questioned why fire department vehicles shouldn't be used for providing first aid, as had been the case for the first twenty-odd years of their existence.

Even though the use of fire department rescue squads was expensive, the key problem was that there wasn't a viable alternative for responding to heart attacks and drownings. Interestingly, even after Winnipeg Ambulance Service was formed, heart attack victims assisted by the fire department's rescue squads had slightly better survival rates than those treated by Winnipeg Ambulance. The fire department, before 1975 maintained a 6.5 percent heart attack survival rate, while Winnipeg Ambulance, after its creation, hovered around 5 percent.[168]

In response, the city's finance committee created a subcommittee on ambulance services. After studying various proposals, in January 1973, they began discussions with the Winnipeg Ambulance Association to build a municipal service. In Winnipeg tradition, the governing rule was that it had to be created "so there would be little or no cost to the City."[169]

As has often been the case in Winnipeg's history, financial considerations have a way of getting results that logic and common sense alone could never hope to achieve. In February 1973, in anticipation of the January 1974 merger of the area fire departments, Charles Chapman, Manitoba's Provincial Ambulance Officer, prepared an internal memo outlining the financial costs of non-action. Mr. Chapman noted that in order to continue to use fire department rescue squads to service ambulance calls in the new Unicity (with its

168 Paterson Report, 8.
169 Coulter Report, 8.

population twice the size of the former inner city), the city would need to spend approximately two and a half million dollars per year on additional equipment and personnel.[170]

Needless to say, if the private ambulance companies couldn't figure out a way to cooperate after three years of mediated talks, designing an entire ambulance system was definitely too large of a request. In the end, there was a divide, with members of the former Winnipeg Ambulance Association (United Rescue Services Ltd, Metro Ambulance Service, Wiley Ambulance and Rescue, and Reliable Ambulance Service) duking it out with the newly formed Unicity Independent Ambulance Operators Association (Astorian-Veterans-Prince Ambulance Service, Seven Oaks Ambulance and Rescue, and Riverview Ambulance Service). While all agreed on the need to amalgamate, there was serious dissention on how to accomplish such.[171]

In May 1973, city council proposed amendments to the *City of Winnipeg Act* to permit it to license and regulate a municipal ambulance service. Then, with no relief from the private ambulance companies, the City of Winnipeg found another source; the Manitoba Blue Cross/ United Health Insurance Corporation (Blue Cross). In contemplation of the amendment the *City of Winnipeg Act,* in the Spring of 1973, Blue Cross was asked to set up a municipal ambulance service. On September 4, 1973, the Act was amended, clearing all but arguably the biggest hurdle: Who was going to pay for it?

Through ongoing discussions behind the scene, an interesting solution arose in November 1974. The province announced that effective January 1, 1975, it would set up a new provincial ambulance program that would provide municipalities with funding to acquire proper ambulance services, ensure ambulances were properly inspected, and provide proper training for ambulance attendants.[172] Through grants, the new program was intended to cover 50 to 75 percent of a municipality's costs for acquiring ambulances, purchasing communications equipment, and running the actual service; essentially what was needed to have a system of decent ambulance services across the province.

---

170 C.C. Chapman, Ambulance Officer, Province of Manitoba. *Unicity Ambulance Service.* File: A1-20-01/1, February 21,1973.

171 David Lee. "Ambulance Operators Call for Amalgamation", *Winnipeg Free Press.* March 14, 1973.

172 "Provincial Ambulance Plan Ready." *Winnipeg Free Press.* November 2, 1973.

As a result of this new grant structure, the Manitoba Health Services Commission announced that, based on a per capita allowance of $1.00 to $1.50 per resident (it is not clear how the formula distinguished the different rates), Winnipeg was entitled to a grant of $535,220.00.[173]

With a sudden influx of cash, in the spring of 1975, Blue Cross was given the go-ahead to actually develop a municipal ambulance service for Winnipeg. As it was obvious that the cooperation of the private owners, to create either a cooperative or a combined service was a non-starter, the option selected by Blue Cross was to buy the assets of existing ambulance providers and set up a new service.

Once the decision was made to act, City Council was ruthless in its timelines. Council initially gave Blue Cross a little over two months to pull a service together. But when staff was not hired until May 15, Council was forced to extend its deadline by two weeks to June 16, 1975. On that date, the only emergency ambulances permitted to operate within the city were those from the Winnipeg Ambulance Service.

The developers of the new ambulance service faced a daunting task. In a two-month period, for a city the size of Winnipeg, they had to develop a service with a minimum of ten efficient vehicles and a trained staff of seventy.[174]

Due to the city's unwillingness to be directly involved, the resulting creation was going to be a nightmare for all involved.

---

173 November 7, 1974 correspondence from E.L. Desjardins, Chair of Manitoba Health Services Commission to Winnipeg Mayor, Stephen Juba.

174 C.C. Chapman, Ambulance Officer, Province of Manitoba. Unicity Ambulance. File: 40.102 Undated memo: 1.

## 1975-2000

# Where Is Home?

Much of the late twentieth century was spent trying to find a home for Winnipeg's ambulance service. While frustrating for staff and politicians alike, it was also a time of extensive growth and development. Winnipeg's emergency medical service employees evolved from rudimentarily trained "ambulance attendants" to advanced life support paramedics—true professionals in their own right—with a comparable evolution of service quality.

Nevertheless, Winnipeg's financial challenges impacted on the city's emergency medical services at every step, affecting the type of service provided, how it was provided, and by whom.

## Unicity

By 1975, Winnipeggers were learning to live with their new urban reality. The Unicity merger created a city with twice the population and three times the area but without the corresponding tax revenue per square kilometre ratio of the former inner city. With the formation of Unicity, Winnipeg instantly morphed from 246,246 to 535,233 inhabitants, with an almost three-fold land area increase, going from approximately 177 square kilometres to 464 square kilometres. Seven of the twelve municipalities that merged to form Unicity (Fort Garry, North Kildonan, Old Kildonan, Transcona, Charleswood, West Kildonan, and Tuxedo) had populations of less than 25,000 people[175]. Prior to the Unicity merger, these cities already had low tax bases, with minimal services. Put another way, there were 150 fewer taxpayers per square kilometre, going from

175 Figures from De-Amalgamation of Winnipeg: https://skyscraperpage.com/forum/showthread.php?t=227673, accessed November 25, 2023.

1,391 taxpayers per square kilometre in the former inner city to 1,154 in the new Unicity, creating a significant revenue drop for the entire area.

To garner support for the merger, Mayor Stephen Juba indicated that all 535,000-plus residents would get the same level and types of services previously enjoyed by the 246,000-plus residents of the former inner city. The city needed to provide the same services to a land mass almost three times the size but with only twice the number of taxpayers. It appears that the planners of Unicity didn't have an understanding of basic economics.

While a significant benefit to the residents of the surrounding municipalities, without enough revenue, the expanded services created a serious financial drain on the newly merged city. The increased services with decreased income exacerbated the financial struggle Winnipeg was facing; the struggle that started with the 1914 opening of the Panama Canal. It continues to plague Winnipeg today. The struggle creeps into every aspect of city life, including emergency services. The result is an ongoing pattern of reducing costs, avoiding costs, and, when possible, downloading costs onto other layers of government.

## Paramedics and Firefighters Are Not the Same

Since the formation of the Winnipeg Ambulance Service, the economic constraints of Unicity have affected Winnipeg's emergency medical services. Unfortunately, finding a workable solution has been equally challenging. Complicating the issue has been the pervasive myth that firefighters and paramedics have similar personalities. As a result of this myth, there have been repeated attempts within Winnipeg to combine the two services.

It is crucial to understand this line of thinking to understand the evolution of Winnipeg's ambulance service. At first blush, firefighters and paramedics seem compatible because:

- both groups come when people need immediate help,
- both groups arrive in vehicles with lights and sirens, and
- with compassion, kindness, and varied skills, members of both groups do inspiring work helping people cope with what for many is their *worst day ever.*

Adding to the confusion is the fact that firefighters have been providing first aid as part of their core services since 1911. The confusion is understandable if we think of modern paramedicine as seriously advanced first aid. A more accurate and less confusing distinction is to picture first aid as care given until a physician's care can be provided and paramedicine as specialized training bringing physician-like care to the emergency scene.

It helps to understand some of the crucial differences between firefighters and paramedics:

- First, there is a solid but closed brotherhood in firefighting. As a relatively new profession, paramedics don't have the same bond. When the two professions merge, paramedics are often excluded, or *feel* excluded, creating a we/them environment.
- Second, the two professions have different, typically incompatible, decision-making processes. Firefighting is a team effort with top-down direction. Generally, *mavericks* or *lone wolves* are strongly discouraged in the fire service and often disciplined. On the other hand, paramedics need to work independently, making quick, individual decisions regarding patient care. This distinction can lead to friction when the two groups work under joint command. For example, in Calgary, when EMS was part of the fire department, paramedics were typically unwilling to take direction on patient care from a captain with "just a first aid certificate." Conversely, many fire captains, assuming they had scene command, were perplexed as to why paramedics were ignoring them.[176]
- Third, an oft-overlooked factor is that EMS is typically provided on a fee-for-service basis, with patients being charged for the response. Firefighting services, with exceptions—such as special events and out-of-jurisdiction calls—are generally provided on a no-charge basis to the public. As a result, when the two services are merged, there can be conflicts in service delivery.

With these distinctions in mind, let's look at how Winnipeg Ambulance survived its creation.

---

176 Duncan (2019): 57.

## Winnipeg Ambulance Service

Time was of the essence!

After Blue Cross hired Patrick Johnstone, a manager from Toronto's ambulance service as Winnipeg Ambulance's general manager, it went to work hiring staff for the new ambulance service. Starting on May 15, from 217 applications (including one woman) the newly evolving Winnipeg Ambulance hired seventy four driver-attendants.[177] They came from a collection of soon-to-be former employees of the city's private ambulance services—including the bulk of staff from Wylie Ambulance—medical students, a group that Johnstone had recruited from Toronto, and a few miscellaneous Winnipeggers who responded to the newspaper advertisements.

While the original plan was to have seventy ambulance attendants trained by the June 16 start date, things didn't quite work that way. Winnipeg Ambulance found that as of its official start date it did not have properly trained personnel.[178] The idea was to utilize the province's new five-week, 160-hour course for ambulance staff, on material created by St. John Ambulance, the Health Sciences Centre, and the Provincial Ambulance Officer. At the time that the new ambulance service was set to begin operations, the first course had not been completed. The first class graduated the following day—June 16, 1975—and there were two additional classes after that to prepare the initial seventy ambulance attendants.

It's interesting to note that at a time that Winnipeg was struggling to get its ambulance attendants to take a 160-hour course, both Calgary and Montreal had their municipal ambulance attendants qualifying as advanced life support paramedics, requiring 1200 hours of training.[179]

The problem of not having enough trained staff on the start date was eclipsed by not having enough ambulances! The City of Winnipeg's plan was to revoke the private ambulance licenses as of June 16,

---

177 Alan Christie. "Ambulance Owners Hit City Takeover." *Winnipeg Free Press.* June 11, 1975.

178 M. Hawrysh. "Winnipeg Ambulance Service Response to the Ad Hoc Committee Report." Winnipeg Ambulance Service: June 28, 1976.

179 Paul Pihichyn. "Better Training Urged For Ambulance Staff." *Winnipeg Free Press.* February 21, 1975.

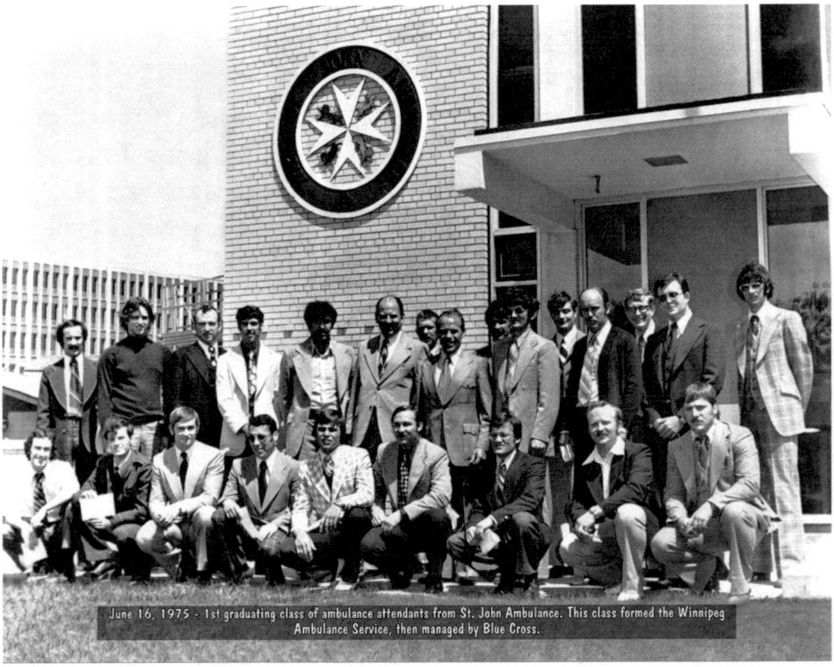


*Winnipeg Ambulance's first class of ambulance attendants; graduated on June 16, 1975. The front row: Randy Morgan (or Gerry Desjalais?), Wayne Grisewood, Chris Bruce-Smith, Brian Gross, Ken Maurin, Dan O,Malley, Norm Traughton, George Oldry (or Oldroid?), Jim Dzikowski Back row: Derek White, Doug Redden, John Wylie, Don Miller, Marty Kramer, Trevor Bachelor (SJA Instructor), Gerry Leach, (SJA Instructor), Doug James, Dave Campbell (Manitoba Health–Ambulance Services Director), Les Harden, Wayne Gould, Lloyd Wally, Al Sangster (or Mike Munroe?), Stan Stone (Courtesy of St. John Ambulance, MB, NWT, & NU Council). Special thanks to Derric Boles, Chris Bruce-Smith, Greg Ford, Barry Guttormson, Sandy Schoofs, and Stan Stone for help in identifying this group—it was a challenge!*

1975 and have Winnipeg Ambulance[180] fully operational and ready to roll. Having spent $250,000 of its $535,000 provincial start-up grant to purchase ambulances from the private operators and having them turned over to the ambulance service on the eve of June 15, 1975,[181] the city presumed that it had the initial equipment needed to operate.

---

180 While the service has been formally named "Winnipeg Ambulance Service" and the "Winnipeg Ambulance Department" at different times, City staff and the media consistently ignored the current titles. Hence, I will refer to the municipal organization providing Winnipeg's ambulance service as "Winnipeg Ambulance".

181 Alan Christie. "Ambulance Owners Hit City Takeover." *Winnipeg Free Press.* June 11, 1975.

The purchase of the private ambulance companies' equipment was controversial. When Blue Cross structured the purchase agreements, there was no negotiating with respect to the price. As private ambulances would be banned as per the new city bylaw, if not sold to Blue Cross, they became useless. Hence, the private owners received offers on a "take it or leave it basis," creating animosity and in some cases, ongoing dissention.

In fairness, the owners' frustrations were understandable. Most went into the ambulance business as a result of Winnipeg's ongoing refusal to create a proper municipal ambulance service. They then acquired state-of-the-art ambulances, often at great cost to themselves, in an effort to provide adequate ambulance services to Winnipeggers. Due to free services provided by the police and fire departments, the city declined to make it cost efficient for private operators to run their companies. This resulted in ambulances that did not necessarily get proper maintenance. Then when city council decided to reverse a seventy-year policy of not providing a proper public ambulance service, the private operators were forced to sell their equipment at a reduced price, with the buyer—the city council—claiming the units were substandard. It's not hard to appreciate the private ambulance providers' frustrations.[182]

In an effort to be efficient, the city purchased available units from private owners on an "as is" basis. As mentioned earlier, there had previously been complaints about the condition of many of the private ambulances. It is not a major surprise that on the appointed day, four of the purchased units were found to be unroadworthy and were scrapped, and many others were in need of significant repairs. Ultimately, only five of the twelve ambulances were fully functional.[183] It appears that some of the private ambulance service owners had misrepresented the condition of their units. Through repairing some of the original units and purchasing additional, used units, by November 1975, Winnipeg Ambulance was hobbling along with fifteen ambulances.[184]

In hindsight, at the time of Winnipeg Ambulance's creation, the idea of the province inspecting ambulances had just been announced. Even in 1980, six years later, the provincial ambulance office advised that "Officials admit that sometimes they have to turn a blind eye because suspending

182 Taken from 2004 discussions with John Wylie, September 2024 notes from Garry Leach, and multiple 1975 newspaper articles.

183 Coulter Report: 8.

184 Coulter Report: 8.

a license means leaving a community without ambulance service… the province has never suspended an ambulance license although the department knows that many operators skirt the law daily."[185]

## Where to Put it All

There were other problems. Perhaps most surprisingly, the City of Winnipeg's bureaucracy had not given serious thought as to where to house the vehicles or staff. The grand idea of "operating out of the hospitals" fell apart when the city's hospitals announced that they had neither the interest in housing ambulances nor available facilities or space. After further negotiations, the city agreed to let the Winnipeg Ambulance use abandoned fire halls for their ambulance stations. These stations were in a deplorable condition, having been closed and sitting empty for over a year in part because they were already deteriorating.

In fact, *deplorable* was an understatement. Besides being full of cobwebs and mildew, they had been built from stone in the mid-1910s, so the stations had minimal insulation and insufficient heating. In some of the stations, ambulance attendants needed to use the kitchen oven as their main source of heat. With only hard wooden chairs, and no couches, beds, or showers, it was extremely difficult to get any kind of rest. The crews at Ambulance Station No.1 at Lipton and Westminster would fight over the six-inch by four-foot wooden bench found at the station—it was the only place to lie down! The other stations didn't even have this *luxury*. The irony is, being severely understaffed and underequipped meant that ambulance attendants spent most of their time in warm ambulances, sitting in reasonably comfortable seats as they rushed from one call to the next.

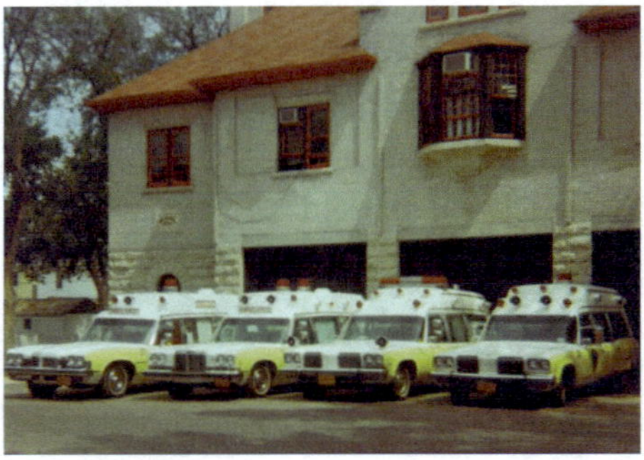

*Some of the original units acquired from the private ambulance operators in front of a make-shift station – the former sixty-year-old Lipton Street fire hall. The custom-built, automobile-chassised units tended to fair better than the newer home-built and truck-chassised ambulances. (Courtesy of Peter Adsten @ EMS Classics)*

185 Maureen Brosnahan. "Loose ambulance rules create risks." *Winnipeg Free Press.* October 14. 1980.

The fledgling service initially used five fire halls and an ambulance based at Grace Hospital[186] to cover the city. Besides the station at 161 Lipton Street, which was also used as the training centre, Winnipeg Ambulance used abandoned fire halls at 325 Talbot (in Elmwood), 600 St. Mary's Road, and 524 Osborne Street, as well as a former service station at McGregor and Liela. While not an ambulance station, the former Winnipeg fire hall at 1066 Dorchester was also used for training. As all of these halls were built from stone between 1906 and 1914, they were drafty and cold.

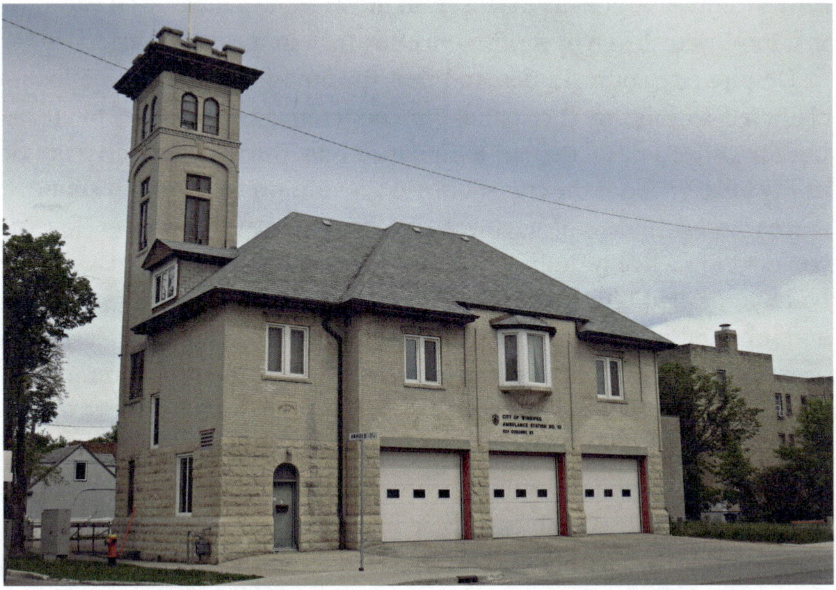

*EMS Station #4 (now WFPS EMS Station No. 30), at 524 Osborne Street. Built in 1913 for the WFD, it is the only original Winnipeg Ambulance station still in active service. (Courtesy of Gordon Goldsborough, Manitoba Historical Society)*

Despite the *Winnipeg Free Press*'s suggestion that there was an ambulance station at Grace Hospital, it really only consisted of a white telephone installed in the hospital ER's waiting room that ambulance crews were supposed to answer.[187] Grace Hospital staff quickly tired of ambulance attendants sitting in the waiting room, and as a result, personnel relocated to either sitting in the ambulance at Sturgeon Creek, or driving around the West End/St. James. As there was no ambulance station on

186 "City ambulance service wants extra $3 a ride." *Winnipeg Free Press.* April 10, 1976.
187 Online interview with Stan Stone, September 5, 2024.

the west side of Winnipeg until the mid-1980s, crews often were parked on street corners and in parking lots, waiting for calls.

If this doesn't capture the early staff's dedication, it's worth noting that at the time, minimum wage in Manitoba was $2.30/hour, jumping to $2.60/hour in late 1975. The starting wage for Winnipeg Ambulance was around $3.18/hour. Some early ambulance attendants sold their homes in order to survive on their Winnipeg Ambulance income. While people who work in the emergency response industry typically don't do it for the money, with early Winnipeg Ambulance staff, given the working conditions it was clear that most were driven by motivators other than money or prestige.

Despite city council's demand that the ambulance service be financially self-sustaining, it remained uncooperative with respect to allowing for collection of unpaid ambulance bills through property tax or utility bills. Without the city willing to provide any oversight or support, there were significant obstacles arising every step of the way. By November 1975, after five months of operation, Winnipeg Ambulance already had 600 unpaid bills and $11,500 in uncollected ambulance fees. While a number of nonpayers were seniors who couldn't afford the fees, there were also a number of users who provided false identification and/or left the hospital as soon as they were delivered.[188]

As is often the case with new businesses, the only way that Winnipeg Ambulance survived the first year was through the dedication, perseverance, and enthusiasm of its staff. Ambulances were often staffed by people taking classes during the day and working the night-shifts, and supervisors doing double-duty to ensure that a basic service could be provided. The service was also augmented by fire department rescue squads, which responded as they had before Winnipeg Ambulance's creation. Once Winnipeg Ambulance had enough trained staff and roadworthy ambulances, WFD ceased regularly responding to EMS calls.

## Infighting, Debt, Unionization, and Departure from Blue Cross

By March 1976, the infighting and disharmony at Winnipeg Ambulance was so severe that the Manitoba Health Services Commission launched

188 "$11,500 arrears claimed." *Winnipeg Free Press.* November 26, 1975.

an investigation into the service's management.[189] The following month, the $11,500 had morphed to an estimated $91,000 in uncollectible bills. City council refused to permit a $3 raise of ambulance rates to try to recoup some of the losses.[190] By the end of June 1976, the uncollectible bills were up to $236,816.[191]

The morale was such that the driver/attendants had already unionized; represented by the Manitoba Emergency Medical Technicians Association.[192] The ambulance supervisors, in turn, sought representation by the International Association of Machinists and Aerospace Workers.[193] By June 1976, it was clear that the management of Winnipeg's ambulance service via Blue Cross was not working. While many sources suggest that city council was unhappy with Blue Cross, the reality is that both sides were frustrated at not getting what they believed they had bargained.

With Blue Cross being a private, profit-driven company and the city being unwilling to assist in collecting unpaid ambulance bills, Blue Cross was unhappy from a business perspective. Almost half (43 percent) of Winnipeg's ambulance bills were going unpaid.[194] While Blue Cross was entitled to annual compensation of 3 percent of Winnipeg Ambulance's operating budget,[195] given the uncollected bills. it was next to impossible to cover the service's basic expenses and get the agreed compensation.

The city urgently needed another solution. The city's finance committee recommended that the city take over the running of the service and created a task force to formulate a plan.[196] After considering whether a merger with the fire department was viable, the task force ultimately decided that a separate municipal department was the best option.

Hence, in October 1976, council passed resolution to terminate the agreement with Blue Cross. The termination was sweetened by contracting with Blue Cross to continue to manage Winnipeg Ambulance until

---

189 "Ambulance probe launched." *Winnipeg Free Press.* March 25, 1976.

190 "City ambulance service wants extra $3 a ride." *Winnipeg Free Press.* April 10, 1976.

191 Alan Christie. "Defence of private ambulances fails to convince civic committee." *Winnipeg Free Press.* June 30, 1976.

192 "City ambulance service wants extra $3 a ride." *Winnipeg Free Press.* April 10, 1976.

193"Ambulance supervisors seek union." *Winnipeg Free Press.* June 17, 1976.

194 "Almost half of Winnipeg ambulance bills went unpaid in 2022, report says." CBC News. May 1, 2023. https://www.cbc.ca/news/canada/manitoba/winnipeg-ambulance-costs-1.6828949. Accessed November 1, 2023.

195 "Takeover urged for ambulances." *Winnipeg Free Press.* June 23, 1976.

196 "Takeover urged for ambulances." *Winnipeg Free Press.* June 23, 1976.

a new service could be established. At same time, a bylaw was passed to establish a public ambulance service in Winnipeg, as required under the province's *Municipal Act.*

In December 1976, effective January 7, 1977, the city scrapped its ambulance advisory committee and established the Winnipeg Ambulance Board. Such was needed to oversee the ambulance service's transition to a separate municipal organization. Jack Litvack, CEO of St. Boniface Hospital, chaired the Board, and it had a combination of twelve city councillors, physicians, Blue Cross representatives, and private citizens as directors.

Moving toward a complete departure from Blue Cross, in February 1977, the province amended the City *of Winnipeg Act* to permit Winnipeg to establish an Ambulance Commission and to run an ambulance service.

In the midst of the infighting, in January 1977, Winnipeg Ambulance general manager Patrick Johnstone quit.[197] Ultimately, Johnstone had become the scapegoat for everybody; staff, supervisors, and city council. In reality, having been given minimal resources by city council to run the service, it was impossible for Johnstone to do a decent job.

## City Run Version of Winnipeg Ambulance

After obtaining the legal authority to run an ambulance service, in March 1977, the city hired John Farrington to manage the new city-operated version of Winnipeg Ambulance. Farrington had originally joined Blue Cross in March 1976 as the accounts manager. After the ambulance service was transferred to Winnipeg, given he understood the operations, Farrington joined the city's staff. Having a civic employee responsible for overseeing ambulance operations, Winnipeg could now run its own ambulance service. On June 20, 1978, the city's new eight-person Ambulance Commission was established, chaired by Councillor Jimmie Ray Ragdill, to oversee the city-run service.[198]

Almost before the ink was dry on the Ambulance Commission's appointment, it became painfully clear that Winnipeg didn't have the resources, or wasn't willing to allocate the resources, to run a proper ambulance service.

---

197 "Johnstone quits ambulance post." *Winnipeg Free Press.* January 22, 1977.

198 Also on the Commission were: B. Chornopyski, W, McGarva, G. Savoie, L. Hutcheon, J. Litvack, a Mr. Cox, A. MacDonald, and Drs. H. Krahn and J.W. O'Toole.

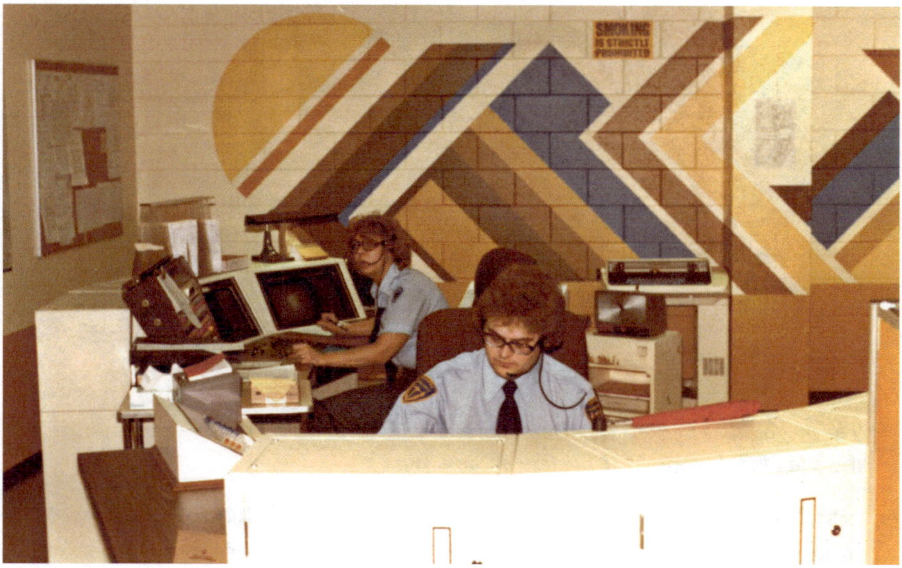

*The new Winnipeg Ambulance dispatch centre, circa 1977. Everything about this picture screams 1970s; the only thing missing is a disco ball. (Courtesy of Stan Stone)*

For starters, Winnipeg didn't have enough ambulances for the new Unicity area. Further, many of the units purchased from the private ambulance services were falling apart. The city had fifteen units but needed eighteen. Within an ambulance service, some units are used full-time, some are used during peak hours, some are used for non-emergency inter-hospital transfers, and some are needed as spares/to cover special events. Most of the existing fifteen were patched up remnants from the 1975 purchase of the private ambulance companies' equipment: many of which were *already* in a less than pristine condition at the time of acquisition.

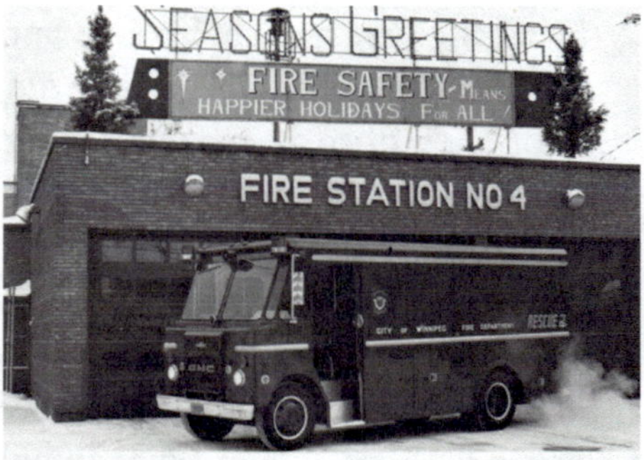


*Early 1970s WFD Rescue Squad provided back-up ambulance service during Winnipeg Ambulance's transition to a city-run service. (Courtesy of FFHSW)*

Between 1977 and 1980, Winnipeg Ambulance upgraded its fleet. Recognizing that modular ambulances were the wave of the future (as well as more cost efficient to replace/upgrade), in 1977, it acquired four new, almost identical units: two Superior-Chevrolet 61-M models from the Superior

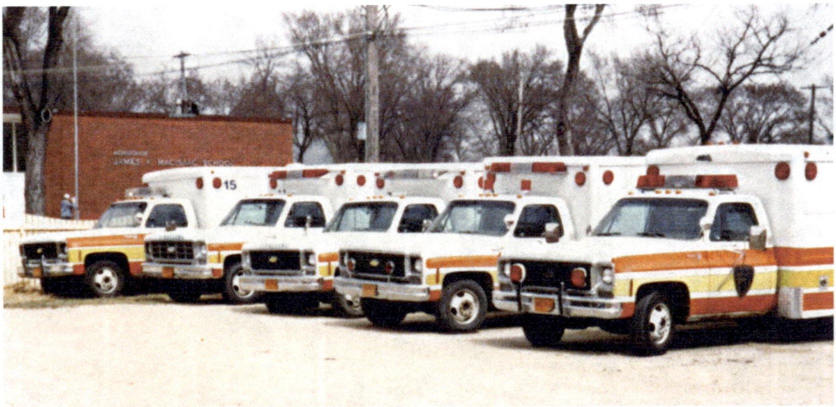
*The originally acquired 1977 Superior and Wayne modular ambulances – toward the end of their careers. (Courtesy of Stan Stone)*

Coach Company in Lima, Ohio, and two Wayne-Chevrolet Lifeguard models from the Wayne Corporation in Richmond, Indiana. As the new ambulances had been "demonstrators" from two companies, each came with somewhat different configurations. As these were new models for their respective manufacturers, many demonstrators had likely been produced for promotional purposes. The availability of the slightly used demonstrators enabled Winnipeg to get modern, well-built ambulances at a lower cost than normal.

After purchasing the four demonstrators, in 1979, the city acquired a two-year-old, used type I modular unit[199]. Built by the Modular Ambulance Corporation of Dallas, Texas, it was hailed as the first Modular Ambulance Corporation product sold in Manitoba. The reason for being the first quickly became apparent; as it was built for the warm Texas climate, Winnipeg's unit didn't have enough insulation and the floor often froze during winter mopping.[200]

Winnipeg also purchased a new Ambucraft/Crestline-Ford modular ambulance. As Saskatoon's Crestline Coach had recently acquired Ambucraft, their products were released under either name. However, having been built in Saskatchewan, it was compatible with Winnipeg's climate.

Winnipeg then purchased several relatively poor-quality Superior-Dodge Type II (van-type) ambulances from Sheller-Globe in Morris, Manitoba. While the Sheller-Globe company in Morris was part of the

199 "Ambulance purchase okayed by committee." *Winnipeg Free Press.* December 20, 1978.
200 Online interview with Stan Stone, August 13, 2024.

Superior Coach Company's operations, the units made in Manitoba were of poor quality[201] and only lasted a few years.

With extremely limited funds, Winnipeg Ambulance was doing the best it could to acquire much-needed new equipment. By 1977, it had six Dodge vans, six modulars, and six car-based remnants from the private ambulance period. When staffing permitted, thirteen units were operated on the day shift and ten at night.

While twelve new vehicles[202] were needed to replace the decaying vehicles and increase its fleet size, in 1979, Winnipeg Ambulance asked the city for nine new ambulances to replace existing units. Even after noting that the units had a wear-out rate of four per year, the city's finance committee approved the purchase of three new ambulances.[203] At this point, Winnipeg Ambulance had neither sufficient ambulances nor staff to provide twenty-four-hour service in the East Kildonan-Transcona area. The problem of response times in Transcona would continue for decades.

## Problems with the Vehicles

In 1980, Winnipeg found the funds to order five Crestline-Ford Type III modulars from Crestline Coach; both Winnipeg's and Crestline's first multi-unit order.[204] With the new batch of five modulars, the remaining car-based and van ambulances were phased out. This enabled Winnipeg Ambulance to have eight to ten functional ambulances to cover the 75 to 100 calls per twelve-hour shift.[205] Unfortunately it did nothing to provide relief for peak hours or stabilize the city's underequipped EMS.

The new Crestline-Ford ambulances had a small problem. Like the Ford Pinto, the modulars had a propensity to blow up. With the fuel tank being placed too close to the exhaust system, the fuel expanded as the exhaust system heated up, causing the gas tank cap to blow off and spray fuel. The hot exhaust system then set the fuel on fire; an even more serious problem for vehicles equipped with oxygen tanks. Shortly after the new ambulances arrived, one of their gas caps blew

---

201 Both Adsten (2008):76, and Stan Stone (Interview November 12, 2023), describe these units as being of "inferior quality."

202 "Ambulance purchase okayed by committee." *Winnipeg Free Press.* December 20, 1978.

203 "Ambulance cuts called medieval." *Winnipeg Free Press.* February 23, 1979.

204 Peter Adsten (2008): 45.

205 Michael Hoffman. "A 'Quiet' Friday for the five-minute men.'" *Winnipeg Free Press.* June 20, 1979.

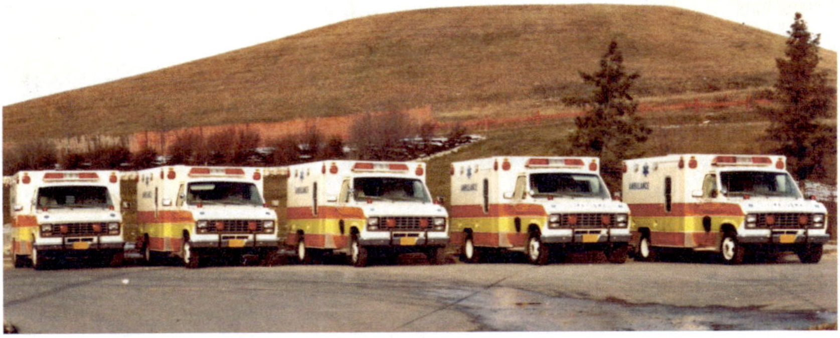

*The 1980 Crestline-Ford fleet order. (Courtesy of Peter Adsten @ EMS Classics)*

off in front of the Health Sciences Centre. Then in January 1981, one of the new modulars caught fire.[206] As the city could neither afford to purchase more ambulances nor "park" the new modulars, staff were instructed to only partially fill the gas tanks. The following year, Winnipeg Ambulance bought two Modular Ambulance Corporation Fords, one propane and one gasoline, from Crestline. Presuming the expanding fuel line was a common problem, it can be speculated that

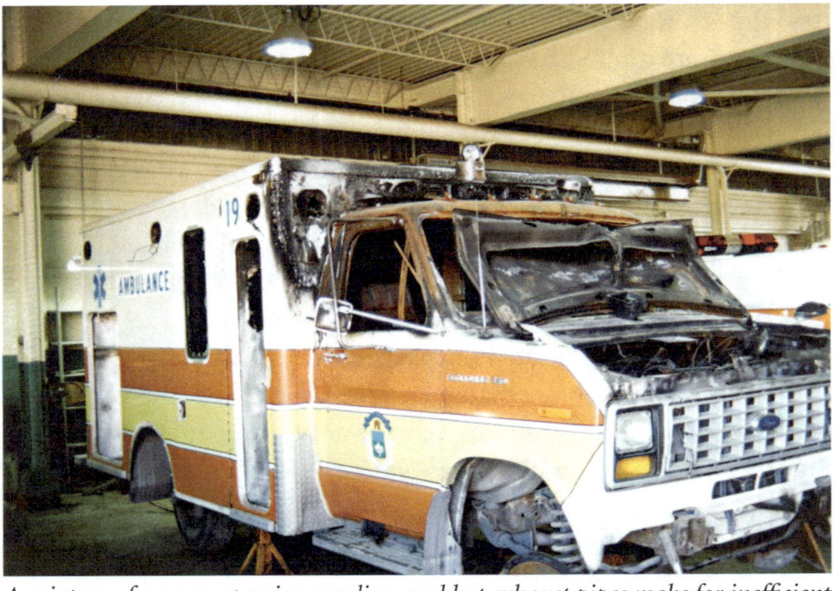


*A mixture of oxygen, spewing gasoline, and hot exhaust pipes make for inefficient ambulances. (Courtesy of Stan Stone)*

206 David O'Brien. "Faulty ambulances stay on road." *Winnipeg Free Press.* November 6, 1981.

Winnipeg got the units on sale. Subsequent ambulance purchases had either the more expensive diesel or propane engines, or gas engines with a Chevrolet chassis. The Chevrolet chassied units didn't have the same propensity to blow up.

## Lack of Training

Equally disturbing to exploding ambulances was the level of training for Winnipeg ambulance attendants. While Calgary, Montreal, and Vancouver (as well as many American cities) were already using advanced life support (ALS) paramedics (with up to 2,000 hours of training), and Toronto's Basic Life Support ambulance crews had 1,200 hours of training and would have fully trained ALS paramedics by 1981,[207] Winnipeg was still in the EMS *dark ages*. Despite rapid growth in the North American emergency medical industry, Winnipeg still used the six-week, 140-hour ambulance attendant training program developed by the province in 1974. In essence, it was a glorified advanced first aid course. The city was "five years behind comparable services in other Canadian cities and 20 years behind its American counterparts."[208]

Even heart defibrillators, an essential tool that paramedics in other parts of Canada had been using for years to revive cardiac arrest patients, weren't used by Winnipeg Ambulance. These wouldn't be purchased for another four or five years. While deplorable for Winnipeggers, it was incredibly frustrating for Winnipeg's ambulance attendants. They saw the fabulous lifesaving results that their colleagues in other cities were delivering, yet the training, equipment, and legal authority to get the same for Winnipeggers weren't available.[209]

## More Training Arrives

In 1977, Winnipeg Ambulance appointed Derek White as its training supervisor. By coincidence, or not, this was a fascinating time for emergency care in Canada. The year before, in 1976, the Canadian Heart and Stroke Foundation (CHSF) had decided to get heavily into the promo-

207 Newton (2015): 188-192.

208 Hoffman, Michael. "A 'Quiet' Friday for the five-minute men." *Winnipeg Free Press*. June 20, 1979.

209 Hoffman, Michael. "A 'Quiet' Friday for the five-minute men." *Winnipeg Free Press*. June 20, 1979.

tion and teaching of CPR to the public. Recruiting some cardiologists in Toronto to assist in developing a national program and then seeking help from the American Heart Foundation for training, the CHSF soon had a national CPR program.[210] A number of Winnipeg's ambulance attendants got involved in teaching, both as instructors and instructor-trainers for the CHSF. This was crucial in getting Winnipeg's ambulance staff quickly trained in CPR.

There had been minimal training for staff since 1975, when four ambulance attendants volunteered to be training coordinators. White began teaching additional EMS skills to staff, such as CPR, patient stabilization, and oxygen therapy, from the Canadian Medical Association's EMT-200 (Basic Life Support) curriculum.

The following spring, given the greater breadth of training being given to ambulance attendants in other Canadian jurisdictions, Winnipeg Ambulance management realized that a more in-depth training program was needed. As a result, Barry Guttormson was added as the Assistant Supervisor of Training and began teaching the six-week Emergency Medical Technician course to Winnipeg Ambulance staff. To augment their meagre skill sets, many of Winnipeg's ambulance attendants also started taking the University of Winnipeg's first year anatomy and physiology course, while White and Guttormson took three months of the intensive care nursing course at St. Boniface Hospital.[211] Using the skills acquired through this program, the training officers began providing Winnipeg Ambulance staff with day-long seminars.

The lack of training and equipment was a severe detriment to ordinary Winnipeggers. The Ambulance Commission began proposing that Winnipeg Ambulance get the Canadian Medical Association's EMT-300 Advance Life Support (ALS) paramedic training in 1978; at a cost as high as $5 million.[212] City Council responded to the request by increasing Winnipeg Ambulance's budget by $1,071 for 1979.[213] Acknowledging a funding issue, Winnipeg increased its ambulance service fees by 50 percent, going

210 Heart and Stroke Foundation: https://www.heartandstroke.ca/articles/the-amazing-story-of-cpr, Accessed August 30, 2024.

211 Telephone interview with Barry Guttormson, August 28, 2024.

212 Ingeborg Boyens. "Departments to Justify Expenses." *Winnipeg Free Press.* November 3, 1978.

213 "Ambulance cuts called medieval." *Winnipeg Free Press.* February 23, 1979.

from $40 to $60[214]. It's debatable how effective this solution was, given that almost half of the city's ambulance users weren't paying the fees anyway.

In 1978, four years after British Columbia started its own provincial ambulance service, Derek White was recruited to assist with its staff training. Given his twelve years experience running a private ambulance service, combined with his work as a training officer with Winnipeg Ambulance resulted in him being offered the position of manager of EMS training—teaching BC Ambulance staff—at BC's emergency services college, the Justice Institute of BC (JIBC). This subsequently provided the opportunity for several of Winnipeg Ambulance's supervisory staff to take the EMS Educator's course at the JIBC. Guttormson also earned a Manitoba Certificate in Adult Education. With Guttormson then promoted to Supervisor of Training and Chris Bruce-Smith as his assistant supervisor, over the next few years the training program curriculum was written into a proper educational format. This would prove very helpful when Winnipeg Ambulance began seeking program certification from the Canadian Medical Association.

To highlight the need for better training, in 1980, Winnipeg doctors Gerry Bristow and Arnold Tweed did a study of 840 Winnipeggers whom, between 1978 and 1979, had suffered cardiac arrests outside of a hospital. They found that only thirty-three, or 6 percent, had survived. The doctors suggested the obvious; If Winnipeg had paramedics armed with defibrillators and proper emergency drugs, and more citizens were given training in cardiopulmonary resuscitation, the survival rate would jump to 25 percent.[215] However, this wasn't happening, given Winnipeg's finances. The numbers speak for themselves, but without money what was the answer?

## A Merger?

On January 1, 1978, Jack Coulter became Winnipeg's new fire chief. As the chief administrator, Coulter had a vested interest in creating work for the fire department. With fire calls decreasing yearly, it became harder to justify the fire department's budget. Coulter also understood the bigger picture of improving emergency medical care. He recognized that firefighters, in *some capacity*, provided the answer to faster response for medical emergencies and began lobbying the city council accordingly.

---

214 "Ambulance cuts called medieval." *Winnipeg Free Press.* February 23, 1979.
215 Maureen Brosnahan. "MDs rap heart attach care." *Winnipeg Tribune.* February 15, 1980.

Hearing Coulter's suggestions, and likely the stinging media criticisms of the ambulance service's response times, in 1979 the city's finance committee began investigating a better system. In particular, they started examining ways to cut costs by jointly using the facilities and services of the fire department and the ambulance service. The following March, the finance committee asked Coulter to report on the potential amalgamation of the two departments.

While saving money was at the forefront, the ultimate goal was to create a system that would keep city residents who had gone into cardiac arrest alive. One immediate problem was that ambulance response times in Transcona and Charleswood were abysmal. A solution was needed, given that city council was committed to providing the same level of service to all areas of Unicity. To accomplish this, Winnipeg needed to develop an EMS system that would have cardiopulmonary resuscitation started in less than four minutes, and an Advanced Life Support level of emergency care on scene in less than ten minutes.

By way of explanation, when evaluating civilian emergency medical services, out-of-hospital cardiac arrest survival rates are seen as the "litmus test" for assessing the effectiveness of the service. Cardiac issues are the one condition that regularly occur in virtually every community, are connected to many other medical emergencies, and are easy to measure. For example, it's fairly straightforward to determine how many people in a given community go into ventricular fibrillation (cardiac arrest) outside a hospital and subsequently walk out of the hospital with good brain function. For comparative purposes, in the United States, in the early 2010s, the bookends for assessing emergency medical services were Omaha, Nebraska with a 3 percent survival rate, and Seattle, Washington, with a 45 percent survival rate.[216]

As mentioned, Coulter had a significant challenge as fire chief to maintain the fire department's budget. Over the previous decade, fire-related responses had significantly dropped. Thanks to the increased use of smoke detectors and sprinkler systems, a decrease of people smoking in bed (as well as a better awareness of other high fire-risk activities), and more recently, the removal of street corner fire-call boxes—decreasing calls to the fire department (mainly false—ie. no actual fire) by about fourteen per day—it was getting harder to justify the fire department's budget. The

216 Bell (2009): 338.

reality is that whether there are ten fires per day or ten per month, to keep fires in check, the fire department still needs to be able to arrive at each fire within four minutes. Hence, regardless of the number of fires, there needs to be sufficient numbers of firefighters to get anywhere in the city quickly. This was especially challenging given Unicity's vast area.

## Chief Coulter's Plan

Jack Coulter began his study by comparing Winnipeg with Edmonton, Alberta, where fire and EMS were separate, cooperating services; Calgary, Alberta, where fire and EMS services had been combined; and Seattle, Washington, the "Blue Ribbon Service," where firefighters provided some (but not all) EMS services. All cities were roughly the same size and covered the same approximate area as Winnipeg.

Shortly after Coulter was assigned his task, in February 1980, the province announced that Winnipeg's 1980 ambulance subsidy would only increase by $55,000, despite the fact that the city needed to purchase nine new ambulances. The city needed to find $1.8 million to cover the ambulance service.[217] A serious issue, given that they had only increased the budget by $1,071 the year before. If the city couldn't afford its existing ambulance service, bringing it up to the desired advanced life support level of care was not going to happen.

In reviewing options for Winnipeg, Coulter provided four different models for integrating fire and ambulance services:[218]

- Alternative 1: Keep the current system, separate ambulance service, no involvement of the fire department in EMS, and no ALS. Existing cardiac arrest survival rate: 4.5 percent.
- Alternative 2: Keep separate ambulance service with the fire department providing initial first response/first aid services, with no ALS. This was compared to Edmonton, Alberta, which didn't start its ALS program until 1982.[219] Existing cardiac arrest survival rate: 6 percent. Edmonton's program was bolstered by having members of the fire department, on a limited basis, teaching CPR to members of the public.

217 "City's Pleas for Money Net $55,000." *Winnipeg Free Press.* February 5, 1980.
218 J.T. Coulter. "Proposal for Fire/Ambulance Amalgamation". April 22, 1980.
219 Plumbtree (2011): 266.

- Alternative 3: The two services would be separate divisions of the fire department, where each had their own uniforms and staff, with joint management. The ambulance service would provide EMS services with ALS, while the fire department provided initial first response/first aid services. This was compared to Calgary, Alberta. Existing cardiac arrest survival rate: 12 percent.
- Alternative 4: A fully amalgamated service, with all frontline staff cross-trained as both firefighters and emergency medical technicians (a forerunner of a "paramedic"), with ALS. This was compared to Seattle, Washington. Existing cardiac arrest survival rate: 19 percent. Seattle's program was bolstered by having members of the fire department teaching CPR to the public.

Coulter ultimately found that Alternative 1 would be expensive to maintain, with little improvement in service. Alternatives 2 and 3 would significantly improve services, at a similar cost to Alternative 1. He further noted that Alternative 3's problem was that the two departments would be competing for the same resources, which could lead to frustrations. Alternative 4, full amalgamation, was recommended as the most effective use of personnel and resources. However, it was a long-term project. Still, once implemented, the operating costs allegedly would not increase. It was coincidentally, the most beneficial model for maintaining the fire department's resources.

Alternatives 2, 3, and 4, with the ambulance service providing ALS and firefighters teaching CPR to the public, would result in out-of-hospital cardiac arrest survival rates increasing to 12 to 19 percent. Ultimately, there was no simple answer, other than that the current model was not sustainable, especially if the goal was to improve the cardiac arrest survival rates in Winnipeg.

## Consultant Hired

To get better direction as to what was needed for the next step, in September 1980, the city's finance committee hired consultant Jack Paterson. Paterson's job was to provide direction on how to proceed with the options that Chief Coulter had provided.

Paterson claimed that a 25 to 35 percent survival rate was possible with a combination of basic life support and advanced life support ambulances, based on the experiences of Seattle, Washington.[220] At the risk of over-simplification, Paterson concluded that the only way to accomplish this was through collaboration between the fire department and the ambulance service. Like Coulter, he advised that having both services within the same department, but as separate agencies would cause a lot of friction. Therefore, Paterson's opinion was that the only viable, long-term solution was the complete merger of both departments with full cross-training of staff.

The bulk of Paterson's report was a model of how the two departments could be merged. He also emphasized that proper training, with field experience, for dispatchers and call-takers was crucial. Paterson also addressed the need to separate non-emergency patient transfers from emergency patient transportation, noting that using emergency ambulances for non-emergency patient transfers (between hospitals, clinics, and care homes) unnecessarily ties up ambulances, making them unavailable for emergency response.

Early in the new year, on January 13, 1981, the ambulance commission prepared a report, recommending that Paterson's report be accepted, that the number of ambulances operated by Winnipeg Ambulance be doubled, and that the Winnipeg Ambulance Commission be responsible for the overall amalgamation process. Two months later, on March 3, 1981, the city's finance committee accepted both reports and recommended that Winnipeg move toward a full amalgamation of Winnipeg Ambulance and the city's fire department.

Immediately, it became apparent that things were not as *rosy* as Coulter's, Paterson's, and the Commission's reports suggested. Winnipeg Ambulance's general manager, John Farrington explained that it would take at least eighteen months to train the first paramedics and five years for an advanced life support system to be fully operational. On cue, Winnipeg's new fire chief, Lloyd Moist piped in that there would be no "short-term savings" and what was being proposed "was not a cheap service."[221]

There were also some conflicting numbers. The city's administrative steering committee estimated that the capital costs of the amalgamation

220 J.E. Paterson, et al., Ambulance and Fire Services Study, Quotation No. 590-80 "Emergency Medical System". December 19. 1980: 5.

221 "Single ambulance, fire service urged." *Winnipeg Free Press.* March 4, 1981.

would be $933,000, and the annual operating costs would be $765,252. The finance committee was convinced they would have $80,000 in capital savings for administration costs, and $275,000 savings due to staff reductions; using cross-trained staff.[222] At best, it seems that different advocates, those who were for or against the merger, were picking numbers that supported their side.

For example, the reports all indicate that an additional seven or eight staffed ambulances needed to be added to the fleet to accomplish the target response times. However, other than the cost of purchasing/staffing two additional fire department rescue squads, the cost estimates of these additional ambulances were noticeably absent from both reports. Similarly, the Commission's report suggested that ambulance attendants would not be paid on parity with firefighters until they were cross-trained, yet there was no proposed budget for the extra pay once cross-training was completed.

The biggest problem, the solution for which was absent from both reports, was how to get the ambulance attendants to agree to a significant change in their job description. Coulter and Paterson both assumed that the men and women hired to provide emergency medical care would suddenly agree to become firefighters. Also no one seems to have noticed that while there were a few female ambulance attendants, there weren't (and wouldn't be for another seven years) female firefighters. Both reports were oblivious to the employment relations component, which would ultimately lead to the merger's downfall.

Despite the seemingly contradictory numbers, two weeks later, Winnipeg City Council approved the merger, with the caveat that details needed to be *worked out*.[223]

City councillors, and likely city staff, were repeatedly confusing a number of different issues. At the time, the city only had eight ambulances staffed twenty-four hours per day.[224] It was fairly obvious that there needed to be more ambulances and faster response; likely by using firefighters to aid with medical calls, and better training for ambulance attendants, but all magically delivered in a cost-efficient manner. Somehow, this would be accomplished by merging with the fire department.

222 "Single ambulance, fire service urged." *Winnipeg Free Press.* March 4, 1981.
223 "Fire, ambulance, merger a step closer." *Winnipeg Free Press.* March 19, 1981.
224 "Single ambulance, fire service urged." *Winnipeg Free Press.* March 4, 1981.

None of the reports provided this "magic solution," and there was no indication that councillors wanted any kind in in-depth study: evidenced by their stipulation that the "details were to be worked out."

At this point the debate amongst city councillors and the fighting between the two unions went into high gear. Unfortunately, the two separate topics, giving emergency medical technicians (at some point during the process, ambulance attendants began being referred to as EMTs) proper training and merging or amalgamating the two departments, became so intertwined that the real issue—improving the survival rate of Winnipeggers having heart attacks—got lost in the confusion.

General disharmony evolved. Civic politicians saw the merger primarily as a way for the city to save money. Fire department officials saw it as a way to keep their budget while retaining the same staff levels. Ambulance personnel were frustrated at the idea of being turfed out of a job unless they took on new, unwanted tasks as firefighters. The unions were fighting tooth and nail. The firefighters' union balked at having to work with EMTs, rejecting the idea that the head of the ambulance service should be given deputy chief status. There was also a concern that firefighters would lose promotional opportunities if EMTs were included in the bargaining unit. Ultimately, the firefighters' union had difficulties comprehending that providing emergency medical care was anywhere as demanding as firefighting. What was lost in the discussions was the need, merger or not, to increase the quality of prehospital emergency care for the citizens of Winnipeg.

Despite the infighting, there was acceptance that regardless of the outcome, firefighters would need to assist with emergency medical response, in some capacity, for the foreseeable future. With the ambulance service's severely limited resources and the obvious need for rapidly improved response times, there was no other option.

Between the various reports and city council's dithering, before retiring, Chief Coulter kept pushing for a combined service. In 1979, illustrating Coulter's belief that a combined service would eventually happen, the fire department opened the new No. 13 station at 799 Lilac Street. Reflective of the prevailing mood, or hopes, it had three apparatus bays and was designed to accommodate both the fire and ambulance services.

## On With It

Despite the disharmony around the merger, it was recognized that firefighters would need to play some type of formal role in providing emergency care, more than the ad hoc first aid and inhalator services they had been providing since 1928. Once the city and the province reached an agreement that firefighters would be trained as first responders, research started to find appropriate training. A three-week American fire-based first responder course was selected, and then the weekend before the course was to start, training officer Barry Guttormson received new instructions from the manager of Winnipeg Ambulance to provide the fifteen firefighter recruits with a six-week Emergency Medical Technician course. Upon completion, even though the firefighters had been taught by Winnipeg Ambulance staff, it was still difficult for Winnipeg's ambulance personnel to accept firefighters' assistance.

Even after receiving their new first responder training, firefighters were rarely used on medical calls. During the 1981 judicial inquiry into the death of Timothy Sarna, a youth who died as a direct result of poor response times, the evidence showed that first responder trained firefighters were not requested by Winnipeg Ambulance unless every ambulance in the city was busy. In essence, WFD's first responders were deemed to be a last resort.[225] This significantly increased the time that life sustaining care was being withheld from Winnipeg's sick and injured.

After the firefighters began their first responder training, there was a stalemate. Winnipeg's ambulance service couldn't proceed with paramedical training until a medical director was hired, and the medical director couldn't be hired until a formal proposal for merged EMS services was approved.[226] By June 1982, it had reached the stage where both the chair of the city's ambulance committee and the mayor, Bill Norrie, were proposing that the city scrap the merger plans. It seems that by now, both the firefighters' union and the ambulance employees' union were fighting the merger, and the logistics of the merger having a positive outcome seemed increasingly less promising.

---

225 Pamela Fayerman. "Fire crews seldom attend to medical calls, inquest told." *Winnipeg Free Press.* July 22, 1981.

226 Joe Rubin. "Fire, ambulance merger could begin in August." *Winnipeg Free Press.* June 2, 1982.

As the merger idea waned, the fire department formally implemented its first responder program. Two additional Winnipeg Ambulance training officers, Jim Brennan and Brian Gross were recruited for the process, and their first task was to run twelve, three-week EMT classes for firefighters. In the end, including the initial trainees, 159 firefighters had either their Emergency Medical Technician 100 or Emergency Medical Attendant 50 certificates. Another 256 were recertified in first aid and cardiopulmonary resuscitation. After an additional week's delay, the Winnipeg Ambulance Commission claimed that the fire department hadn't gotten proper authorization from the Manitoba College of Physicians and Surgeons,[227] the first responder program finally got rolling on September 6, 1982.[228] Ultimately, this ensured that the citizens of Winnipeg received faster emergency care.

Subsequently, several firefighters were certified as first responder instructors, and all new fire department recruits received either the EMT 100 or EMA 50 course: each involving about eighty hours of training. Both courses had similar medical content, but the EMT 100 course focused on transporting casualties, while the EMA 50 course, similar to today's First Responder course, focused on stabilizing the casualty at the scene.

While initially using the WFD's four rescue squads, by 1993, with 546 firefighters having the necessary training, twenty pieces of frontline fire apparatus (rescue squads and pumpers) were equipped for first responder duties. The basic supplies include a heavy-duty first-aid kit or "trauma kit," oxygen, a bag valve mask ventilator, an obstetrics kit, burn packs, saline solution, blankets, splints, and a scoop stretcher. In 1999, semi-automatic external defibrillators were added to the first responders' arsenal.

Ambulance service personnel gradually started accepting the fire department's help, and firefighters became more receptive of the EMTs' role. In 1982 the fire department made 337 first responder calls. The following year, this jumped to 1,957 calls as Winnipeg Ambulance began requesting and accepting assistance. It is worth noting that during this period, a fire department vehicle arrived before the ambulance in roughly 75 percent of all first responder calls.[229]

---

227 Patrick McKinley. "Troubled emergency service plan to start." *Winnipeg Free Press.* August 30, 1982.

228 Margot Chester. "City's "first responder' units go into service." *Winnipeg Sun.* September 15, 1982.

229 Bjarnason (2005): 108.

## Merger Scrapped

An event 1,330 kilometres away provided the final impetus for Winnipeg to scrap the merger plans. By late 1981, the cracks in Calgary's merged fire-EMS service were becoming major fissures, with paramedics all but refusing to work with firefighters and fire halls becoming chasms of hostility. Calgary hired clinical psychologist Dr. Gerry Belton to do an independent evaluation of the merged Calgary Fire Department.

The Belton Report[230] did a detailed study of both Calgary's existing system and other EMS systems across Canada and the US. As part of his report, Belton reviewed Winnipeg's proposed merger with some disdain, summarizing Winnipeg's cost estimates as *wholly unrealistic.* Ultimately, he concluded that *anything* was better than the current structure in Calgary. After a review of the report by a task force of Calgary firefighters, paramedics, union and city representatives, Calgary decided to scrap the merger and separate EMS from the fire department.

The Belton Report made its way to Winnipeg. After the civic finances committee reviewed it and got input from Edmonton's medical director, who claimed: "… amalgamated services often bring about lower morale among participants, and don't always produce the anticipated savings,"[231] the entire question of a merger was referred back to the Ambulance Commission for reevaluation.

By January 1983, a city task force was recommending that the merger plan be scrapped.[232] Despite multiple recommendations from the city task force, the ambulance workers' union, and the Belton Report to scrap the merger, a group of ad hoc city councillors who supported the merger demanded yet another inquiry. Mayor Norrie best captured the anti-merger sentiments, saying: "There is no point in forcing reluctant employees into an amalgamated service which will not be happy from the outset... the city should decide the issue so needed improvements in the ambulance service, such as the introduction of paramedics, can go ahead."[233]

---

230 G.P. Belton. *Organization Review Project.* Report, Fire Department, Ambulance Division. City of Calgary. 1982.

231 Fred Youngs. "Ambulance, fire merger at square one." *Winnipeg Free Press*". October 27, 1982.

232 Patrick McKinley. "Report urges City scrap merger plan." *Winnipeg Free Press.* January 14, 1983.

233 Patrick McKinley. "Ambulance plan gets yet another look." *Winnipeg Free Press.* February 2, 1983.

The long smoldering merger debate was finally quashed, for the time being, on March 16, 1983. Despite the strong pro-merger faction, councillors agreed to scrap the two-year merger proposal with a unanimous vote. In the same meeting, Council voted to make the Winnipeg Ambulance Service into a municipal department, the Winnipeg Ambulance Department, which would give it the same corporate status as the fire department. Council also voted to hire a medical director, a required step for initiating Winnipeg's paramedic training program. Finally, they voted to fully fund the first responder program, enabling the fire department to provide initial medical response in Charleswood (Station 18 on Roblin Boulevard) and Transcona (Station 21 on Pandora Street), where existing ambulance response times were abysmal.[234]

## Medical Director and Paramedic Program

Based on City Council's resolution, the medical director would be employed by the University of Manitoba's Medical School as a professor, but under contract to the City of Winnipeg to provide medical training/supervision to the ambulance service's emergency medical technicians and firefighter first responders.

Following the advice of the medical advisory committee that spring was the best time to do a job search,[235] the city started advertising in May 1983. In the Fall of 1983, Winnipeg hired emergency room physician Dr. Ken McKenzie as its first medical director. Perhaps because it was a new position, Dr. McKenzie wasn't as well-versed in prehospital emergency care as one would have hoped, and his public comments help illustrate why his tenure was short-lived.

In the spring of 1984, addressing the idea of training ambulance attendants to use defibrillators, something that other Canadian ambulance services had been using for twelve years, Dr. McKenzie commented: "Unofficially, it's a darn good possibility. I think we're very clearly disposed to getting something like that going."[236] Training the ambulance attendants would ultimately require legislative

234 Patrick McKinley. "City Scraps Ambulance Amalgamation." *Winnipeg Free Press.* March 17, 1983.

235 "Ambulance, fire services link on Jan. 1." *Winnipeg Free Press.* October 13, 1982.

236 Maureen Brosnahan. "Fatal heart attack rate remains high." *Winnipeg Free Press.* April 26, 1984.

changes and consent from the College of Physicians & Surgeons of Manitoba because it involved performing medical procedures.

## SUVs

Fortunately, despite Dr. McKenzie's weaknesses, Winnipeg Ambulance worked to upgrade its equipment and improve the training of its personnel. With four training officers there was a concerted effort to find new techniques and equipment. The training officers would often work the day shift and then in the evenings, head out (on their own time) in their station wagon (and later, SUV) to attend calls and test new ideas, equipment, and procedures. Again, this was illustrative of how, even when the system was flawed, individual employees worked to find solutions. The level of dedication from Winnipeg Ambulance staff was beyond reproach.

As an aside, the switch from supervisors and training officers driving station wagons to SUVs has a story. On the weekend of November 7-9, 1986, Winnipeg had a crazy blizzard—with more than thirty centimeters of snow. The accumulation was so great that Winnipeg's snow removal equipment stopped trying to plow the streets, and were assigned to assist fire, police, and ambulance with emergency calls; clearing paths for emergency vehicles. To reduce the strain on ambulances, training officers assisted by responding to low-priority medical calls, with the goal of cancelling as many as possible. After an assessment and a phone discussion with the patient's family physician, in many cases it was determined that a trip to the hospital wasn't necessary. Adding to the overwhelming number of calls were an inordinate number of new babies deciding they needed immediate delivery.

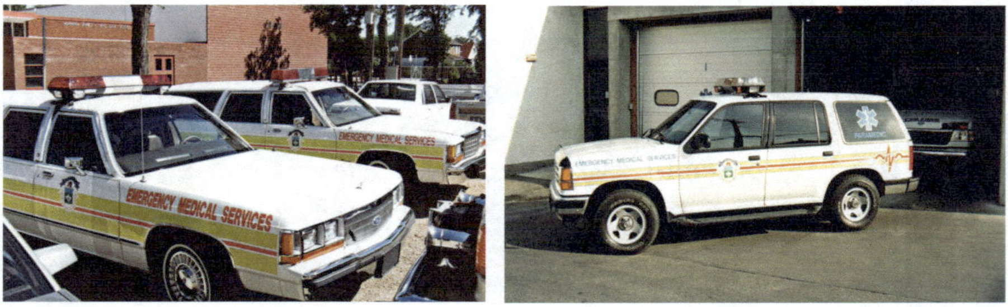


*Mid/late 1990s supervisors' vehicles versus the new 1991 Ford Explorer ALS units. The four-wheel-drive Explorers were much more efficient for responding to calls during Winnipeg's winters. (Courtesy of Stan Stone)*

Once the snow had cleared, Winnipeg Ambulance determined that given Winnipeg's climate, four-wheel-drive SUVs were a more practical choice for supervisors' and advanced life support vehicles. While it took a few years to get the extra budget, the SUVs were finally acquired in 1990 and used in conjunction with the ALS paramedic pilot project.

While using non-patient transport vehicles for supervisors and ALS paramedics had a number of benefits, an incident a few months before the 1986 blizzard captured one of the downsides. On a frosty evening in March 1986, there was an altercation—okay, a small riot—on Main Street, between a group of about twenty residents and four off-duty Winnipeg police officers. When two of the officers were stabbed, one seriously, the mob converged on the officers. Ambulance supervisor Gunter Dorno drove his supervisor's truck through the crowd, lights and sirens, and rescued the four officers.[237] Then, despite having two ambulances on scene, Dorno drove the most seriously injured officer to the Health Sciences Centre in his non-transport equipped truck. While heroic, it also created a small problem. In the cab of a Ford F-350, there was no room to provide medical treatment. As a result, Dorno's "rescue" wasn't really much different than ambulance services provided seventy five years before; A ride to the hospital but with no treatment.

Winnipeg Ambulance's administration was not impressed, and suspended Dorno for four days without pay. This created a public backlash, with the police union hailing Dorno as a hero, the press criticizing ambulance administration, and even dissention within the ambulance supervisors' union.[238] In the end, Dorno was reimbursed by the city for his lost wages and the discipline notice was removed from his file.[239] Regardless of whether his conduct was appropriate or not, the incident captured the downside of using non-patient transport vehicles within the EMS system. Some emergency medical services have paramedics and supervisors driving SUVs, providing greater maneuverability, while others have them driving fully equipped ambulances; giving the option of providing transport. There's no right or wrong answer, just different implications.

237 "Stabbing sends police to hospital." *Winnipeg Free Press.* March 17, 1986; Paul Rodgers. "Hard-Luck Hero." *Winnipeg Sun.* March 20, 1986.

238 Heidi Graham. "Brawl rescue provokes spat within union." *Winnipeg Free Press.* March 21, 1986.

239 Shirley Muir. "Hero's reward." *Winnipeg Sun.* March 23, 1986.

## CPR Training

Not surprisingly, Winnipeg's EMS state was reflective of EMS throughout the province. In June 1984, Manitoba's *Public Health Act* only required that ambulance attendants have a basic, eight-hour first aid certificate. At the time, basic first aid didn't include CPR and so there wasn't even a mention of such training. There was no requirement that an ambulance be staffed by two attendants; only a driver was needed. The requirement of a designated driver is both reassuring and perversely disturbing. Who else would drive, the patient?

After woman in Selkirk—a community north of Winnipeg—died, Manitoba's manager of ambulance services issued a directive recommending two attendants answer all calls and CPR be started on all unconscious victims.[240] While interesting, it begs the question of how ambulance attendants could follow the recommendation when there was no legal requirement for them to know CPR? To round things off, Manitoba ambulance attendants were only required to have a Class 4 driver's license, but with no specific driver training. At the time, Winnipeg Ambulance was giving its attendants a six-week course, which contained some defensive driving techniques.[241]

Three weeks after the provincial directive for ambulance attendants to use CPR came out, lightning hit and killed a Winnipeg soccer player. After taking twenty minutes to arrive, the two Winnipeg ambulance attendants allegedly asked the teammates whether "anyone knew cardiopulmonary resuscitation." A teammate ultimately ended up performing chest compressions, while two others did mouth-to-mouth resuscitation.[242] A preliminary inquiry found that the ambulance attendants had recently recertified in CPR, they still asked bystanders to help and were unable to initially insert an airway.[243] While there was no explanation as to why fire department first responders weren't present, it's worth noting that this was in the period where Winnipeg Ambulance staff were hesitant to request fire department assistance. Ultimately, this scenario captured the still-insufficient level of training.

---

240 Maureen Brosnahan. "Death of woman prompts new ambulance rules." *Winnipeg Free Press.* June 2, 1984.

241 Julia Necheff. "Ambulance speed, driver training unregulated, official says." *Winnipeg Free Press.* July 26, 1984.

242 Don Retson. "Ambulance response criticized." *Winnipeg Free Press.* June 22, 1984.

243 Patrick McKinley. "Ambulance response satisfies City." *Winnipeg Free Press.* June 27, 1984.

## LifePak 5 Defibrillators

While unfortunate, the incident provided the needed push for change. Four months later, in November 1984, Winnipeg Ambulance got its first twelve defibrillators; Physio Control LifePak 5s, the electric gadgets designed to get the rhythm of a human heart recalibrated.

By way of background, the LifePak 5 was first introduced in 1976. As it was both light (8.25 lbs./3.7 kg) and advanced for the time, it remained the industry standard until the early 1990s. After eighty ambulance attendants were given a three-day course on detecting heart problems and using the LifePak 5, and the College of Physicians & Surgeons of Manitoba provided consent, the defibrillators went into service in selected city ambulances in December 1984.

Acquiring defibrillators was the ambulance service's first step to providing an appropriate level of emergency care to Winnipeggers. It also gave Winnipeg emergency medical technicians a crucial tool to help save lives.

In response to this advancement, Winnipeg Ambulance's medical director Ken McKenzie stated that: "training ambulance attendants to defibrillate will cost hundreds of thousands of dollars less than developing a paramedic team."[244] Given that defibrillators were a basic tool needed to restart a heart, and only one of many tools that paramedics can use to correct heart irregularities, it appears that Dr. McKenzie didn't understand the role of defibrillators, advanced care paramedics, or much else in the EMS field. Despite the introduction of improved emergency care tools such as MAST pants, defibrillators, and bag valve masks or "Ambu-bags" (a rubber, hand pumped resuscitator which enables paramedics to manually force oxygen into a non-breathing casualty), Winnipeg's EMTs were still only receiving six weeks of initial training.[245]

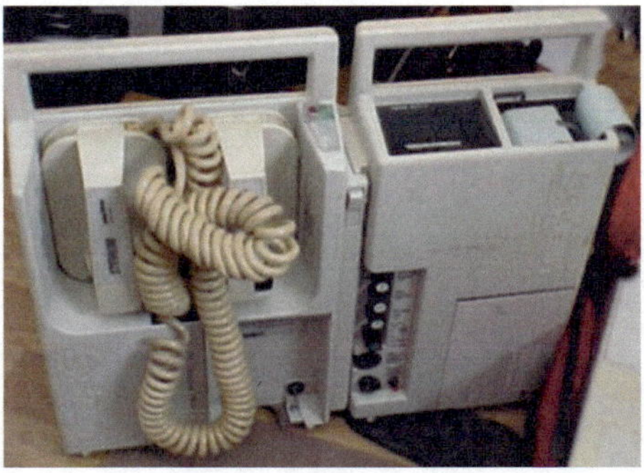

*Physio Control LifePak5s: The industry standard for portable defibrillators when acquired by Winnipeg Ambulance in 1984. (Courtesy of the National EMS Museum)*

244 "Ambulances to get heart defibrillators." *Winnipeg Free Press.* November 28, 1984.
245 Barbara Robson. "Blood and Guts." *Winnipeg Free Press.* November 26, 1985.

As an aside, the MAST pants, "Military/Medical Anti-Shock Trousers," quickly went out of vogue in Winnipeg. They were introduced into Winnipeg Ambulance's repertoire in the early 1980s as a tool to deal with severe shock. However, as they force the casualty's blood into their chest area, they can be deadly if used on a person with a serious chest wound. After the tragic death of J.J. Harper in 1988, who died of a chest wound after ambulance attendants applied the MAST pants, it seems that Winnipeg Ambulance ceased using them.[246]

## A Positive Wave of Changes

A positive wave of changes within Winnipeg Ambulance finally started in 1986. In August 1985, after nine years as director, John Farrington left for adventures in Australia. At about the same time, Ken McKenzie was relieved of his duties as medical director. With Jake Enns appointed as the new director of Winnipeg Ambulance, and Dr. Moe Lerner appointed as Winnipeg's new EMS Medical Director in early 1986, the ambulance service gained the momentum needed to move forward.

While Jake Enns' predecessor was essentially a bureaucrat or paper pusher, Enns was the antithesis. As a former police officer, as well as an emergency medical technician, he was used to working on the street and understood his staff's needs. Working with the Board of Commissioners, he advocated for those things that would enable Winnipeg's EMTs to have better working conditions, such as stand-alone ambulance stations, as well as skills and equipment necessary to get the job done: newer ambulances, better training—including extrication and trench rescue skills—for EMS staff, and more practical uniforms (wearing ties and oxford shoes when doing extrication was extremely dangerous). Perhaps most importantly, because of his background, human resources-wise, he understood the needs and issues of EMTs; crucial for improving morale within the ambulance service.

At the same time, Dr. Lerner arrived with both an interest and a deep understanding of prehospital emergency care. This, combined with his engaging personality, enabled him to connect with staff in a more positive way than his predecessor. Both during and after his tenure as Winnipeg Ambulance's medical director, he served as an

246 Heidi Graham. "Use of pressure pants up to attendants, inquest told." *Winnipeg Free Press.* April 20, 1988.

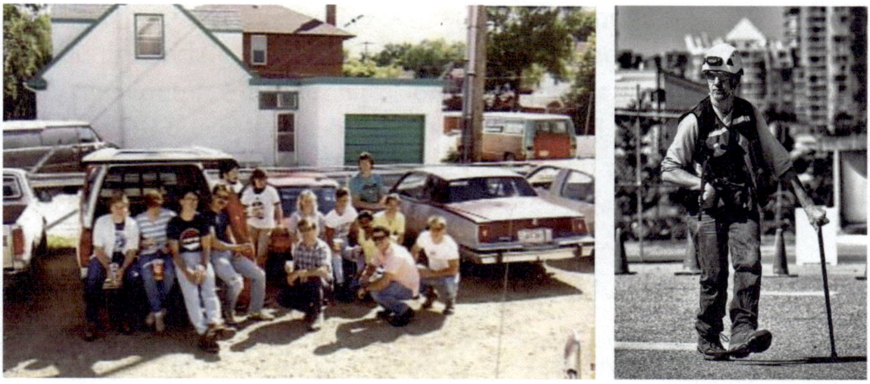

*The Class of 1988 dressed for extrication training—t-shirts and jeans. (Courtesy of Sandy Schoofs.) Contrasted with the author at a more recent extrication practice with Vancouver Fire Rescue Service's NEAT program: helmet, eye protection, protective vest, gloves (in pocket), and steel-toed boots. (Courtesy of Vancouver Fire Rescue Service.)*

adjudicator of British Columbia Ambulance's advanced life support competitions.[247]

One of Dr. Lerner's strongest skills was giving feedback to crews. For example, he provided formal memos to staff whenever a Winnipeg Ambulance EMT performed a defibrillation.

> THE CITY OF WINNIPEG
> AMBULANCE DEPARTMENT
> CARDIAC ARREST CRITIQUE
> TO: BARRY GUTTORMSON, DON DACQUAY & SANDY SCHOOFS
> FROM: M. LERNER, M.D. MEDICAL DIRECTOR
> RE:INCIDENT #25948
> DATE: 1988-06-28
>
> I have reviewed this tape concerning a 70-year-old male who was discovered in cardiac arrest. The past medical history and circumstances of arrest were not on the run sheet, however I believe this was an unwitnessed situation. The patient presented with a slow ventricular standstill in EMD. Apparently, the patient was cardioverted three times but unfortunately remained in asystole.

247 Online interview with Lynn KleIn, BCAS. January 1, 2024.

> You worked well as a team, assisting with intubation, drug administration and safe but rapid transport. Although this patient did not survive, I know that his family appreciated your efforts. Dealing with sudden death is one of the most difficult tasks involved in being an EMT. Continue to study and practice and I am sure that you will enjoy greater success in the future.
>
> —M. Lerner, M.D., Medical Director

A March 1986 heart attack death in Transcona again highlighted that Winnipeg had neither enough ambulances nor an adequate EMS response. Winnipeg had the same number of emergency ambulances, transfer ambulances, and EMTs as nine years before, despite the city's aging population and higher call volume. While the seventeen fire department first-responder vehicles provided initial response within Winnipeg, they could not provide the necessary enhanced medical response nor transport patients to hospitals. In an attempt to rectify, the city hired three more EMTs.[248]

In response to the March heart attack, in July 1986, Lerner initiated the city's first Advanced Life Support Pilot Project. While not the full-scale paramedic program that Winnipeg needed, it was a start.

With limited resources, Lerner's pilot project demonstrated that advanced life support paramedical services would be a significant benefit to Winnipeg. Under the project, training officers Barry Guttormson, Jim Brennan, and Brian Gross were trained and equipped to administer specialized, advanced prehospital cardiac care, including endotracheal intubation, intravenous access, and epinephrine.[249] Under the pilot project, when a Winnipegger suffered a cardiac arrest, firefighters provided initial first response services, including starting CPR; ideally within four minutes. This was followed by basic life support EMTs in ambulances with defibrillators, ideally within nine minutes. Then, as availability permitted, a training officer would arrive and start administering advanced cardiac care, including drugs.

248 Don Retson. "Heart victim's death linked to tight ambulance budget." *Winnipeg Free Press*. March 23, 1986.

249 Dr. Moe Lerner to All EMTs and Supervisors, City of Winnipeg Inter-Office Memorandum Re: Advanced Life Support Pilot Project. July 13, 1986.

As part of the project, ambulance supervisors also carried the cardiac care kits in their vehicles. However, as the supervisors were not given the same hands-on training and practice as the training officers, they typically did not use the equipment.

Moe Lerner left the medical director's role in 1988, amidst some unspecified concerns over patient care.[250] While the actual reasons haven't been identified, Dr. Lerner left shortly after the inquiry into J.J. Harper's death. During the inquiry, Winnipeg Ambulance's policies on the use of Military/Medical Anti-Shock Trousers ("MAST pants"), which had been used for almost ten years, were brought into question.

One possible explanation of Lerner's departure was that the roles of the EMS Medical Director and the Director of Winnipeg Ambulance had overlapping jurisdiction, without clear boundaries. As a result, Lerner and Enns, while both dedicated to improving Winnipeg Ambulance, were both new to their jobs and in an ongoing turf war. They were at constant loggerheads, often with training officers stuck in the middle. This led to a difficult relationship that more likely than not, contributed to Lerner's early departure.[251]

Change can sometimes be a blessing in disguise. After Lerner's departure, the city hired Dr. Linda Nugent, an anesthesiologist and dynamo, as Winnipeg's new Emergency Medical Director. Over the next thirteen years, she took Lerner's initial work and propelled Winnipeg Ambulance's programs forward, eventually equipping Winnipeg with a nationally accredited advanced care paramedic program.

In 1989, shortly after being hired, Nugent commenced a two-year pilot project, training eight EMTs as advanced life support paramedics. Under the training officers, and using the Canadian Medical Association's EMT 300 protocols, the soon-to-be paramedics received sixty weeks of training in advanced care; significantly more than the training officers received in the 1986 pilot project. The training included spending significant amounts of time in hospital emergency, intensive care, and obstetrics wards, observing and providing hands-on assistance. Going beyond the cardiac care that was the focus of the 1986 pilot project, the EMT 300 training included identifying and treating such diverse conditions as:

250 Terry Weber. "MD quits ambulance advisory board." *Winnipeg Free Press.* January 24, 1989.

251 Telephone interview with Barry Guttormson, August 28, 2024.

- hypoglycemia (low blood sugar);
- anaphylaxia (serious allergic reactions);
- bradycardia (extremely slow heart rate);
- unstable angina (lack of oxygen to the heart);
- respiratory failure (poor or absent breathing);
- bronchospasm (wheezing);
- status epilepticus (continued seizures); and
- obstructed airway.[252]

Many of which are conditions which, if not treated immediately, can result in death before the casualty reaches a hospital.

Under the 1989 pilot project, two ALS paramedics were assigned per shift. While they were assigned an ambulance, it was typically not used for patient transport. By using the Basic Life Support ambulances for transport, it ensured that the ALS paramedics were not tied up at the hospital, enabling them to immediately respond to their next call.

While the program was working well, pay for the new paramedics became a typical City of Winnipeg challenge. As the paramedics had volunteered for the new roles, they were only paid their EMT wages during training. However, once qualified as ALS paramedics and accredited by the Canadian Medical Association, despite promises to the contrary, Winnipeg refused to pay their extra $2.50/hour wages. Nevertheless, the new paramedics continued to work voluntarily at the BLS level.[253] Such reflects the ongoing commitment of Winnipeg's emergency medical personnel. Despite silliness at the political level and despite limited resources, Winnipeg's EMTs worked to provide the city with the best emergency medical services possible.

After five years of pilot projects, it was clear that the ALS program was saving lives, even in its most rudimentary form. As a result, in 1991, Winnipeg Ambulance asked the province for $6.5 million to create a full-scale paramedic program.[254] The proposal was to hire twenty four

---

252 Aldo Santin. "Lifesavers Baffled." *Winnipeg Free Press.* August 17, 1992.

253 Heidi Graham. "Paramedic loss would be deadly, City woman warns." *Winnipeg Free Press.* March 30, 1992.

254 "Paramedic service tag $6.5 million." *Winnipeg Free Press.* September 10, 1991.

additional paramedics (allowing for three, two-person paramedic units per shift), acquire four paramedic SUVs, and build a world-class ALS program over the following five years.

## Extrication

In the midst of trying to formalize the ALS program, a fight over extrication jurisdiction erupted, capturing the tenuous relationship between Winnipeg's ambulance and fire departments.[255] As mentioned in the last chapter, Hurst's hydraulic extrication tools (and a variety of high-quality copies), a.k.a. the "Jaws of Life," revolutionized motor vehicle accident rescues. While originally designed for auto racing rescue work, through superb promotion by the Hurst company, these tools became the benchmark for mitigating auto and industrial accident entrapment.

Winnipeg Ambulance acquired its first set of Hurst tools in the fall of 1977. For the next decade and a half, it provided the primary accident extrication service in the city. About forty times a year, one of the two supervisors' trucks, equipped to carry the extrication tools, would respond to automobile or industrial accidents where

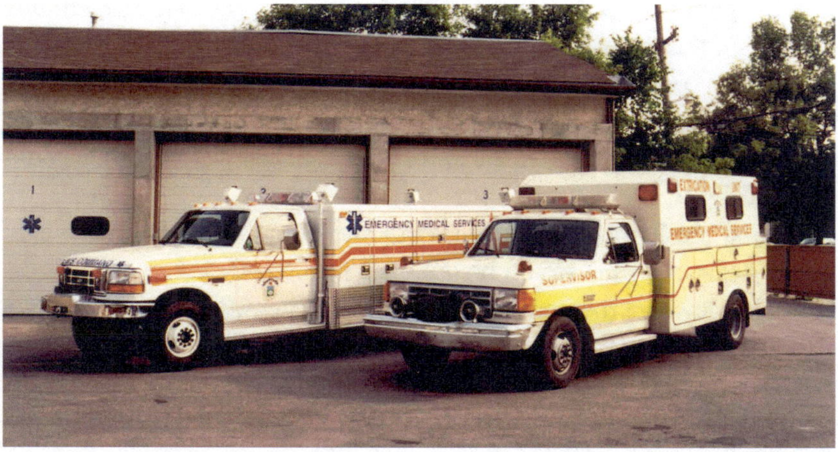


*Winnipeg Ambulance's second and third extrication units. The third unit (one the left), based on a 1993 Ford chassis, was the last unit acquired before fire department rescue squads became responsible for extrication. (Courtesy of Brian Schuff.)*

---

255 Donald Campbell. "Ambulance workers rip firefighters over jaws of life." *Winnipeg Free Press.* April 2, 1990.

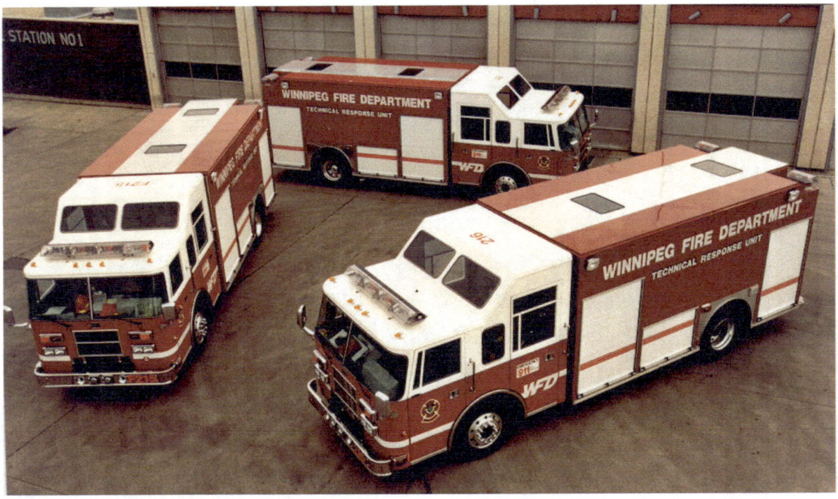


*During the 1997 Winnipeg Emergency Response Service merger, the fire department acquired specific Technical Response/Extrication Units, assuming responsibility for extrication. (Courtesy of FFHSW)*

people were trapped. Trained ambulance personnel would do their magic freeing them.

In 1988, the fire department bought its first set of Hurst's Jaws of Life,[256] and by 1990, had all four rescue squads equipped with Hurst hydraulic tools.[257] At that point, the fire department administration began suggesting to city council that firefighters should have primary responsibility for vehicle extrication. In response to the ambulance service's claims that they had jurisdiction for extrication, the WFD claimed that they could respond faster.

At first blush, the debate seems odd; one would think that when lives are at stake, everyone would be onboard with the fastest rescue process possible. However, the underlying rationale is interesting. There were two issues at play. First, the fire department needed to get more work to maintain their budget. As shown in 1980, fire calls were dropping when then-fire chief Coulter was vying to take over Winnipeg's EMS. There were even fewer calls ten years later. Going to car accidents was more business, as stressed by then-fire chief Jack Henderson, who observed: "We used to have a policy where we went to all vehicle accidents. I'd like to see that

256 "Rescue unit makes west safer." *Winnipeg Free Press.* August 7, 1988.

257 Kevin Rollason. "Council orders review of policy on use of extrication equipment." *Winnipeg Free Press.* January 8, 1991.

policy reinstated."[258] More *business* helps to justify a larger budget. Second, as a result of the underlying bitterness from previous merger attempts, where EMTs believed that firefighters were trying to take over their jobs, there was no desire, whatsoever, to give up *any* jurisdiction.

This wasn't a new issue. In New York City, the police department's Emergency Service Unit (ESU) carried extrication tools and responded to all traffic accidents. As a result, there was ongoing strife between the NYC police ESU and the Fire Department of New York's rescue squads, which respond to almost every other kind of extrication and rescue scenario in the city. The difference between New York and Winnipeg was that in New York, when the police didn't like firefighters impinging on their extrication jurisdiction, they would arrest them and slap on the handcuffs.[259]

Winnipeg's jurisdictional match came to a head in December 1990 when both departments responded to a serious three-vehicle accident with multiple injuries and a death. While there was no suggestion that any responding emergency personnel acted inappropriately, the incident got before the Civic Protection, Parks, and Culture Committee because of the apparent hostility. There were concerns about it becoming a turf war. After six months of debate, the committee decided to keep the status quo and leave primary responsibility for extrication with ambulance staff.[260] The policy stated that ambulance personnel were responsible for using the extrication equipment, based on what resources were available at the time. The policy occasionally caused flare-ups, such as at a 1996 motor vehicle accident when ambulance personnel decided to wait for their own extrication gear instead of using the on-scene fire department equipment.[261] However, until the city merged the two

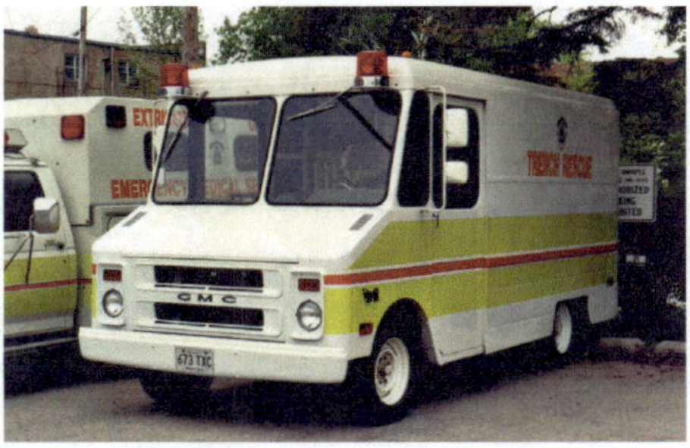

*Winnipeg Ambulance's 1993 Trench Rescue Unit. (Courtesy of Brian Schuff)*

---

258 Kevin Rollason. "Council orders review of policy on use of extrication equipment", *Winnipeg Free Press.* January 8, 1991.

259 Samuel M. Katz. *Anytime Anywhere!* Pocket Books, 1997.

260 Kevin Rollason. "Responsibility for Jaws of Life to stay with ambulance crews." *Winnipeg Free Press.* June 25, 1991.

261 Steven Forbes. "Victim trapped extra 10 minutes." *Winnipeg Sun.* October 4, 1996.

departments, there was the ongoing discourse over funding, which occasionally led to turf wars.

In 1992, Winnipeg Ambulance's industrial rescue capacity was increased when it ran a course on trench rescue; the process of shoring up the sides of a trench and digging a trapped victim out of a collapsed ditch (or other hole in the ground). Using the city's Operations Yard on Roblin Boulevard, Winnipeg Ambulance staff extended their extrication skills to below-ground operations. The ambulance service subsequently purchased a GMC panel truck and set up a trench rescue response truck. While necessary, and part of Winnipeg Ambulance's industrial rescue/extrication mandate, it also put ambulance personnel in direct competition with the Winnipeg Fire Department's technical rescue team.

## Back to ALS

In February 1992, after six months of negotiating, the city and province finally hammered out a funding agreement for Winnipeg's ambulance service. Each of Winnipeg and Manitoba Health would pay 25 percent of Winnipeg Ambulance's $9.4 million operating budget. The remaining 50 percent was to be covered by user fees, which, as previously discussed, were the city's responsibility and often hard to collect.

The ALS paramedic program's start-up costs were another $1.6 million, on top of the $9.4 million base budget. The city was intent on getting the province to pay half of the program. Some city councillors had a concern that if the city paid for all costs related to the ALS program, it would set a precedent resulting in the city losing even more provincial funding.[262]

While it may have been a political game or negotiating strategy, it also suggests that Winnipeg's city council was collectively not as concerned about keeping Winnipeggers alive as one would hope.

After a media campaign by the Winnipeg Ambulance Employee Association—the EMT's union—in September 1992, city council decided to fund the ALS program unilaterally, adding twenty four ALS paramedics to the ambulance service's roster over the next three years.[263] The lobbying

262 Aldo Santin. "City, province playing with lives, union says." *Winnipeg Free Press.* August 17, 1992.

263 Radha Krishnan Thampl. "Proposal breathes life into program." *Winnipeg Free Press.* September 9, 1992.

occurred on the eve of the municipal election. Refusing to support the ALS paramedic program would have placed current council members in a poor light. This aided in getting the program approved. This type of pressure is a technique that the firefighters' union had been using for years, but Winnipeg's EMS personnel, being much newer to the game, were just learning effective political maneuvering.

Having ALS-level trained paramedics was a definite step forward from the original 1975, 160-hour ambulance attendant's course. By accepting the Canadian Medical Association's standards, Winnipeg Ambulance's training program increased to 870 hours for the EMT/Level I program. It then took an extra 340 hours of training for the Intermediate Paramedic/Level II program, and a 780-hour internship. Once the Level II program was completed, it took a further 1,115 hours of training as well as an additional 620-hour internship in one of the city's hospitals, with clinical rotations in the emergency department, operating rooms, psychiatric and obstetrical areas, respiratory therapy, dialysis, and cardiac and intensive care units to acquire full ALS Paramedic/Level 3 status. Winnipeg's ALS Paramedic level was almost identical to the Canadian Medical Association's Critical Care Paramedic standards.

At the time, Winnipeg Ambulance's training supervisor, Barry Guttormson had been the president of the Paramedic Association of Canada. As part of this role, along with Winnipeg's EMS Medical Director Linda Nugent, he sat on the CMA's Committee on Conjoint Accreditation. With Winnipeg Ambulance Operations Supervisor, Al King, Guttormson surveyed numerous paramedic programs, including those at the Southern Alberta Institute of Technology, Saskatchewan Polytechnic, St. John's, Newfoundland, Charlottetown, PEI, and Fredericton, NB. As a result, Winnipeg Ambulance had a team with decent working knowledge of what the CMA was looking for and used this skill to design Winnipeg's inhouse program. Winnipeg's proposed program, eventually expanded into Level 1 (Basic Life Support Paramedics), Level 2 (Intermediate Care Paramedics), Level 2 Advanced (Advanced Care Paramedics), and Level 3 (Supervisors/Critical Care Paramedics), with the Advanced Care program being eventually approved by the CMA in 2002. It was the first Advanced Care Paramedic program to be approved in Canada, making it the "Gold Standard" for paramedic programs.[264]

264 Online interview with Sandy Schoofs, February 5, 2024; and telephone interview with Barry Guttormson, August 28, 2024.

As the medical protocols became more advanced, and Winnipeg's paramedics got greater responsibilities and skill sets, it provided a means for the Winnipeg paramedics' union to negotiate closer wage parody with firefighters. However, this would not occur until the next millennium.

## Merger... Again

While the September 1992 municipal election provided the stimulus for finally getting a complete ALS program in Winnipeg, it also provided stimulus for revisiting the fire-ambulance merger idea; yet again.

As a reminder, the merger idea was not just a political issue. The fire department was hit with significant cutbacks, so its administration wasn't opposed to ideas that would help them maintain their budget. In 1985, city council removed twenty four firefighters' positions, despite increasing call volumes: from 10,498 in 1982 to 13,934 in 1984. These were primarily first responder medical calls, as fires were down to about 4,000 annually.[265] Then in 1991, seventeen additional fire positions were cut, as well as eighty five police positions, in order to partially trim $3 million from the city's annual budget.[266]

In November 1992, almost ten years after being put to rest, the fire-ambulance merger debate was reactivated after Susan Thompson's mayoral election. In order to appreciate why Ms. Thompson would choose to pursue the idea of a fire-ambulance merger so aggressively, it's important to understand both her role and Winnipeg's economic circumstances at the time.

In her autobiography, Thompson succinctly describes the city that she had inherited as mayor:

> "... Winnipeg was a city in decline economically and financially. We had the highest property taxes and the highest per capita city debt, and we had been dubbed the "murder capital of Canada". We had an agjng population and our growth was stagnant... If anything, we were referred to as a "have not" city, as was our province."[267]

265 Patrick McKinley. "Budget proposal to cut 24 firefighters backed." *Winnipeg Free Press*. February 13, 1985.

266 Kevin Rollason. "Board proposes eliminating 102 fire, police jobs." *Winnipeg Free Press*. February 7, 1991.

267 Thompson (2016): 105

The financial picture got worse shortly after Thompson took office. For the first time in thirty years, since the creation of Unicity, property taxes were reassessed, and in many cases, listed property values skyrocketed. Property taxes were hiked by 8 percent, resulting in many property owners appealing their tax bills. In 1993, it ended up costing the city hundreds of millions of dollars in property tax refunds and lost revenue.[268] Needless to say, this placed Thompson in an unpopular position.

Winnipeg has never recovered from this upheaval. As of the city's 2022 budget, it had $1,009,108,000—more than a billion dollars—of actual debt.[269]

While the city was in financial tatters, Thompson had a further obstacle to overcome. Being a woman—the first female mayor of a major Canadian city—a political neophyte, and not being part of the city's well-established "Old Boys' Club," she received very little internal support for doing her job:

> "... whether it was a lack or appropriate protocol shown to me as mayor, sometimes as simple as a welcoming chair at the Board of Commissioners' meeting, or being unavailable for a first meeting between a mayor and chief commissioner, a clear message was being sent to me immediately that I was but one vote in the approval process at city hall and nothing more."[270]

At the same time, Thompson desperately wanted to make a difference in the city. As a politician—and the "face of Winnipeg"—she needed to improve the city's image and financial situation. As an individual, she was driven to increase the number of women employed by the city. From Thompson's subsequent research, she believed that a fire-EMS merger could potentially accomplish all of these objectives.

Shortly after becoming mayor, Thompson raised most civic fees, including ambulance fees, to offset the fallout from the property tax fiasco. Increasing ambulance fees by $5 to $185, it also provided some of the extra funds needed to cover the evolving ALS paramedic program.

268 Thompson (2016): 106.

269 City of Winnipeg. *2022 Annual Financial Report.* 2023: 66.

270 Thompson (2016): 137.

By 1995, it became obvious that something needed to change. In February, Winnipeg Ambulance had nine ambulances in full-time service and ALS paramedics had switched to driving SUVs. This resulted in there being no additional means within the ambulance service to transport patients.[271] When overload occurred, with no available ambulances, fire department rescue squads had to be utilized to transport patients, under the supervision of an ALS paramedic.

In November 1995, Winnipeg Ambulance's fleet was increased to eighteen units, allowing for fourteen to fifteen ambulances to be on duty during the day and ten at night.[272] This would have improved things considerably, except that at the same time, the province closed Winnipeg's community hospital emergency rooms at night. These closures left only the emergency wards at St. Boniface Hospital and the Health Sciences Centre open between 10:00 p.m. and 8:00 a.m., putting a new, additional strain on Winnipeg's EMS. At night, ambulances often had to drive across the city to reach an open emergency room. During the day, ambulances were often either driving around in search of an emergency room that was not overloaded or waiting at busy emergency rooms to hand over their patients. Either way, the nighttime emergency room closures caused Winnipeg's ambulances to be out of service or unavailable for longer periods, creating a need for more ambulances.

To add insult to injury, the following year, when Winnipeg Ambulance needed more resources, City Council slashed the ambulance subsidy by $200,000. In desperation, a $100 per patient service charge was proposed, even when the ambulance was not needed.[273]

While the service fee does not appear to have been implemented, if you want to discourage people from calling for help, this would certainly do it!

In addition to the fact that Winnipeg Ambulance continued to be stretched beyond its capacity, two other catalysts propelled Mayor Thompson and city council to revisit the fire-EMS merger idea.

First, in August 1995, with an upcoming municipal election, the Canadian Federation of Independent Businesses (CFIB) began lobbying

---

271 Michael Thibault. "Ambulances busy, patients ride in rescue trucks." *Winnipeg Free Press.* February 12, 1995.

272 Stevens Wild. "Whole City covered by 10 to 15 vehicles." *Winnipeg Free Press.* November 4, 1995.

273 Aldo Santin. "Ambulance wants $100, even if nobody gets a ride." *Winnipeg Free Press.* November 4, 1996.

for a fire-ambulance merger. Citing Edmonton as a classic example of how well a merger works (this was two years before Edmonton's merger imploded), the CFIB argued that a merger would save money and provide a better service.[274]

Second, in 1996, Gary Richardson, Ottawa's fire chief and former Winnipeg deputy fire chief, completed his thesis for a master's degree in public administration. As Richardson was a friend and former colleague of Thompson, she passionately accepted Richardson's paper as a report on how to merge the fire department and ambulance service and set out to sell it to city council.

The main problem is that Richardson's paper, which was designed to present an academic argument, doesn't stand up in the real world. While his intent was to argue that a merger of the two departments would be effective, it's important to appreciate the flaws in his research in order to understand the difficulties with his recommendations.

In his thesis, Richardson provided the following "case studies" as evidence that *mergers between separate fire departments and ambulance services can be successful.* The reality is slightly different:

- **Seattle, Washington:** Was described as a success because: "While all of the above perceptions (against mergers) create legitimate concerns there is absolutely no basis in fact to substantiate them. One only has to look at very successful examples of fully integrated services to dispel these myths. Seattle, Washington, arguably a high-quality service with statistics to prove it, has been fully integrated for decades."

  REALITY: Put simply, there has never been a fire/ambulance merger in Seattle. The fire department provided, and still provides, fire/rescue services. Private ambulance services provide Basic Life Support transport. In 1971, as the concept of a paramedic was evolving, ALS response was added to the fire department's list of duties, and the department acquired paramedic response vehicles. The fire department also provides first responder services using "aid cars," while private ambulances from either American Medical Response or Tri-Med Ambulance provide BLS ambulance service. Seattle's fire and ambulance services have never merged.

---

274 John Collison. "Emergency alert." *Winnipeg Sun.* August 8, 1995.

- **Lethbridge, Alberta:** Was described by Richardson as a success because: "the fire service can provide top quality, efficiently run EMS Services (sic)."[275]

  REALITY: There has never been a fire/ambulance merger in Lethbridge. In 1912, the fire department took over operating the town's ambulance from the district hospital and has been doing so ever since.

- **Phoenix, Arizona:** Was described by Richardson as a success because: "the fire Service can provide top quality, efficiently run EMS Services (sic)".[276]

  REALITY: As with Seattle, Phoenix has never had a fire/ambulance merger. In 1971, Phoenix began training its firefighters as EMTs. Two years later, their training was upgraded to ALS paramedics. EMTs and paramedics rode on fire apparatus, and private ambulance companies provided patient transportation. In 1985, Phoenix decided to use one ambulance service instead of seven. It opened the provision of ambulance services to a competition, and the fire department provided the winning bid. The previously trained firefighters began driving ambulances newly purchased by the Phoenix Fire Department.

- **Edmonton, Alberta:** Richardson described it as a failure because "… working conditions, benefits, etc., for the newly created organization were not properly addressed. Personal and group agendas, factions, perceptions, turf wars, personality and fear of the unknown all contribute to the creation of the climate within which crucial decisions must be made... many mergers (Calgary and Edmonton) are made without first addressing these concerns."[277]

  REALITY: In 1993, Edmonton merged its Fire and EMS to become the City of Edmonton's Emergency Response Department. It was initially endorsed by Edmonton city council as a merger of the administration functions, with two separate streams. Despite a very critical review in 1995, Edmonton's fire chief unilaterally expanded the merger into integrated training, with a goal of

---

275 Richardson (1996): 82.
276 Richardson (1996): 82.
277 Richardson (1996): 73-74.

cross-training all frontline staff. Under the cross-trained regime, firefighting staff supervised EMS operations. After numerous unsuccessful attempts to reorganize and rectify the hostile work environment, only twenty five percent of the merged department's employees considered the relationship between fire and EMS as positive.[278] In 2009, the combined department separated and EMS became part of the Alberta provincial ambulance service.

- **Calgary, Alberta:** Was described by Richardson as a failure because: "... working conditions, benefits, etc., for the newly created organization were not properly addressed. Personal and group agendas, factions, perceptions, turf wars, personality and fear of the unknown all contribute to the creation of the climate within which crucial decisions must be made... many mergers (Calgary and Edmonton) are made without first addressing these concerns."[279]

  REALITY: Between 1970 and 1984, Calgary's EMS was a branch of the Calgary Fire Department, operating as two services under common management—similar to the current Winnipeg Fire Paramedic Service. It became a separate service in 1984 after the work environment became untenably toxic. Calgary's EMS is now part of the Alberta provincial ambulance service.

- **Norfolk, Virginia:** Was described by Richardson as a success because: "... all of the players were forced to interact and become familiar with both sides in the issue before concrete plans for implementation were made..."[280]

  REALITY: In summary, Norfolk's Paramedical Rescue Service (their ambulance department) didn't have adequate funding, and their fire department was being underutilized. Norfolk gave a batch of firefighters paramedical training and then indicated to the city's existing emergency medical staff that if they didn't want to merge and cross-train as firefighters, they would find themselves out of work. During discussions, police officers were stationed at the door to prevent firefighters and paramedics from leaving the room. In Canada, this would likely constitute

278 Plumbtree (2011): 330.
279 Richardson (1996): 73-74.
280 Richardson (1996): 74.

> an "unfair labour practice," and contains many of the tenets of the Canadian *Criminal Code*'s definitions of "extortion" and "forcible confinement." While Norfolk's merger was successful, the techniques used appear to be illegal in Canada. Hence, it's questionable whether Norfolk is a valid comparison.

Richardson states: "Integrating two services or departments has never been an easy task but many examples exist to demonstrate that it is not impossible."[281] In his thesis, Richardson didn't provide a single example of a successful fire/ambulance merger, despite arguing that such was possible.

In response to Richardson's ongoing promotion of the fire-EMS merger, the *Winnipeg Free Press* ran an article in 2004 describing yet another failed fire-EMS merger, this time in San Francisco, California. In quoting an American expert on emergency health services, the article noted that he was "unaware of any fire-paramedic mergers that have been successful from a human resources perspective... This is an experiment that's been going on for a long time in the States. I'm not aware of any successful outcomes."[282]

In looking at the potential for merging Winnipeg's fire and ambulance services, Richardson claimed that he would: "examine the issue through analysis of several North American municipalities who have followed various models in the attempt to partially merge or fully amalgamate services."[283] While submitting that his evidence shows that a merger in Winnipeg would be successful, as outlined in the above analysis of his studies, in reality, his research shows the opposite. In retracing Richardson's research into the services provided in Seattle, Phoenix, Norfolk, Lethbridge, Edmonton, and Calgary, the more accurate conclusions are that:

- city fire departments where firefighters have historically provided paramedical services appear to be successful; and
- mergers between fire departments and non-fire paramedical services, unless there is quasi-illegal coercion involved, will implode.

Richardson's research shows that a fire-EMS merger like Winnipeg's *wouldn't* be successful; he just forgot to mention it.

281 Richardson (1996): 62.
282 Paul Egan. "Fire, paramedics a poor marriage?" *Winnipeg Free Press*. September 26, 2004.
283 Richardson (1996): 2.

Looking at Richardson's research by analogy, he took a box of apples, a box of oranges, and a can of orange spray paint. After spraying all of the apples with orange paint, he dumped all the fruit in the same box and called them "oranges." You won't immediately notice the difference if you don't taste them.

Using this type of misinformation to rearrange $100 million municipal departments is more problematic. As Richardson passed away in 2005, we will never know whether he was genuinely mistaken, was *willfully blind* to the differences, or intentionally misrepresented the examples to get the results he wanted.

Irrespective of Richardson's paper and his intentions, an unconnected but relevant legislative change happened in Manitoba in the fall of 1997, making the fire-ambulance merger financially justifiable, regardless of whether it would actually work or not. We'll get to that in a moment.

## Women in EMS

Mayor Thompson's interest in a merged fire-EMS service went beyond being a cost-saving venture. At the beginning of her term as mayor, she was clear that one of her objectives was to increase the number of women in Winnipeg's civic employment. At the time of her election, only 23 percent of Winnipeg's civic employees were women[284]. Roughly four firefighters, fifteen paramedics, and two dozen police officers were female; a very small percentage of staffing in their respective departments.

In preparation for Canada's participation in the United Nation's 1975 International Women's Year, the federal Trudeau government had begun looking at ways to improve the existing, somewhat subservient role of women in Canada. The 1972 creation of the National Action Committee on the Status of Women provided a driving force for political change within Canada, with several national conferences over the period leading up to 1975.

This movement led to specific advances in women's employment in non-traditional careers. Possibly to garner more publicity during the International Women's Year, in 1974, the Royal Canadian Mounted Police, Canada's national police force, hired its first female constable. While a seemingly small step, the following year, the District of Halton-Mississauga Ambulance Service in Ontario hired the first female career

284 Telephone interview with Susan Thompson, April 23, 2021.

emergency medical technician in Canada.[285] Also in 1975, it appears that there was also a female applicant to the newly formed Winnipeg Ambulance Service, although she was not hired.

In response to Canada's commitment to the International Women's Year, Winnipeg city council's Executive Policy Committee (EPC) made a decision to address the issue of gender inequality in municipal employment. In 1975, the EPC ordered the city's Board of Commissioners to investigate the status of employment of women and to "recommend a goals and guidelines policy to bring about a greater utilization of women within the employ of the City of Winnipeg."[286] When the Board of Commission's report came out in 1977, it showed that Winnipeg's civil service was comprised of only 17.39 percent women.[287]

While there is no indication of the Blue Cross-run ambulance service hiring women, the city hired Judy Mader shortly after it took control of the service in 1976. Unfortunately, Ms. Mader passed away in 2016, so her experiences were not documented. However, given that Ms. Mader continued with Winnipeg Ambulance for thirty years, it suggests that she found a relatively supportive environment.

Louise Stitt's experiences support this assumption. Ms. Stitt was hired a year after Ms. Mader, in 1977, as a Winnipeg ambulance attendant. While there were foreseeable hiccups in the first few months, for example, not having a uniform for the first six weeks because women's sizes didn't exist, Ms. Stitt indicates that the attitudes of her co-workers were not an issue. If anything, she found herself on a bit of a pedestal, but support was always there.[288]

A bigger problem was the initial concerns from co-workers' wives and girlfriends about their partners spending nights in ambulance stations alone with Ms. Stitt.[289] The perception is somewhat amusing given that Winnipeg Ambulance was so understaffed that there was often little time for staff to have personal interactions. However, as Ms. Stitt discovered, as did early female Winnipeg firefighters who found themselves in a similar situation,[290] these types of unnecessary biases

285 Hanna (1982): 82.
286 *The Status of Women in the Civic Service.* City of Winnipeg, 1977: 4,
287 *The Status of Women in the Civic Service.* City of Winnipeg, 1977: 10.
288 Telephone interview with Louise Stitt, January 19, 2024.
289 Telephone interview with Louise Stitt, January 19, 2024.
290 Bjarnason (2005): 124.

quickly disappeared by maintaining high professional standards and building trust with all involved.

Winnipeg Ambulance management's attitude toward female staff is aptly captured in a 1979 scenario. Winnipeg had just opened its first purpose-built combined fire-EMS station: Number 13, on Lilac Street, which housed both an ambulance and an engine company. Ms. Stitt was assigned to work at that hall, but on the day before her transfer, Winnipeg Ambulance supervisor John Farrington was called by fire department administration and told that "perhaps he should consider not assigning a woman to a fire station." The call came to an abrupt end when Mr. Farrington responded: "On the day I can tell you where to put your firefighters, you can tell me where to put my EMS staff."[291]

Ms. Stitt reported to Station 13 as scheduled, with no notable issues. While there were minor inconveniences—for example the hall had no facilities for women—when there are committed staff, solutions surface. In this case, similar to when Winnipeg's fire department began hiring women, the station captain's private washroom became the women's shower area until proper co-ed facilities could be built.

Respecting women in the EMS field, the next challenge that arose was in 1982, when Ms. Stitt became pregnant. There were no policies in place and no precedents. The first female paramedic *anywhere* was Dianne Rechle, who in 1972, worked at a private ambulance service in Palm Springs, California.[292] However, as Rechle and her husband were the owners of the ambulance company, presumably she faced few employer-related issues.

With two female EMTs in Winnipeg and a handful across Canada, the issue of an emergency medical responder getting pregnant had not arisen. To Ms. Stitt's benefit, her ambulance partner was also the union president. Both the union and Winnipeg Ambulance had a vested interest in developing a proper policy. In addition to no precedents for a maternity leave policy, there was no research on the specific risks to pregnant EMTs. Ultimately, Ms. Stitt's personal physician advised that a twenty-week-old fetus was a fully intact child and, as a result, could potentially be affected by a workplace injury. With nothing else to go

291 Telephone interview with Louise Stitt, January 19, 2024.

292 "Crashing the Party: Women of EMS." feminem, February 20, 2018, https://feminem.org/2018/02/20/crashing-party-women-ems. Accessed January 25, 2024.

on, Ms. Stitt was placed on short-term disability at twenty weeks and then got six weeks of maternity leave (a good amount of time during that time period) after becoming a mother. The issue of maternity leave arose again in 1989 with EMT Sheri Crighton.

There have since been numerous Winnipeg Ambulance staff who have gotten pregnant, and the practice of utilizing light-duty/maternity leave, as needed, has become well-established. While it is still managed on a case-by-case basis, the current Winnipeg Fire Paramedic Service's stores branch now works with pregnant employees to ensure relatively proper-fitting uniforms. When one of Winnipeg's paramedics become pregnant, she is either supported by getting an existing uniform properly (and comfortably) altered to fit over her growing body or reimbursed for the purchase of suitable alternate uniform items.

Despite becoming one of the city's first female EMTs, having a triple shooting as her first medical call, and being the first paramedic to need a maternity leave policy, Ms. Stitt was undeterred. She went on to have an impressive forty-year career in Manitoba's emergency medical system.

After Ms. Mader and Ms. Stitt were hired, over the next decade fourteen other women were employed by Winnipeg Ambulance as emergency medical technicians. A more proactive approach began in 1986-87, as there was a push to hire female career firefighters in Canada. The Canadian emergency response industry was facing a curious problem; While women had been employed as career firefighters by American fire departments since 1974, there wasn't a single female career firefighter in Canada.

Firefighters and paramedics require similar levels of fitness. However, in the firefighting industry, where Canadian winters require the strength to maneuver frozen fifty-foot lengths of hose and potentially rescue an injured partner, whom, while wearing protective gear, can easily weigh 250 to 300 pounds, firefighters require an exorbitant level of strength. This is something that few women *or* men possess.

Several cities began wrestling with this issue, and Winnipeg's approach was to develop a specialized recruitment program under the auspices of the Core Area Initiative. In 1986, from a core group of forty applicants, four highly fit women were selected as having the potential to be firefighters. After a six-month training program that included serious fitness routines, and learning firefighter-related and first responder medical skills, the four applied to the Winnipeg Fire Department.

The city hired Brenda Boyd as Winnipeg's first female firefighter, coincidently a few months after Toronto hired its first female firefighter; the first female career firefighter in Canada.

The decision to actively recruit women as firefighters appears to tie into the city's overall decision to diversify its workforce, as was apparent from the hiring practices of Winnipeg Ambulance. With Boyd joining the fire department in the fall of 1987, Lori Shoemaker and Heather Freeland were recruited for Winnipeg Ambulance; given that Winnipeg Ambulance training officers provided the program's first responder training. The remaining participant was hired for another challenging position within Winnipeg's civil service. The following spring, Winnipeg Ambulance ran another EMT training class which had five women and four men from non-white ethnic groups, reflecting the city's desire to, at least in its frontline services, diversify its workforce.

It was a few years after this point that Susan Thompson's term as mayor began. While impossible to conclusively assess the effectiveness of Thompson's efforts to increase women's roles in Winnipeg's public service versus societal changes generally, it appears that Thompson's efforts on the gender employment issue had a positive impact. By 2004, six years after Thompson left office, roughly 25 percent of the city's paramedics were female.[293] At the time of writing, 41 percent of paramedics in Manitoba are female,[294] and while precise numbers are not available, informal statistics suggest that close to 50 percent of Winnipeg's paramedics are female.

## Susan Thompson and the "Need" for a Merger

While Winnipeg's employment of women was low, more troubling was the fact that at the time of Thompson's election, there was only a six percent increase in the number of female civic employees from 1977, sixteen years *after* city council made a formal decision to start addressing gender inequality in Winnipeg's civil service.

Thompson was committed to fixing this inequity. Shortly after being elected, she went on a fact-finding trip to Phoenix, Arizona—a city with one of the highest numbers of female firefighters in North America and

293 Patti Edgar, et al. "Fire hall fiasco divides unions." *Winnipeg Free Press*. September 22, 2004.

294 Government of Canada, "Job Bank", accessed January 19, 2024: https://www.jobbank.gc.ca/marketreport/outlook-occupation/4402/MB

one of the first female fire chiefs. What Thompson found was a system with a high number of female employees. She sensed that it was the nature of the department—providing both fire and EMS—that permitted the higher gender balance.[295]

Hence, Thompson saw the ambulance service and the fire department as perfect targets for potentially increasing, in a publicly visible way, the ranks of women in Winnipeg's civil service.

During Thompson's first three years as mayor, she had worked closely with Gary Richardson in his role as Winnipeg's deputy fire chief. After reviewing Richardson's thesis, with its strong bias toward merged departments, Thompson got the sense that the merger idea would also create a more cost-efficient service. With her two main objectives covered, hiring more women and saving Winnipeg money, Thompson was hooked. Richardson's 1996 thesis gave her the strategy she needed.

Once she decided that Richardson had the answer, Thompson adopted an aggressive approach to accomplishing the fire-ambulance merger. After getting city council's permission to hire Richardson as a consultant to assess the potential for a merger, she then directed him to oversee the merger. When questioned, her response was:

> "Nobody's come up with a better solution, in my opinion. The first step of change is denial and resistance. I'm sick and tired of stonewalling. We're still stuck in this rut where other cities of the same size and larger are switching …"[296]

At the time, Winnipeg's fire chief, Barrie Lough, the ambulance department's director, Jake Enns, and Derric Boles, president of the Winnipeg ambulance employees' union, all expressed significant concerns about the proposed merger.[297] Despite detractors, Thompson pushed ahead. In hindsight, Thompson's tendency to ignore detractors was reasonable. Thompson often faced multiple detractors for everything she did, so the negative reaction to her merger proposal was pretty consistent with her other experiences. With the history of regular opposition she faced as mayor, it is foreseeable that

295 Telephone interview with Susan Thompson, April 23, 2021.
296 Randy Turner. "Plan cuts City 100 jobs." *Winnipeg Free Press.* February 17, 1997.
297 Randy Turner. "Plan cuts City 100 jobs." *Winnipeg Free Press.* February 17, 1997.

she viewed the negativity as directed at her as opposed to the idea of the merger itself.

By April 1997, Richardson announced he had already been instructed to come to Winnipeg and start the merger process, albeit without a signed contract.[298]

## The Flood!

Things didn't move as quickly as Thompson and Richardson had hoped; Winnipeg's infamous blizzards and floods intervened. On April 5, 1997, copious amounts of snow started falling on Winnipeg. The following day, snow covered the city that was so deep that ambulances and other emergency vehicles could only navigate city streets when preceded by a snowplow.

While the snow itself severely hampered emergency services, perhaps even more serious was the fact that the volume was so great that as it melted, it doubled the amount of the average spring run-off.

As the melt started, Richardson announced his new role in the merger. Within weeks, Winnipeg became engrossed in the "Flood of the Century," threatened with water levels higher than ever recorded before. This put the fire-EMS merger and almost every other ongoing, non-urgent civic issue on hold.

Winnipeg Ambulance was not used to water-based responses, and as a result, new systems and procedures were often developed on the spot. The swollen Red, Assiniboine, and Seine Rivers created numerous real and potential issues for Winnipeg's emergency services to mitigate.

Winnipeg Ambulance modified its services for two and a half weeks from April 21 to May 8, as floodwaters ravished the city and surrounding areas. Coordinated by Wayne Mirrlees for EMS and Ken Sim for the fire department,[299] an ALS paramedic was assigned on a 24/7 basis to the fire department's rescue boat (or hovercraft, as needed). This unit responded to any situation where ALS support was required but inaccessible by land.

For non-life-threatening medical emergencies, the Winnipeg Harbour Master provided boats at whatever land access point was required

298 Aldo Santin. "Emergency Services Merger Set to Begin." *Winnipeg Free Press.* April 26, 1997.

299 City of Winnipeg History – Civic Emergency Program during the 1997 Flood, https://legacy.winnipeg.ca/History/flood/emergency_program/default.stm. Accessed December 31, 2023.

to get paramedics to the casualty. As the Harbour Master had positioned boats at all points along the rivers where the water was too high to navigate under the bridges, boats were plentiful and accessible.

Where boats could not accomplish the needed task, the Canadian Armed Forces (CAF) brought a plethora of helicopters into and around the city to assist. These were dispatched as the need arose. A helicopter would meet the ambulance at the closest point of land access to a patient and fly the ambulance crew to the patient. After stabilization, the CAF crew would fly the paramedics and patient to a temporary helipad set-up at William Avenue and Tecumseh Street. From there, a land-based ambulance would transport the patient a couple of blocks to the Health Sciences Centre's emergency department.[300]

Given the number of apartment buildings along the Red and Assiniboine Rivers, flooded basements and parking garages became a common problem. With most buildings' mechanical services being below ground level, the flooding often resulted in elevator and other system failures, trapping residents. Winnipeg Ambulance staffed two special "flood duty units" during the peak period. These units responded with the fire department to all flood-related evacuations, assisting residents, particularly seniors and people with disabilities, and transporting them to a hospital as needed.

During the flood's peak, the biggest fear for Winnipeg was the collapse of the "Z-dike". As the flood waters were rising, city and provincial engineers quickly realized that the Winnipeg Floodway, the mammoth basin built in 1966 to prevent future floods, did not have the capacity to hold the 1997 flood waters. As a result, the Z-dike, a 24-kilometre zigzag dike heading west of the intersection of Highways 305 and 330: thirty kilometres southwest of Winnipeg, was quickly built to divert water from Winnipeg. It also made the lives of many farmers in the area miserable as their newly seeded fields turned into newly formed lakes.

Once built, the Z-dike accomplished its job. During the flood, only 9,000 Winnipeggers—about 3,000 homes—needed to be evacuated. However, the concern was that if the Z-dike broke, there would be the potential evacuation of 125,000 city residents. If the evacuation was nec-

300 Joe Kowal. "Prepared to Move the sick, the infirm and the elderly to safety." https://legacy.winnipeg.ca/History/Flood/emergency_program/ambulance.stm. Accessed December 31, 2023.

essary, the biggest worry was how to move the 1,200 patients from the hospitals and personal care homes located along the city's riverbanks.

In conjunction with Manitoba Health, Winnipeg Ambulance developed a plan, creatively named "Operation Evac," in which sixty ambulances from outside of Winnipeg were placed on standby to assist city ambulances in moving these patients to safety. For coordinating any evacuation, a Special Operations Command and Communication Centre was established at the then-ambulance headquarters at 2000 Portage Avenue. Given that the command centre was only a couple of blocks from the then-raging Assiniboine River, staff had a good view of the evolving situation.

Fortunately, the Z-dike held and Operation Evac was never implemented. However, the cooperative planning effort with Manitoba Health allowed the development of a large-scale joint operational plan, suitable for use in similar situations. This planning proved useful the following year, as Winnipeg's preparations for hosting the 1999 Pan Am Games shifted into high gear.

Once the flood waters receded, the province announced that it was changing how EMS would be delivered in the province, hinting that a regional or hospital-based ambulance service might be in the works. As a result, the city's Protection Committee, which oversaw Winnipeg's ambulance service, held back on ratifying Richardson's contract.[301]

## Responsibility Changes Hands

In the fall of 1997, the Manitoba *Regional Health Authorities Act* came into force, shifting the legal responsibility for Emergency Medical Services from municipalities to the local Regional Health Authority. Correspondingly, the section of the *Municipal Act* which permitted municipalities to operate ambulance services was repealed. Henceforth, if Winnipeg wanted to provide emergency medical services, it needed to contract that role from the Winnipeg Regional Health Authority (WRHA) and get paid accordingly.

As a result, the City of Winnipeg and the WRHA entered into an agreement, similar to the 1992 agreement between the city and the province, whereby 25 percent of Winnipeg Ambulance's annual budget came from the city, 25 percent came from the WRHA, and 50 percent came from service fees (ambulance fees charged to the patient).

---

301 Aldo Santin. "Merger Contract on Hold." *Winnipeg Free Press.* June 13, 1997.

Under this new funding model, merging Winnipeg's fire and ambulance services, cross-training firefighters as paramedics, and using fire apparatus staffed by paramedics as first response emergency medical vehicles suddenly became financially advantageous. It enabled the city to recategorize some of its fire-related expenses—such as firefighter first responders—as EMS costs and reclaim those expenses from the WRHA. Under the 25-25-50 funding model, Winnipeg received an extra $7.1 million in annual fire-related reimbursements from the WRHA[302]. The payments for fire-related disbursements had increased to $10 million by 2018.[303]

For a municipal politician to not pursue these additional funds would be akin to negligence, irrespective of whether the evidence used to rationalize the merger, the "Richardson Report," was factually correct or not. On point, in a 2015 newspaper article, former Winnipeg fire chief John Lane bragged about how the fire department had accessed these additional funds by way of the fire-ambulance merger.[304]

With the new funding schedule in place, in October 1997, the city formally retained Richardson to provide a report on the different options for merging fire and EMS.[305] This one is a bit odd, given that the fire-EMS merger options had already been explored in detail by both Coulter and Paterson in 1980. However, as has been repeatedly the case in Winnipeg politics, why make a decision when you can do more research?

It's unclear whether Richardson was asked to study the merger proposal or start the merger implementation process. In either case, once hired:

- he set up a committee—the "Integration Research Team"—made up of representatives from the firefighters' and paramedics' unions, the Winnipeg Regional Health Authority, and Dr. Linda Nugent, Winnipeg's EMS medical officer,[306] and

302 Reg Toews. *Manitoba EMS System Review.* Ministry of Health, Government of Manitoba. 2013: 21.

303 Aldo Santin. "Paramedic transfer would save City $3M: chief." *Winnipeg Free Press.* April 12, 2018.

304 John Lane. "Winnipeg's integrated EMS-fire model is working." *Winnipeg Free Press.* March 19, 2015.

305 Nancy Westaway. "Ambulance service in critical condition: paramedics." *Winnipeg Free Press.* January 4, 1998.

306 Kim Guttormson. "Dept, merger sparks fiery debate." *Winnipeg Free Press.* July 7, 1998.

- there was disagreement amongst city councillors as to his actual role in the process.[307]

It's worth noting that besides all of the other previously discussed reasons used to rationalize the merger, the process was also part of Mayor Thompson/City Council's larger goal of combining a number of civic departments and removing redundant management. Ultimately, Council wanted to merge eight municipal departments into four and cut out redundant middle-management positions. By March of 1998, this process had cut thirty six civic management jobs.[308]

Unfortunately, as part of Thompson's/City Council's process of cutting "redundant" management positions, Winnipeg Ambulance director Jake Enns was terminated. As characteristic of the process, he was terminated before the city council formalized a replacement to jointly manage fire and EMS. As a result, the three ambulance supervisors, Jim Brennan, Doug Major, and Joe Kowal, with the assistance of Dr. Linda Nugent, were stuck managing Winnipeg Ambulance until an official replacement, someone with both firefighting and paramedic experience, could be hired.

As part of this process, in March of 1997, fire chief Barrie Lough was asked by Mayor Thompson to figure out a way to trim $24.5 million from the fire department's budget over the next six years. While Lough accomplished Thompson's request, his plan required Winnipeg to cut 173 firefighters.[309] Such did not endear Lough to the firefighters. Similarly, when the fire-EMS merger details were being solidified, Lough, following city council's direction to cut management positions, alienated the paramedics by proposing that district fire chiefs (with no medical training) take over the role of EMS supervisors.

After significant delays, Richardson presented his amalgamation report to council on July 15. 1998. A week later, on July 22, it was accepted by city council and the merger formally approved, creating Winnipeg's Emergency Response Service. The city then put the implementation on hold until a new chief operating officer could be hired for the combined departments. By following Thompson's directions, Lough alienated both firefighters and paramedics.

---

307 Kim Guttormson. "Dept, merger sparks fiery debate." *Winnipeg Free Press.* July 7, 1998.

308 Aldo Santin. "City cuts 18 middle-management jobs." *Winnipeg Free Press.* March 11, 1998.

309 Kevin Rollason. "Firefighters hope to extinguish cuts." *Winnipeg Free Press.* March 11, 1997.

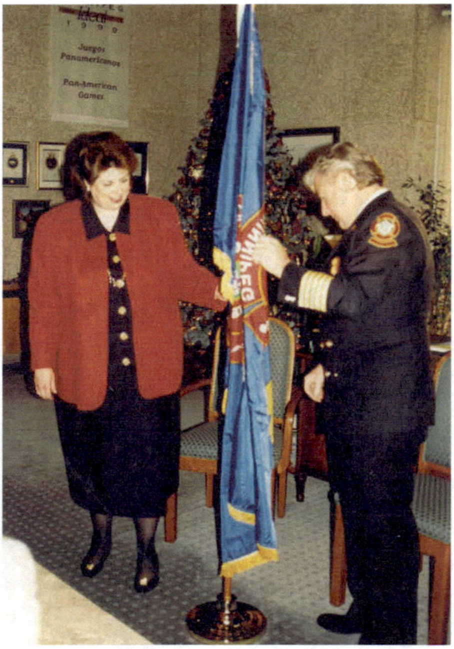


*Mayor Susan Thompson and Chief Barrie Lough, two of the key participants in the Winnipeg Ambulance-WFD merger. (Courtesy of FFHSW)*

Sometimes, life is truly unfair. By following his employer's directions, Lough put himself out of a job.

The challenge was that, as with previous merger attempts, there was no definite plan for how the merger would proceed. Richardson kept putting the fear of God into city council, repeatedly reminding them that if the departments didn't merge, Winnipeg would need to purchase four more ambulances and hire fifty more staff; something required anyway. At the same time, Richardson reminded Council that if the merger happened, the city would somehow save $4 million and provided vague suggestions about potentially making money.[310] It was pretty difficult for Council to not approve the merger.

Council decided that as it was creating a new system, it should be led by someone who did not have roots in either branch of the service. At the same time, they needed to hire a chief who could both understand and work with both firefighters and paramedics. In September 1998, the city's first externally recruited fire chief, Wesley Shoemaker, was hired as the new chief operating officer of both services. While Shoemaker was both a firefighter and a paramedic, he was an odd choice given that he was the deputy fire chief in Edmonton during its disastrous attempt at merging fire and EMS. Nevertheless, it seems that Winnipeg's administration believed that this past experience would help him to understand the current issues.[311]

---

310 Kim Guttormson. "Councillors hear presentation on fire, ambulance merger." *Winnipeg Free Press.* July 16, 1998.

311 Kim Guttormson. "Hamilton chief to merge City's fire, ambulance." *Winnipeg Free Press.* September 22, 1998.

Despite his experience, Shoemaker began questioning whether a merger was even possible almost immediately after his November 23, 1998 start date. In May 1999, the CBC reported:

> "... City hall has been moving slowly toward a merged fire and ambulance service for a couple of years now. But while there is now one chief, some administrative functions have merged and some paramedics work out of fire stations ... there are really still two departments on the ground ... And Wes Shoemaker says that may not change: "it ranges from the status quo to a totally integrated workforce. We may well end up somewhere in between", Shoemaker says.[312]

When the Chief Operating Officer, hired because of his experience in the same type of merger, expressed doubts five months into the job, it seemed curious the council would keep pushing forward. Possibly the potential for saving money in a city that has very little is an effective motivator for hope, regardless of how remote.

Ultimately, it was all about money. Council believed that it could eliminate sixty-one positions within the combined services, save the city an annual $4 million, and still provide a quality service.[313] The added $7.1 million in extra funds, coming from the WRHA for using firefighters likely didn't hurt the desire to push forward. During this period, there appears to have been minimal discussion about why the emergency services were more appropriately combined, except as a cost saving measure.

But then, it got more confusing. After Glen Murray's November 1998 mayoral election, he recommended slowing down the fire-ambulance merger to save money and reduce the city's financial bleeding.[314] If former-Mayor Thompson believed the merger was needed to save money, Mayor Murray believed the merger was unnecessarily costing money, and with no precedent because no other Canadian city had successfully merged their fire and EMS, who was correct?

---

312 "Shoemaker cautious about full-scale fire, ambulance merger." CBC News. May 24, 1999. https://www.cbc.ca/news/canada/shoemaker-cautious-about-full-scale-fire-ambulance-merger-1.177760. Accessed December 22, 2023.

313 Kim Guttormson. "Amalgamation cuts 61 jobs." *Winnipeg Free Press.* July 15, 1998.

314 Keith McArthur. "Road repairs may be put on back burner." *Winnipeg Free Press.* November 28, 1998.

Murray's decision to apply the brakes on the merger process created another issue. When the city first announced the merger, one of the big selling points (for the paramedics) was the potential for paycheques comparable to those of firefighters. By merging the administration, but then not moving on response operations, it meant that the discussions about wage increases for paramedics fell flat.

Respecting the wage increase issue and the merger efforts in general, the paramedics realized that their existing union, the International Association of Machinists and Aerospace Workers, wasn't adequately promoting their interests. As a result, in October 1998, the paramedics voted to form their own association; the Emergency Response Services Employee Association of Winnipeg (ERSEAW).[315] At the start, the paramedics were supporting the merger. While paramedics received significantly less pay than firefighters, there was an underlying belief that if merged, all emergency responders would be paid at the same scale.[316] As salary negotiations had been put on hold pending the merger, the paramedics had not had a contract since February 1996.

Given that city council was intent on saving money with the merger, in hindsight, the idea of increased wages seems like a pipe dream, but at the time, the paramedics were into *positive thinking.*

By May 1999, ERSEAW decided to take matters into their own hands. Working in conjunction with other provincial health care providers, it demanded an increase in wages, irrespective of the merger process.[317]

One of the curious things about Manitoba's labour laws at that time was that unlike police officers, firefighters, doctors, and nurses, the province's *Essential Services Act* did not include paramedics. Hence, they were legally permitted to strike if given such a mandate by their union's membership. The challenge was that the ERSEAW's president, Derric Boles, hesitated to push for a strike mandate. By applying the same logic as was behind the rule that fire and police can't strike, he was concerned about public safety.[318] Boles' underlying rationale for

315 "City paramedics win costly battle to form new union." *Winnipeg Free Press.* November 7, 1998.

316 "Rescue staff seek divorce from union." *Winnipeg Free Press.* September 2, 1998.

317 Glen MacKenzie. "It's payback time, union members say." *Winnipeg Free Press.* May 17, 1999.

318 Keith McArthur. "Paramedics in turmoil days before the strike vote." *Winnipeg Free Press.* May 15, 1999.

not striking was that if paramedics were on strike and a Winnipegger died as a result of a delayed response, the ERSEAW would be vilified. Such was not great for public image purposes. It was a no-win situation. While a strike was necessary to get the wage increase, if anything went sideways, the union, and possibly the paramedics themselves, would potentially face the ire of Winnipeggers and get zero subsequent support.

While meritorious, public safety is not a union president's primary mandate. It's the municipality's (or health region's) job to ensure there's adequate EMS coverage. The union and its president's role are to protect its members' interests. As a result, during the May 17 strike vote, the ERSEAW's membership also demanded a non-confidence motion for Boles' removal.

The ERSEAW had a successful vote on May 17 with the membership voting overwhelmingly in favour of striking, demanding wage parity with firefighters and improved working conditions; namely, more ambulances. The membership also voted overwhelmingly to terminate Boles as president and elected Don Fotti as his replacement.

Immediately after the vote, the city requested that the province declare paramedics as essential service workers; mandating that they were prohibited from striking during a labour dispute and, upon taking a successful strike vote, were required to enter into binding arbitration. The provincial government rejected this request to amend the *Essential Services Act*, as the paramedics hadn't formally set a strike deadline. At the same time, the city began preparing contingency plans in case of a full strike.

One of the more baffling ideas that city staff allegedly came up with, which was quickly nixed by the firefighters' union, was transporting patients on the backs of fire department pumpers.[319] While an interesting story, I can't find any independent confirmation of this allegation. Given that it came out during a very heated fight between the city and paramedics, it defies logic and appears to be nothing more than a rumour.

Rather than immediately going on strike, following Boles' proposition, Fotti and the ERSEAW began negotiating with the city. By late June, the province had appointed a mediator, Paul Teskey, to find a solution. On June 29th, the mediator recommended that Winnipeg's paramedics receive a wage increase of 10 percent over five years.

---

319 Keith McArthur. "City's paramedics crying foul." *Winnipeg Free Press*. June 30, 1999.

Murray immediately responded that the "City probably can't afford that kind of wage increase."[320] It appears that Murray may have been slightly bluffing. After all, it was a negotiation. On July 7, the city and ERSEAW agreed to the mediator's recommendations. While the paramedics got neither wage parody with firefighters nor additional ambulances, they did end up with significantly better wages—with retroactive increases of 3.5 percent for 1998, and increases of 3 percent in 1999, 2 percent in 2000, and 1.5 percent in 2001.[321] A definite coup for the new ERSEAW. The union's timing was superb; with the Pan Am Games coming to Winnipeg in July, it was the perfect time to threaten job action.

The ERSEAW eventually became the Professional Paramedic Association of Winnipeg ("PPAW"). In 2004, the bargaining unit became Local 911 of the Manitoba Government Employees Union and has remained the same as of the time of writing, with Ryan Woiden at the helm.

While great for the city's paramedics, it started another round of fights between the city and the province over the provincial contributions toward Winnipeg's ambulance services. When the WRHA took over funding of ambulance services in 1997, the city and the WRHA agreed that the province would be responsible for twenty-five percent of Winnipeg EMS's $11.2 million budget. Unfortunately, with the increased paramedics' wages, the province was only paying twenty-two percent of the budget. Also, while Winnipeg needed fourteen peak-time ambulances, it only had ten,[322] as noted by ERSEAW during negotiations. The province responded by stating that the city's 1999 ambulance service grant had been increased by $300,000. Again, the ongoing problem was that neither the city nor the province could commit sufficient funds to support a proper ambulance service. Manitoba was making the lowest expenditures in terms of percentages of provincial health dollars for ambulance services in Canada and the second lowest (next to Prince Edward Island) for per capita provincial spending on ambulance services.[323]

---

320 Keith McArthur. "Paramedics turn up the heat on the City." *Winnipeg Free Press.* May 19, 1999.

321 Keith McArthur. "Paramedics' dispute with City may be over soon." *Winnipeg Free Press.* July 3, 1999.

322 David O'Brien. "Ambulances in trouble: mayor." *Winnipeg Free Press.* September 14, 1999.

323 Paramedic Association of Manitoba. *Manitoba's Quiet Crisis.* May 2007: 8.

Mayor Murray responded by advising the WRHA that as of mid-August, Winnipeg Ambulance would cease providing non-emergency ambulance transfer service.[324] Given that the WRHA was already paying private transfer services higher fees than it was paying Winnipeg Ambulance, this appears to have been another negotiation strategy.

Despite the preoccupation with the merger and paramedics getting wage parody with firefighters, as the twentieth century came to an end, some new changes improved emergency care and Winnipeggers' cardiac arrest survival rates.

## Pan Am Games and Timing of Changes

In February 1999, Winnipeg Ambulance began preparing for the upcoming Pan Am Games. In doing so, it adopted some old and new technology. First off, it started acquiring bicycles to be used by ALS paramedics in crowded areas.[325] Carrying about seventy pounds of equipment, including oxygen, an AED, an airway kit, a basic medication kit, and first aid supplies, the bikes enable paramedics to respond to medical emergencies in crowded areas where ambulances often have a difficult time maneuvering. Bike paramedics were a relatively new concept; Toronto's ambulance service created their bike squad in 1996, and the London (England) Ambulance Service didn't start experimenting with bikes until 2000.

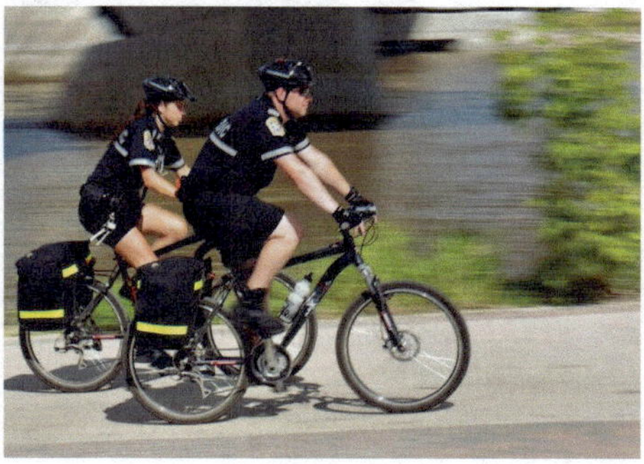

*Members of Winnipeg Ambulance's bike squad, patrolling downtown. (Courtesy of Gus Black)*

Winnipeg's ambulance bike squad would become a formal WFPS program in 2002.

The second thing that Winnipeg Ambulance acquired for the Pan Am Games was two Major Incident Response Vehicles ("MIRVs").[326] The

324 Keith McArthur, et al. "Ambulance service cut blamed on underfunding." *Winnipeg Free Press.* May 14, 1999.

325 Catherine Mitchell. "Buses, bikes being outfitted for paramedics' use." *Winnipeg Free Press.* February 6, 1999.

326 Catherine Mitchell. "Buses, bikes being outfitted for paramedics' use." *Winnipeg*

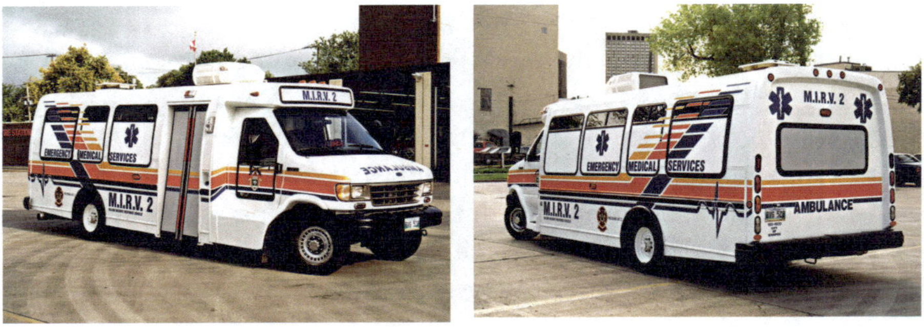


*Winnipeg's 1997 Major Incident Response Vehicle #2, initially built for the Pam Am Games. (Courtesy of Stan Stone)*

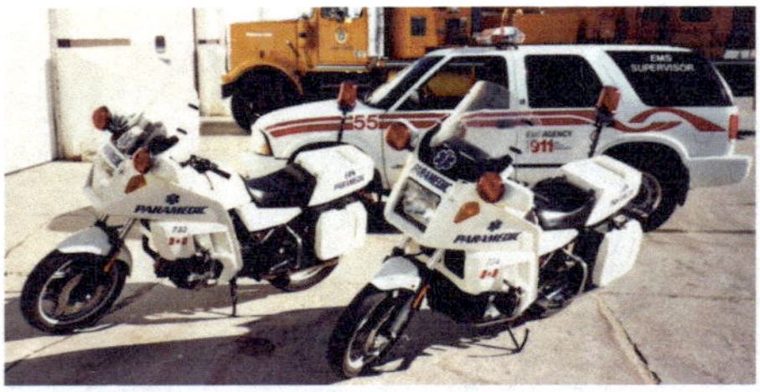


*Ex-WPD BMW 750 motorcycles converted to paramedic units for the Pam Am Games. (Courtesy of Stan Stone)*

vehicles were created by taking two of Winnipeg Transit's front wheel drive Overland ELF (Economical Low Floor) buses, gutting the interiors and re-equipping them as large ambulances, each capable of carrying three stretchers. The idea was to either use them as base stations to provide onsite treatment at major incidents or, when needed, to transport multiple patients to a hospital. In 2008, these units were upgraded to a large, transit-bus-style ambulance, capable of carrying eight stretchers. Unlike using bikes for paramedics, which was a new concept, major American cities, such as New York City and Portland, have been using converted transit-type buses as disaster/multi-casualty units since the late 1930s.

A third innovation created for the Pan Am Games was paramedic motorcycles. Acquiring a couple of surplus BMW 750 police motorcycles from the Winnipeg Police Department (WPD), Winnipeg Ambulance outfitted them with the same medical gear as the paramedic bicycles. While the motorbikes permitted paramedics to move quickly through traffic, they were not a versatile as bicycles and required additional drivers' licenses to operate. As a result, their use was discontinued shortly after the games.

---

*Free Press.* February 6, 1999.

## More Accessible AEDs

In March 1999, utilizing grants from the Medtronic Foundation Heart-Rescue Program and the provincial government, and taking funds from the Emergency Response Services' budget, the city raised $450,000 to purchase new defibrillators. In all, Winnipeg acquired twenty-seven semi-automatic external defibrillators for all of the fire department's first responder units, as well as fifteen more sophisticated ambulance-based defibrillators.[327] Winnipeg's ambulances had been equipped with defibrillators since 1984. However, by placing AEDs on first responder apparatus, Winnipeggers experiencing cardiac arrests could now be defibrillated within four minutes as opposed to the nine minutes it took for an ambulance to arrive. Given that a person's survival rate drops by roughly 10 percent for each minute that they don't receive proper cardiac care, this was a huge step forward.

The introduction of defibrillators got a further boost in October 1999, when Winnipeg's casinos acquired AEDs. In a move hinting at Manitoba's future public AED program, Manitoba Lotteries realized that a lot of their senior customers were having cardiac-related issues at casinos. With ambulances being called to casinos on a regular basis, Manitoba Lotteries decided to invest in defibrillators, permitting trained security staff to start emergency cardiac care almost immediately.[328] The installation of AEDs in high-use public areas represented a huge but necessary step in the process of increasing heart attack survival rates in Winnipeg.

The twenty-first century was going to bring some exciting changes.

---

327 Mike McIntyre. "City firefighters armed for war on heart attacks." *Winnipeg Free Press.* March 9, 1999.

328 Kim Guttormson. "Casinos getting cardio-smart." *Winnipeg Free Press.* October 31, 1999.

## 2000–PRESENT

# Providing the Best Care Despite the Obstacles

In many ways, the evolution of Winnipeg's emergency medical system in the new century is two separate stories. Fortunately, both have good endings.

In one sense, it's a complex story of firefighters and paramedics merging operations; something that historically hadn't been done before successfully. In another, it's a fabulous story of how, despite limited funding and a less-than-ideal working environment, Winnipeg's EMS staff, collectively and individually, strove to provide the best prehospital emergency care possible. It's about a profession that is continually becoming more specialized, and following national and international trends, developing new ways to bring quality emergency health care to Winnipeggers, whenever, wherever, and however it's needed.

When I started researching this book twenty-five years ago, the Winnipeg Fire Paramedic Service (WFPS) merger was in its infancy. There was a lot of hostility and a lot of hope; human beings in a new working environment were being typical, infallible, contrary creatures. My initial research question was, "Is the merger a good thing?"

The answer remained elusive until the mid-2010s; with family business to tackle, and as an excuse to show my young son the beauty of Western Canada, we drove from Vancouver to Winnipeg. It was a breath-taking trip, but upon arriving in "the 'Peg," my body stopped working. That's right, I couldn't move an inch without pain shooting everywhere. After being helped to a friend's bed, all I could do was writhe in pain and try to convince my ten-year-old son that *things weren't as bad as they looked.* At that point, a call to 911 brought in the cavalry: an assortment of ALS, BLS, firefighter-paramedics, and firefighters. As I watched, I noticed that:

- Each team member was genuinely concerned about figuring out how to help me be as comfortable as possible and get me the medical help I needed. They were working together, each sharing his or her respective skillset and knowledge, and
- I didn't care whether they were driving fire trucks or ambulances, were members of the UFFW or the MGEU, or had come from a firehall or a dedicated EMS station. All I wanted was someone to help me get whatever medical help I needed and to convince my panicking young son that "things were under control."

Fortunately, the WFPS team that arrived did these two tasks in spades. As I watched, I saw a team of professionals, each with a different skill set, working together to determine how best to get me help. While no one could figure out what was wrong with me (no reflection on their combined skill levels—it took the ER doctors another two days of tests to find a diagnosis), I was intrigued at how they worked together to keep us safe; they kept my son calm, and got me the medical help needed.

As I've mulled this experience since then, I've realized that the answer to my initial question: "Is the merger a good thing?," doesn't matter.

In a world with dozens of different models to deliver EMS, the real question is, does it work? Does the city's population get the emergency medical help it needs when it needs it? In Winnipeg's case, the answer is a resounding "yes." Is it perfect? No, it's expensive. But are people kept alive? Yes! Perhaps equally important to staying alive, does the current model reduce the number of trips to the hospital ER while continuing to provide the needed care? Yes!

## Why Does Winnipeg's Current Model Work?

The EMS model that has evolved in Winnipeg works. Let's look at the last quarter century of its evolution.

The Belton Report outlined how mixing firefighters and paramedics is a bad combination; unstable unless properly handled.

To make this portion of Winnipeg's EMS history digestible, and help you to understand and appreciate today's system, I've divided it into the following sections which will cover the merger (or not)!, getting enough ambulances, and getting improved emergency care to Winnipeggers.

## The Merger, or Not!

It took me a long time to appreciate that merging a group of career firefighters with a group of non-fire paramedics is a good thing. At first blush, it doesn't seem logical. The firefighting profession has evolved into an agency that mitigates emergencies; whether it be a fire, a chemical spill, a car accident, or a Ski-Doo going into a not-so-frozen Red River. Whatever the problem may be, if a person or property is trapped or in danger, more often than not, firefighters will have an immediate solution.

On the other hand, paramedics are evolving into an extension of the hospital emergency room physician, but with a twist. As the profession evolves, paramedics often substitute for hospital staff. While part of a paramedic's job is emergency response, an increasingly larger role is that of a stand-alone, community-based healthcare provider.

With the firefighters' involvement, a reasonably logical connection exists; if you view paramedics as emergency responders. In Winnipeg, since the early 1900s, firefighters have been providing first aid services as part of their job. Hence, it's not a total stretch to go from using a resuscitator, to administering CPR, to using an AED, to providing the drugs needed to correct an irregular heart rhythm. Expanding their skill sets is easily foreseeable—if you narrow the scope of a paramedic to that of an emergency responder. However, the catch is that only about 10 percent of EMS calls are true medical emergencies, so the role of a firefighter as an emergency medical responder only captures a small portion of a modern paramedic's job.

For paramedics, it is a different issue. In a nutshell, paramedics' training extends the services of doctors (and nurses—whose roles are also expanding), to environments where doctors don't typically go. Hence, a paramedic's job is to use clinical analysis and drugs to rectify emergent medical problems outside of established medical facilities. The paramedic's expanded role includes determining that a health issue isn't an emergency but still requires appropriate care, and providing that care. For example, if a community paramedic escorts a patient to their doctor's appointment, as will be shown, it may result in a dozen or so fewer 911 calls. While attending the doctor's appointment is not an emergency, the paramedic's work has a noticeable, positive impact on the healthcare system. With the initial merger proposal, which included full integration, paramedics were being asked to drag hoses and ventilate burning buildings; tasks entirely unrelated to their original job description.

Further, the training needed for a merged role often doesn't provide the necessary skills to treat the patient without a trip to the hospital. Why would paramedics want to do a new set of unrelated duties: especially when the new skill sets do not help them to provide better medical care? Ironically, it's similar to seventy-five years ago, when Winnipeg Police provided an ambulance service. At the time, there was little interest in modifying police duties to provide adequate emergency medical transport.

This disconnect between firefighters and EMS-paramedics became apparent early in the new century. Nobody seemed happy with the original name of the merged departments: Winnipeg Emergency Response Service (ERS). It was too non-descript. Given that the police department's Emergency Response Team had no connection to the ERS and the city's emergency waterworks response team wasn't part of the ERS, the name was confusing. However, on September 20, 2000, when the combined service became the Winnipeg Fire Paramedic Service (WFPS), the United Firefighters of Winnipeg were equally nonplussed.[329] It appeared that nothing short of reverting to the name "Winnipeg Fire Department," as used for the past 120 years, would satisfy the firefighters.

Unfortunately, the name "Winnipeg Fire Department" didn't acknowledge the addition of paramedics; something that wasn't of particular concern to the firefighters' union. The WFD had not-so-subtly been suggesting that firefighters take over from the paramedics for the previous twenty-five years. It took a few more years for a solution to arise that would placate the firefighters.[330]

Unsure how to proceed with the merger—one of the problems with City Council's decision to "work out the details later"—in November 2003, Deputy Chief Ken Sim started testing different models for deploying cross-trained staff. Since the start of the merger, Winnipeg had hired 150 cross-trained firefighters and 30 cross-trained paramedics.[331] The process of utilizing cross-trained staff was complicated by not having wage parity between firefighters and EMS-paramedics. In a nutshell,

329 Helen Felding. "Union fights renaming fire dept." *Winnipeg Free Press.* September 8, 2000.

330 "What's in a name?" *Winnipeg Free Press.* September 21, 2000.

331 Patti Edgar. "Fired up over merger." *Winnipeg Free Press.* March 6, 2004.

employees with the same training, working for the same municipal department, got paid a different wage depending on whether they were sitting in an ambulance or a fire engine.

The policy also severely impacted basic operations. For example, in March 2004, city council put aside $459,000 to hire twelve new paramedics to staff two additional peak-period ambulances. However, WFPS delayed the introduction of the additional ambulances because there wasn't enough cross-trained staff.[332] In trying to follow the new policy, it appeared that the WFPS was refusing to use already available singly trained paramedics.[333]

The WFPS started hiring cross-trained firefighter-paramedics. New hires typically had their Public Fire Paramedic Program Diploma from the Manitoba Emergency Services College in Brandon or similar training from another college. After trial and error, new hires without previous EMS experience were assigned to Winnipeg EMS. The idea was that given both branches of the WFPS were primarily doing medical calls, spending time responding to medical calls in one of Winnipeg's busy ambulances was a great way to get quick clinical experience.

The problem was that without wage parity, firefighters were being paid significantly more than EMS-paramedics. At the same time, with forty-odd fire vehicles, as opposed to as few as twelve ambulances responding to medical emergencies, EMS-paramedics had to work significantly harder for less pay. As a result, unless a new employee was committed to pursuing advanced paramedicine, it made little sense for new employees to stay with Winnipeg EMS. As soon as new recruits were hired, cross-trained firefighter-paramedics immediately transferred to the Winnipeg Fire Department—creating a seemingly revolving door for staff at Winnipeg EMS.[334] The problem was so severe that three years after implementing the hiring policy of only cross-trained personnel:

- 39 percent of Winnipeg ambulance paramedics had less than three years experience;

332 "Staff shortage delays plan for additional ambulances." *Winnipeg Free Press.* May 8, 2004.
333 "Paramedics dispute staff shortage." *Winnipeg Free Press.* May 11, 2004.
334 Interview with Stan Stone, March 4, 2024.

- 51 percent of Winnipeg ambulance paramedics had less than five years experience;
- 50 percent of paramedics hired by WFPS in the past three years transferred to the Winnipeg Fire Department from Winnipeg EMS, and
- when Winnipeg EMS hired fifteen paramedics in 2006, four resigned, eleven transferred to the Winnipeg Fire Department, three retired, eight were promoted to management, leaving Winnipeg EMS with eleven fewer paramedics.[335]

With firefighter-paramedics not being permitted to operate ambulances, and if newly acquired ambulances could only be operated by cross-trained staff in the EMS branch, it was no wonder that Winnipeg couldn't get additional ambulances on the street.

In February 2004, the United Firefighters of Winnipeg filed a grievance that the proposed merger process breached their collective agreement.[336] A key issue was that firefighters didn't want to have to operate ambulances.[337] This was finally settled in March 2005, when a labour arbitrator determined that it was a breach of the firefighters' collective agreement to have firefighters responding in ambulances.[338] The upshot it, it's pretty hard to have a merged emergency response service when the employees can't use one another's vehicles.

As firefighters and paramedics squabbled, the silliness was captured in a September 2004 interview with the creator of Mayor Thompson's merger report, Gary Richardson. Richardson chastised the current management for trying to get the agreement of the unions with respect to the merger.[339] Yet, in his report, he emphasized the need to get the unions onboard. This helps to explain why many

---

335 Paramedic Association of Manitoba. *Winnipeg's Emergency Medical Services in Critical Condition*. Media Release. October 19, 2006.

336 Patti Edgar. "Firefighters try to extinguish merger." *Winnipeg Free Press*. February 21, 2004.

337 Patti Edgar. "City hears first of firefighters grievances." *Winnipeg Free Press*. October 1, 2004.

338 Patti Edgar. "Firefighters claim a win in amalgamation fight." *Winnipeg Free Press*. March 8, 2005.

339 Paul Egan. "'Pussyfooting' blamed for poisonous relations." *Winnipeg Free Press*. September 25, 2004.

of Richardson's recommendations didn't work. It is so easy to make recommendations, until you're stuck trying to implement them.

With a touch of irony, the day after reporting on Mr. Richardson's bleatings about failure to control the unions, *Winnipeg Free Press* reporter, Paul Egan, wrote an article about San Francisco's merged fire and EMS departments self-destructing.[340] It seemed that everyone was getting tired of the non-merger.

While simmering for a few years, the merger finally blew-up in 2004. It's hard to tell who or what was main instigator. However, with firefighter-paramedics getting paid more than EMS-paramedics, and EMS-paramedics getting little downtime: 70 percent of calls were medical and EMS-paramedics were being worked off their feet,[341] it's easy to speculate the issues. Combined with power differences—the firefighters' union in both numbers and political savvy was running circles around the paramedics' union—it was easy to identify the roots of growing frustration.

The simmering discontent finally erupted during the summer and fall of 2004 when allegations of misconduct from both paramedics and firefighters were being levelled against each other. In July 2004, there was an incident where four young women, after leaving the bar next door, made late-night visit to the Osborne Street firehall. The women were subsequently chauffeured to their homes in a fire truck. Then, other incidents began surfacing publicly, such as: pornography in firehalls, paramedics' personal vehicles being damaged, and paramedics being threatened after waking firefighters when returning from late-night calls. In response, firefighters' union president Alex Forrest blamed "the vitriolic nature of the charges aired on TV on disgruntled workers who are jealous of firefighters' higher wages."[342] There were obvious problems, but it seemed that the root—financial inequality—was being ignored.

A further issue riling the firefighters' union at the time was control. Historically, the United Firefighters of Winnipeg (UFFW) had the power to affect the fire department's budget. Then, just before the merger of Winnipeg's fire and EMS, in 1997, the province took over control of EMS

340 Paul Egan. "Fire, paramedics a poor marriage?' *Winnipeg Free Press.* September 26, 2004.

341 Patti Edgar & Kevin Rollason. "Fire hall fiasco divided unions." *Winnipeg Free Press.* September 22, 2004.

342 Kevin Rollason and Alexandra Paul. "Fire hall anger bubbles over." *Winnipeg Free Press.* September 23, 2004.

in Manitoba. This reduced Winnipeg's control over the ambulance service's budget. The province reduced municipal control even more when, in 2001, Manitoba's Vehicle and Equipment Management Agency took over the acquisition and maintenance of all ambulances in the province. It created a provincial fleet program, providing ambulances to all EMS purveyors in the province.

As a result, the UFFW lost any power it had to influence Winnipeg's EMS budget. While it was still adept at pressuring Winnipeg's City Council over the fire department's budget, with the majority of emergency calls to the WFPS being related to EMS and ambulances, this loss of power would have been truly frustrating. Put bluntly, with most ambulance funding coming from the province, hence out of the city's control, if amalgamated, and the city wanted to cut the department's budget, the only part they could cut was fire suppression. Combined with the inequality in wages, it was easy to understand the growing tensions.

In an effort to encourage equality—and likely to ensure that there were enough cross-trained paramedics—in January 2006 the city began offering Level 1 firefighting training to current paramedics. This effort further angered firefighters,[343] given that the firefighters' union's objective was to protect *firefighters'* jobs. The risk was that in cross-training current paramedics, it reduced the number of employment opportunities for firefighters. Firefighters were now competing directly against EMS-paramedics for jobs within the WFPS!

In a move that was clearly a tit-for-tat, but ultimately created an environment that ensured a full merger would never occur, the firefighters' union organized a "fact-finding mission" in March 2006. Mayor Sam Katz, Chief Shoemaker, and UFFW President Alex Forrest, without any paramedic representation, examined municipal fire and EMS departments in Los Angeles City and San Diego, California, as well as Tucson, Arizona. Besides not inviting paramedics to be in the delegation, interestingly, none of the cities selected had departments which had merged firefighters with non-fire EMS-paramedics. Firefighters were providing EMS in each city visited.

With the Los Angeles City Fire Department, firefighters had provided the ambulance service since 1927[344]. In San Diego, there was a combination of

343 Jason Bell. "Training draws fiery response." *Winnipeg Free Press.* December 29, 2005.

344 Bill Wells. "There When You Need Them: A Detailed History of the City's Emergency Medical Services." *Alive.* July 2004:22.

municipal and private ambulances, with the paramedic-trained firefighters riding on fire trucks. In Tucson, the fire department trained its firefighters as paramedics, bought ambulances, and then started competing directly against private ambulance services.[345] When questioned by the media about the merits of excluding paramedics, Mayor Katz stated that the trip was to try and build bonds with firefighters.[346]

The result was that the paramedics immediately ceased supporting the merger and stopped cross-training as firefighters.[347] In a curious twist, Alex Forrest had managed to get the paramedics' union into the same mindset as the UFFW; fighting the merger.

In an effort to rectify some of the damage, in 2006 the city applied to Manitoba Labour Board to have unions merged. While it's dubious whether such an application would have been successful, given the animosity between the two bodies, the application was suspended in May 2007.[348]

While the application for a merger of the unions was probably a non-starter, Wesley Shoemaker's announcement in late 2006 that he was leaving Winnipeg and his role as WFPS's chief the following year created a means for temporary amicability between the unions.

As a result of Shoemaker's pending departure, James Brennan was appointed acting WFPS Chief and COO in December 2006. Unlike Shoemaker, who was selected because of his alleged experience with merging departments, Brennan had spent his entire career in EMS. However, as one of Winnipeg Ambulance's training officers, he had spent a lot of time working with both paramedics and firefighters. Having been involved with providing first responder training to firefighters in the mid-1980s, many of the same firefighters were now in officer positions, Brennan had the connections to both fire and EMS. He also had the experience of helping to manage Winnipeg Ambulance before Shoemaker's arrival. As Mayor Katz was convinced that the merger was still the best deal for Winnipeg, Brennan's charismatic, jovial personality, when combined with his past

345 Al Ring and Bob Ring. *Tucson Fire Department Emergency Medical Services.* Greater Tucson Fire Foundation. 2016.

346 Mary Agnes Welch. "Paramedics not invited on mayor's fire hall tour." *Winnipeg Free Press.* March 15, 2006.

347 "Paramedics left behind on amalgamation tour." CBC News, March 16, 2006. https://www.cbc.ca/news/canada/manitoba/paramedics-left-behind-on-amalgamation-tour-1.622975. Accessed March 5, 2024.

348 Bartley Kives. "Firefighters' deal with paramedics praised by mayor." *Winnipeg Free Press.* April 27, 2007.

experience, made him the right person to bring all of the players together.

Wasting little time after his appointment, on April 27, 2007, Brennan hammered out a tentative agreement with the fire and ambulance unions regarding the department merger.[349] It was ratified by both of the unions and city council on May 16, 2007, creating a dual system under one department. Ironically, the terms of the agreement also contradicted the advice provided by virtually every consultant hired by the city over the preceding thirty years.

At the same time that the merger negotiations were being finalized, the arbitration hearing over EMS-paramedics' wage increases wrapped up. It resulted in a new wage contract for paramedics—something they had been asking for since February 2004. While it didn't give the long sought after four-year 24 percent increase for wage parity with firefighters, it provided a 9.5 percent wage increase with an 8.7 percent premium increase for Advanced Care Paramedics.[350] While not perfect, increased wages helped to make the wage disparity a bit more palatable.

It kind of makes you wonder why the city hired the half dozen consultants over the previous three decades when it ignored the one piece of advice that all had agreed on. In a nutshell, under the new deal:

- firefighter-paramedics could respond on fire trucks, but not in ambulances;
- EMS-paramedics could respond in ambulances, but not on fire trucks;
- firefighters would work for the "Winnipeg Fire Department" which is a branch of the Winnipeg Fire Paramedic Service;
- EMS-paramedics (but not Firefighter-paramedics) would work for "Winnipeg Emergency Medical Services" which is a branch of the Winnipeg Fire Paramedic Service;
- there would be more ambulances staffed by advanced care paramedics: sixteen within four years (up from four to six units);
- there would be thirty-six pieces of fire apparatus staffed by firefighter-paramedics (up from eleven) within the next four years;

349 Bartley Kives. "Firefighters' deal with paramedics praised by mayor", *Winnipeg Free Press.* April 27, 2007.

350 Shaun McLeod. "Paramedics to get raises", *Winnipeg Free Press.* April 3, 2007.

- firefighter-paramedic staffed apparatus would respond to non-life-threatening emergencies (as well as provide first responder service for life threatening calls) and ALS ambulances to more serious calls; and
- there would be joint administration, such as the COO/Chief and the medical director, but otherwise the two departments would operate as separate entities.[351]

The new structure made both the firefighters' and paramedics' unions temporarily happy, resulting in general harmony in the stations. However, as predicted by every consultant hired by the city, within a year of Brennan's merger deal, and continuing until 2021, there was ongoing strife between firefighters and paramedics.

As a result of the friction and the infighting, there were cases of relative silliness which could have been avoided. For example, even when it would make more sense for a firefighter to drive an ambulance to the hospital so that more highly trained/experienced medical personnel can work on the patient, they can't. They can assist with patient care, but pursuant to the agreement, an EMS-paramedic must drive the ambulance.

Similarly, in 2008, when the city acquired its new Major Incident Response Vehicle, being on a full-sized bus chassis, it required the operator to have a Class 1 driver's license with an air brake endorsement. As there were not sufficient paramedics with a Class 1 license (one needed a Class 4 license to drive an ambulance), whenever the MIRV was needed, it was taken out on a "training exercise" and driven by a firefighter. As a lawyer, I've often been curious about what liability issues would have arisen if the MIRV had been involved in an accident, while transporting real casualties from a real emergency but driven by a properly licensed, but unauthorized driver. Fortunately, it never happened, so I can happily continue to sit and speculate.

Hence, it begs the question: What is the benefit of a partially merged fire and EMS?

I found the answer in Surrey, British Columbia, a few months before this book was published. As a quick recap, under Winnipeg's current system, ALS paramedics in ambulances handle serious calls,

---

351 Bartley Kives. "Firefighters, paramedics deal to become official." *Winnipeg Free Press.* May 16, 2007.

and firefighter-paramedics on first responder units handle minor calls. In contrast, in Surrey, ambulances are staffed by Basic Life Support paramedics (same as a primary care paramedic). ALS paramedics arrive separately in either ambulances or SUVs—they use both. Municipal firefighters provide first responder service, but only as requested by BC Ambulance. On a Saturday night in September 2024, my friend, Susan (name has been changed) had a panic attack at a local supermarket. As she was having difficulty breathing, staff at the store called 911. They then called me, and I went to join Susan. It was deemed a low priority call, and all of the seventeen ambulances assigned to Surrey were on higher priority calls. After sitting outside for two hours I finally drove Susan to the closest hospital's emergency department. As I suspected, as soon as the cardiac technician ran an EKG and explained to Susan that "everything looks OK," she immediately calmed down, her panic attack ceased, and she was fine. However, in the process, we used up five hours of the ER's time and met with about a dozen staff.

If the same thing had happened in Winnipeg, a firefighter-paramedic would have been on the scene in five to eight minutes, Susan's vitals would have been assessed, and being told she seemed "OK," she may have been able to calm down seven hours earlier without giving further work to the over-burdened hospital emergency staff. While I prefer my friends to not get sick, if they do, having a system that reduces the use of emergency services while ensuring quick treatment has both significant economic and practical benefits.

This comparison is not intended, in any way, to criticize frontline emergency workers. My experience has been, at least in Canada, people who genuinely want to help others are drawn to the firefighting and paramedicine professions. Speaking to friends who are Vancouver firefighters, I'm told they would love to have PCP training. With their basic first responder, or sometimes emergency medical responder training, they often lament that they don't have more skills to use when assisting with a medical emergency.

It provides justification for maintaining fire department staffing levels, a benefit for quick responses to the diminishing number of fire calls. However, when the fire department budget is roughly ten times that of the EMS budget, and yet EMS calls account for 80-90 percent of all calls, it raises questions. In models where firefighters and paramedics can be cross-trained, it provides a means to both reduce staff and increase the number of ambulances on the road during peak periods. However, this will likely never happen in Winnipeg because of the collective agreement restrictions.

By 2009, the "love affair" between Winnipeg firefighters and EMS-paramedics was clearly over. The UFFW was back to emphasizing that firefighters responded to 56,400 of the city's 71,039 medical calls in 2008, and "by firefighters going to these calls, firefighters are cancelling [ambulances] they're going to calls by themselves." The paramedics' union responded by pointing out the obvious, but overlooked point: Ambulances are still needed to transport in most cases—fire trucks are not so equipped. While many firefighters are entry level paramedics, EMS-paramedics bring a much higher level of skill, experience, and equipment.[352]

The UFFW was back to hinting that EMS-paramedics were a redundant luxury. In reality, only about 10,000 of the 71,000 medical calls in 2008 could be handled by firefighters without EMS-paramedics and ambulances, while 15,000 were handled by EMS-paramedics without firefighters. The remainder of the calls, about 46,000, involved firefighters providing a "first responder" role—providing stop gap services until EMS could arrive—with EMS-paramedics providing more advanced care and transport.[353]

However, a significantly larger number of calls could be handled by EMS-paramedics alone, if the city had adequate numbers of ambulances and EMS-paramedics. Put another way, of the 70,000-odd medical calls received in 2008, roughly 60,000 people were transported to hospital.[354] By 2016, due to a slight increase in the number of ambulances, there was a small increase in the number of calls handled by firefighter-paramedics on their own (13,063 as opposed to 10,000 in 2008), slightly fewer first responder calls (38,396 as opposed to 46,000 in 2008), but a sizeable increase in the number of calls handled solely by EMS-paramedics (20,414).[355]

This discourse captured the problem of the "combined, but not really combined" fire-paramedic service. At the time, both divisions were so busy trying to justify their own existence that they overlooked the obvious—that both play a vital role in assisting the sick and injured, but in most cases at

352 Gabrielle Giroday. "Firefighters' union cites hectic year." *Winnipeg Free Press.* January 21, 2009.

353 Gabrielle Giroday. "Firefighters' union cites hectic year." *Winnipeg Free Press.* January 21, 2009.

354 "A new Focus." *Winnipeg Free Press.* October 17, 2008.

355 Larry Kusch. "Tension Smoulders as Flames Fade." *Winnipeg Free Press.* December 23, 2017.

that time, transport by ambulance was still a primary role of EMS and the key reason why most people call for help.

Looking at the examples of firefighter-paramedic animosity over the next fifteen-odd years, the divide increased significantly after the initial euphoria from reaching an agreement on the quasi-merger. This suggests that a working merger requires more than just a written agreement. Unfortunately, an old maxim that we often use in the legal profession became apropos: *The more mud one throws at others the more one gets on him/herself.* I provide the following as a snapshot of the type of antics that evolved as firefighters and EMS-paramedics tried to make each other look stupid:

- As previously mentioned, in July 2004, a number of young women visiting the pub next door to the Osborne Street Station were given rides home by firefighters in a fire department vehicle. When researching *We Hold Thee Safe*, published by the Firefighters' Historical Society in 2005, I found numerous examples of this type of conduct. While there's little doubt that this conduct was inappropriate, and discipline has been meted out as appropriate, what was different in this case was that the incident received front page news coverage, discrediting the whole WFPS.
- In September 2004, the UFFW's newsletter contained such comments as: "firefighter close to being demoted to an ambulance job," etc.[356]
- In December 2006, one EMS-paramedic played a prank on another EMS-paramedic, a regular, acceptable occurrence in fire halls, by leaving white powder laying around. For whatever reason, the WFPS's Hazardous Materials Response Team was called. As it turns out, the witnesses were all firefighters, with the firefighters recommending that "criminal ramifications" be taken against the paramedics.[357] Ultimately, there was no discipline.
- In September 2009, there were accusations that a firefighter at the Osborne Street Station took a drunk woman into the shed behind the station and had sex. Other firefighters had allegedly

356 Patti Edgar. "Firefighters' newsletter jokes 'unprofessional'." *Winnipeg Free Press.* September 23, 2004.

357 Joe Paraskevas. "Paramedic's practical joke sparks probe." *Winnipeg Free Press.* December 14, 2006.

tried to cover it up.[358] Is this type of on-job conduct appropriate? Of course not! However, ensuring that it got significant media coverage only served to discredit the entire WFPS—hurting both firefighters and EMS-paramedics.

- Women visiting the Osborne Street Station were photographed, partially nude, on fire apparatus.[359] Again, clearly not appropriate, but when EMS-paramedics drag these kinds of details into the public eye, it discredits the entire WFPS.
- Perhaps the most extreme example was an October 2020 medical call where, as a result, EMS-paramedics began publicly accusing firefighters of being racist. The incident resulted in a publicized City of Winnipeg investigation. It also resulted in a firefighter suing an EMS-paramedic for defamation, and the EMS-paramedic counter-suing the firefighter for defamation. Ultimately, the Court dismissed both lawsuits, but the incident[360] discredited the WFPS as a whole.
- Unfortunately, the hostilities also spilled over into the professional realm. In 2015, the paramedics' union began lobbying for paramedic self-regulation: the licensing of individual paramedics and an independent discipline board similar to those already existing in other provinces. The UFFW, seeing this as a further loss of control over firefighter-paramedics, shifted into high gear to lobby against the paramedics' college. At the NDP's 2015 convention, the UFFW brought twenty delegates to aid in political maneuvering. As a result of negotiations at the convention, the firefighters shifted their votes to the premier/new health minister. This appears to have been a significant factor in the delay of a public review of the EMS-paramedics' application for self-regulation.[361] When the application for a Manitoba Paramedics' College got approval in 2020, sixty three firefighter-paramedics quit as paramedics.[362] The UFFW asked

358 Mike McIntyre. "Sex at city fire hall alleged." *Winnipeg Free Press.* September 4, 2009.

359 Mary Agnes Welch. "Misdeeds at fire hall described." *Winnipeg Free Press.* September 2, 2006.

360 Tyler Searle. "Legal dispute between firefighter and paramedic dismissed." *Winnipeg Free Press.* December 11, 2022.

361 "Keep games out of paramedic decision." *Winnipeg Free Press.* March 14, 2015.

362 Joyanne Pursaga. "Dozens of firefighters drop paramedic role." *Winnipeg Free Press.* November 18, 2020.

WFPS to ask the province to extend registration deadline until after the pandemic, as firefighter paramedics didn't know how to register. It remains unclear why the UFFW wasn't assisting its members with the registration process, given that its then-president was a lawyer, skilled in administrative documentation.

- This seemed to aggravate the relationship between the unions even further. In March 2021, the MGEU asked Mayor Brian Bowman to remove paramedics from fire halls, citing that conflicts with firefighters were creating unsafe working conditions. A few days later, the UFFW called for the provincial government to take over ambulance services in Winnipeg.[363]

With both the MGEU and the UFFW demanding that the WFPS be disbanded and the EMS portion be taken over by the province, all seemed lost! Fascinating as it may sound, as 2021 disappeared, and 2022 evolved, it suddenly became apparent that it might be possible to fix the two decades of dissention within WFPS. It is intriguing what changes in personalities and approach can do to an entity.

As a benchmark, in February 2021, the WFPS did a survey of its current staff. Ultimately, it found that the "majority of staff deemed the workplace a passive, defensive environment... characterized by cautious work interactions designed to protect their own security." The report found that 67 percent of WFPS staff (478 staff surveyed—roughly half of all employees) found the workplace culture "oppositional," 86 percent found it triggered "conflict avoidance," and only 22 percent found it supportive.[364] Not a very healthy environment!

In May, 2021 WFPS Chief John Lane announced he was retiring; it appears the stresses from unhappy WFPS staff was weighing heavily on Lane. While Lane did not cause the firefighter-paramedic workplace hostilities, he did little to defuse the situation. At least as reported in the media, Lane often seemed to be siding with the firefighters, perpetuating the imbalance. Early is his tenure as chief, Lane presented at an International Fire Fighters' conference, where it indicated in the conference brochure that he "was going to talk about the threat posed to the firefighter-paramedic model, describing critics as non-fire paramedics spewing

363 Joyanne Pursaga. "On the Hot Seat." *Winnipeg Free Press.* August 19, 2021.

364 Joyanne Pursaga. "Paramedics, firefighters get say." *Winnipeg Free Press.* February 1, 2022.

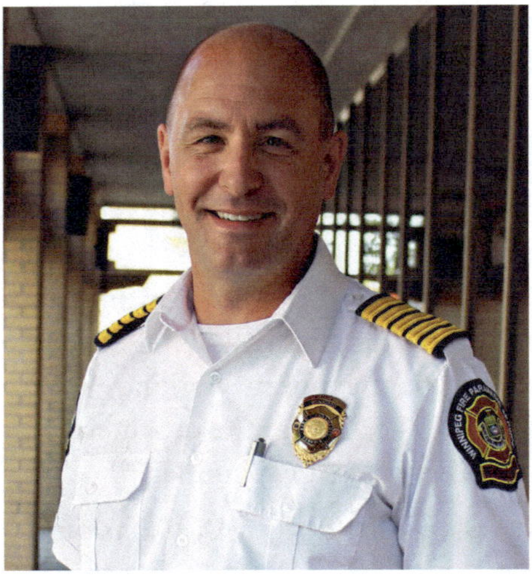

*Winnipeg's new Fire and Paramedic Chief, Christian Schmidt, responsible for taming much of the merger chaos. (Courtesy of WFPS)*

rhetoric..."[365] Lane and the City of Winnipeg were eventually hit with a $115,000 arbitrator's penalty after refusing to apologize to the paramedics. The perception that Lane's loyalties were with the firefighters remained entrenched until his retirement.[366]

The August 2021 appointment of new Winnipeg Fire Paramedic Chief, Christian Schmidt[367] and the spring 2022 retirement of longtime United Firefighters of Winnipeg President, Alex Forrest[368] got the ball rolling for healing and a culture change within the WFPS. While Schmidt came from the EMS branch of the WFPS, he also had the firefighter and 911 communications training, enabling him to see all sides of the discourse. At the same time, all sources suggest that Schmidt's conciliatory but pragmatic nature was precisely what the WFPS needed at that time. Interestingly, as Schmidt started in the new role as chief, he made it clear that his key goal was to improve workplace relations within the WFPS.[369] His diplomatic nature, combined with the February 2021 WFPS survey and subsequent discussion groups, gave Schmidt the tools needed to start a culture change within the service.

As Schmidt was starting his work, Alex Forrest chose to retire as the UFFWs president. The upshot is, as union president Forrest was an enigma. As a firefighter, lawyer, former soldier with the Canadian Forces, as well as a guy with amazing media contacts, Forrest had a combined skillset that enabled him to provide the UFFW with great

365 Aldo Santin. "Fire chief on the hot seat." *Winnipeg Free Press.* March 1, 2018.
366 Joyanne Pursaga. "Fire chief announces retirement." *Winnipeg Free Press.* May 1, 2021.
367 Joyanne Pursaga. "On the Hot Seat." *Winnipeg Free Press.* August 19, 2021.
368 Joyanne Pursaga. "Firefighters union president won't seek re-election." *Winnipeg Free Press.* December 1, 2021.
369 Joyanne Pursaga. "On the Hot Seat." *Winnipeg Free Press.* August 19, 2021.

service. During his twenty five years as president, it's easy to characterize Forrest as one of the most dedicated servants the UFFW and the Canadian firefighting community has had; highlighted by his work on the recognition of presumptive cancer in firefighters under Workers Compensation legislation.[370] Add to this picture Forrest's astute political acumen and a blind dedication to the firefighters he served, he was a force to be reckoned with.

Unfortunately for the WFPS, Forrest's blind dedication to firefighters often made him an antagonist of Winnipeg's EMS-paramedics. Forrest had a tendency to promote Winnipeg firefighters' interests while coming across as downplaying or dismissing Winnipeg's EMS branch. For example, in December 2017, when talking about transferring the ambulance service to the province, Forrest stated: "... firefighter members would be unaffected by the change due to the need to adhere to response time standards, he said. In fact, the role of fire paramedics could be enhanced if the WFPS were to give up its ambulance contract ... Many could be trained to provide advanced life support 'at a very minimal cost for the province."[371] Forrest continued, claiming that "the need for more resources makes it 'the perfect time' for the city to transfer its ambulance service to the province. . .' The province has more resources than the city could ever think of,' said Forrest."[372]

The challenge is that it's difficult to determine whether Forrest's apparent antagonism of Winnipeg's EMS Branch was real or perceived. As the UFFW's president, Forrest did have a fiduciary duty to act in the best interests, and lobby as strongly as possible, for firefighters. With the paramedics' union having neither the membership nor the political acumen of the UFFW, it was often left in the dust when it came to political lobbying against the firefighters.

As a result, in part due to Forrest's positive media connections, he was often perceived as the mechanism of the alienation between firefighters and paramedics. The situation was further complicated in that through the use of the media, it is difficult to tell how widespread the internal

370 Joyanne Pursaga. "Firefighters union president won't seek re-election." *Winnipeg Free Press.* December 1, 2021.

371 Larry Kusch. "Tension Smoulders as Flames Fade." *Winnipeg Free Press.* December 23, 2017.

372 Joyanne Pursaga. "City officials urge ambulance service be transferred to provincial authority." *Winnipeg Free Press.* October 7, 2020.

squabbles were. On the street level, firefighters and EMS-paramedics worked well together—there was never a doubt that the injured or sick Winnipegger was their priority. The bigger question was whether the internal hostility was truly as broad as the media suggested, or whether it was selective political posturing that tended to enrage members of both branches of the WFPS.

Forrest's 2021 retirement corresponded with a number of positive changes within the WFPS' firefighter/EMS-paramedic conflicts. In the spring of 2021, the UFFW elected long-time vice-president Tom Bilous as president. While Bilous came to the office with a similar dedication as Forrest's, he took a slightly different stance: carefully promoting firefighters' interests without targeting paramedics. This reduced some of the angst between the two groups.

The UFFW/WFPS/Fire/EMS-paramedic sometimes-conflict got an additional injection of positivism during the fall of 2024 with the subsequent retirement of Tom Bilous and the appointment of Nick Kasper as the new president of the UFFW. While Bilous took a more moderate approach to dealing with EMS-paramedics, Kasper brought a significantly different approach to the UFFW's president's position. While Kasper had been a Winnipeg firefighter for seventeen years prior to his appointment as president, he has also worked for the Interlake Eastern Regional Health Authority as a PCP, ICP, and ultimately an ACP, as well as an ACP flight paramedic for Northern Manitoba, for an additional seventeen-year period. In addition, in 2021, Kasper was appointed as a paramedic member of the newly created Council of the College of Paramedics of Manitoba.[373]

These experiences give Kasper insight into the hands-on operations and the regulation and governance of both firefighter-paramedics and EMS-Paramedics. In addition to the experiences of being a firefighter and a firefighter-paramedic, Kasper brings to the table a practical, solid understanding—and appreciation—of the range of services that EMS-paramedics provide. As president, while Kasper's fiduciary obligations still are firmly planted with Winnipeg's firefighters, his understanding of the roles of both divisions of the WFPS provides a means to bring connection between the two groups of employees.

Given Kasper's broad experiences as an EMS-paramedic, will having him as president of the UFFW create a long term difference in the

373 Online interview with Nick Kasper. December 13, 2024.

employee-relationships within WFPS? Ultimately, it depends where the Canadian EMS industry goes. If the *Canada Health Act* continues to exclude EMS as a medical service to which Canadians are entitled, then it is likely that to manage costs, WFPS will continue to provide a range of emergency medical services—beyond first responders. Kasper's cross-discipline skillset will likely be invaluable for "keeping the peace." Alternatively, if the *Canada Health Act* is amended to recognize that EMS-paramedic skillsets are well beyond those of emergency responders, and starts reflecting the reality that EMS-paramedics are often used as a substitute for primary-care physicians, it seems more likely that WFPS will not continue to be the best vehicle for EMS-paramedic management. Never-the-less, there will still be a need for firefighters to provide first responder-type services, and Kasper's skillset will still be crucial for bridging the gap between Firefighter-paramedics and EMS-paramedics.

Back in 2021, as Forrest retired, Schmidt went to work sculpting a different type of media relationship. Schmidt managed to eradicate what was becoming a media circus by, encouraging local media to come directly to his desk for the real story, while at the same time, becoming more candid, and at times blunt, with the media. This tended to cut down on the sensationalism and sniping that was becoming common from both the paramedics' and firefighters' unions.[374]

With the help of an institutional culture consultant, Schmidt began attacking the WFPS's misinformation process, cutting the internal discourse. This was cross-pollinated with work at creating a more inclusive culture within the WFPS—addressing perceived racism head-on and implementing increased respect and anti-discrimination measures.[375] Some of the techniques utilized included:

- Providing anti-racism, respectful workplace, and conflict resolution training to staff.
- Creating a diversity and equity firefighter training program.
- Creating more stringent employee workplace complaint procedures.

---

374 In person interview with Christian Schmidt, April 4, 2024.

375 Joyanne Pursaga. "WFPS seeks to improve workplace with 'culture shift plan'." *Winnipeg Free Press*. December 14, 2021.

- A regular, ongoing blog from the chief, outlining current, topical issues within the service.
- A direct, confidential email box to the chief for staff to use—which actually got replies,
- Regular, bi-weekly meetings at various WFPS locations, where Schmidt would meet, talk with, and address concerns of staff.

At the same time as WFPS was working on cleaning up its internal conflict, three of North America's premiere ambulance manufacturers: Demers Ambulances from Beloeil, Quebec, Braun Industries, Inc. from Van Wert, Ohio, and Crestline Ambulances from Saskatoon, Saskatchewan merged into one of North America's largest ambulance manufacturers. While the similarities to WFPS's situation were not immediately obvious, all three of these companies had very distinct cultures. They were involved in the emergency response industry, so were dealing with many similar internal culture issues.

Schmidt, through his affiliation with the Paramedic Chiefs of Canada, was able to speak directly with top executives from Demers and Crestline, allowing him to utilize some of the strategies used by Demers-Braun-Crestline to create greater staff cohesion. This ultimately encouraged positive changes to WFPS's culture.

While it may seem trite, in April 2024, I conducted about thirty interviews with WFPS staff: some organized and supervised by management, some set up but not supervised, and some where I simply dropped by stations unannounced and started talking to staff. During the process, I spoke to employees with experience ranging from six months to thirty-two years, working for both the fire and EMS divisions. What I noticed, consistent in every single interview, was a general respect for the WFPS. With a vast majority of staff, there was also a genuine love of the job. While many employees were willing to express criticism of the WFPS, the criticism was invariably directed toward improving service and better assisting Winnipeggers, as opposed to sniping at the organization itself or members of the "other branch."

These discussions, while neither scientific nor particularly broad, reflected a level of optimism and respect for WFPS that seems significantly higher than the internal fighting and discontent indicated even three years ago via the media and surveys.

Winnipeg's EMS has been constantly evolving over the last 140 years, and there's no doubt it will continue to evolve as the new roles of both firefighters and paramedics unfold. However, it seems that for the time being, WFPS is in a good place.

## Getting Enough Ambulances

For Winnipeg. how many ambulances is enough?

It's probably easier to figure out how many dragonflies Winnipeg will need to control its mosquito infestation next summer or to assess the number of snowplows the city will need for the winter five years hence than to guess how many ambulances are needed.

The challenge is, modern EMS deals with a range of needs, and as the skill levels of paramedics increase, in many cases, the ability to provide solutions for patients that don't involve a trip to the hospital also increases.

Roughly 10 percent of 911 calls are real emergencies: the kind where if advanced medical care is not provided quickly, someone will likely die. This group of patients needs immediate help, and almost always need a quick trip to a hospital. This group typically needs multiple levels of responders: first responders to establish an airway and start CPR, enough responders to continue CPR, responders with advanced medical training to provide drugs and other therapies, and a fast, efficient ability to transport—an ambulance. As with fire calls, these real emergencies are not a significant portion of the workload, but they need immediate response.

The next group of EMS calls, roughly half, require medical assistance—but not necessarily immediately. Dependent on the level of training of responders, they also don't always involve a trip to the hospital. This group of calls involves issues such as broken bones—where a trip to the hospital is often needed—or issues such as the forementioned panic attack, where with a proper assessment and proper counsel, the need for an ambulance ride can be avoided. In the latter scenario, whether the paramedic arrives in an ambulance, in an SUV, or on a fire engine doesn't make a whole lot of difference. For this group of calls, a key factor is often the skill level of the responder—and their ability to provide appropriate onsite care—which determines whether transportation by ambulance is needed.

The third group of EMS calls, roughly 40 percent, are those which don't need emergency medical assistance and definitely don't need an ambulance. However, they may require the skills of people working in the EMS system. These are perhaps the most varied of all calls. This group of callers include folks who genuinely believe they need help, but the issues aren't of an EMS nature, for example, the panic-stricken teenager who can't decide what colour of nail polish will match her prom dress, or the community advocate who believes he may have a panic attack in half an hour. This is where a well-trained call-taker or a triage paramedic can often remove the need for any kind of WFPS response. It may also involve responding to a traffic accident to confirm that there are no serious injuries, or ensuring that the senior who has fallen out of bed has no injuries or the unconscious drug addict on a street corner is simply sleeping. Help is needed, but at a more basic level. Again, a response may be needed, but not with an ambulance.

Finally, there are the calls where medical help is needed, but neither EMS nor an ambulance can provide the solution. For example, in downtown Vancouver, 911 call-takers have received several hundred calls over the past couple of years for a gentleman who, on foot, likes chasing moving cars. He clearly needs mental health assistance and if he is not stopped, he will eventually get hit by a passing motorist. Unfortunately, when the 911 calls come in, *someone* needs to respond and assist, and so it is often left to EMS to come up with a solution.

Given the above, it's evident there are many EMS situations where an ambulance is not required. It becomes even more confusing when one looks at the situations that directly affect the availability of ambulances, but are outside of the EMS's control. For example, when the Manitoba government decides to close half of the hospital emergency departments in Winnipeg, it results in EMS-paramedics needing twice as much time to find an available location to deliver their patient. This significantly reduces the number of ambulances available to respond to emergency calls within the city at any given time. Or conversely, immediately increases the number of ambulances needed, whenever the closures are in effect, to provide the same level of service.

In the end, it's a balancing act. In a moderate-sized city such as Winnipeg: you need to have sufficiently quick firefighter response to quell fires within five minutes, sufficiently quick EMS response to get to medical emergencies within five minutes, sufficient advanced life support EMS response to deal with serious medical emergencies in less than nine minutes, and sufficient resources to respond to significant but non-life-threatening calls within a reasonably short time period.

At the risk of stating the obvious, the fewer non-hospital resources that a city has to deal with minor emergency medical calls means that more ambulances are needed to transport the sick and injured to hospital.

However, the biggest challenge is often just trying to interpret the numbers. In a 1998 exposé, the *Winnipeg Free Press* compared the ambulance services in eight Canadian cities, with the intended objective of showing how Winnipeg's EMS was underequipped and understaffed.[376] The problem was, once you started dissecting the numbers, it showed that there was no real correlation between the number of ambulances and response times.

For example, after highlighting that most Canadian cities had one ambulance for every 34,000 to 40,000 residents, while Winnipeg had one ambulance for every 63,700 residents, the article showed that Winnipeg had one of the fastest response times in Canada—six minutes. Only Regina, a city one-fourth the size, had faster response times. The most intriguing statistic was that while Winnipeg was described as having ten ambulances, and Calgary—a city with only 15 percent more people—was described as having twenty ambulances, they had *identical* response times. Buried in the article was a note that three of Calgary's hospital emergency wards had been closed, which from Winnipeg's experience, we know ties up available ambulances. While there are factors that can affect the efficiency of a city's EMS, the number of ambulances, by itself, does not guarantee either efficiency or fast response times.

## How has WFPS's Ambulance Supply Evolved?

It seems like a simple enough question; how fast does EMS need to be on the scene of a medical emergency? The National Fire Protection Association Standard 1710,[377] establishes a one minute "turnout time" and four minute "travel time" (together, a five minute first "response time") benchmark time goal for not less than 90 percent of dispatched incidents. These "dispatched incidents" include calls where the patient's condition is "urgent" and either potentially or immediately life threatening. Standard 1710 further recommends that ALS arrive within eight minutes of being dispatched.

What does this mean?

---

376 Keith MacArthur. "Emergency!" *Winnipeg Free Press.* January 11, 1998.

377 The Standard for the Organization and Deployment of Fire Suppression Operations, Emergency Medical Operations, and Special Operations to the Public by Career Fire Departments.

As the new century started, Winnipeg needed more ambulances. Irrespective of whether EMS was provided by the Emergency Response Service, a separate municipal ambulance service, or the province, it didn't matter. While the response times were adequate, Winnipeg's ten full-time ambulances could not keep up with demand on a busy night, and with no extra resources, except for the last resort, non-transport equipped fire department rescue squads, more patient transport-capable vehicles were needed.

The problem was captured in February 2000, when the only ambulance in all of Transcona was removed from the area and relocated closer to downtown. In its place was an ALS paramedic "chase car"—a former district fire chief's sport utility vehicle which had been modified to carry carry advanced life support equipment. The problem was, it did not have patient transport capacity.[378] Not only did it not have patient-transport capacity, but previously in the Gunter Dorno case (see page 149), Winnipeg's EMS management had made it abundantly clear that they would not tolerate non-ambulances being used to transport patients. Nevertheless, the city argued that this would provide better service to the area, because unlike an ambulance, it would not be re-deployed to other areas of the city. It seems the city also missed the point that unlike an ambulance, it couldn't transport people—the key role of an ambulance service during that time period.

In response, Mayor Glen Murray put out another of his ultimatums that Winnipeg would stop providing EMS unless the province provided funding for four more ambulances by May 2000.[379] While an obvious political ploy, it didn't help the morale of Winnipeg's paramedics. For a group of professionals, already understaffed and stretched to the limit, being told that they might be fired in two months exacerbated the situation.

Murray's threats also came at a time when the province was undergoing a change in how it supplied ambulances, making immediate supply a bit more of a challenge. In early 2001, Manitoba Health ceased supplying funding for the purchase of new ambulances to service providers such as Winnipeg, and instead, had the province's Vehicle and Equipment Management Agency (VEMA) take over the supply of ambulances for

---

378 Darcy Gillespie. "Paramedics to replace ambulance in Transcona." *Winnipeg Free Press.* February 9, 2000; "New Ambulances." *Winnipeg Free Press.* March 11, 2000.
379 "New Ambulances." *Winnipeg Free Press.* March 11, 2000.

all of Manitoba. The benefit of this process was that VEMA could purchase ambulances in bulk, obtaining better pricing. For example, when VEMA took over ambulance supply in 2001, it immediately negotiated a contract with Saskatoon's Crestline Coach to have 80 ambulances delivered between 2001 and 2002. The obvious downside of this approach (from Winnipeg's perspective) is that VEMA supplies new ambulances on the basis of need. While Winnipeg may need new ambulances, given Manitoba's historical under-funding of EMS, there were areas of the province that were in significantly greater need of new vehicles.

A further benefit of VEMA taking over the management of the province's ambulance fleet was that in addition to purchasing new units in bulk, VEMA was also in the position of being able to take older units—typically twelve to fifteen years on the road—and remount the bodies on new chassis. While being a further cost saving, it also enabled rebuilt units to be reassigned to areas of the province where ambulance usage was lower (including the use as transfer ambulances), creating a much longer lifespan for vehicles.

Murray's threats to stop providing EMS managed to get dialogue going between the city and the province, which ultimately gave WFPS enough funding to staff two additional ambulances, ambulances that had been sitting idle. Whether these were 24-hour or peak-period units is unclear; the newspapers kept flipping between "roughly seventeen full-time ambulances,"[380] and "twelve full-time and five peak-period units."[381] Either way, when the city's 2003 budget was introduced, the

380 "Ambulances aren't new." *Winnipeg Free Press.* January 28, 2003.

381 David Kuxhaus. "Ambulance shortage 'a recipe for disaster'." *Winnipeg Free Press.* January 4, 2005.

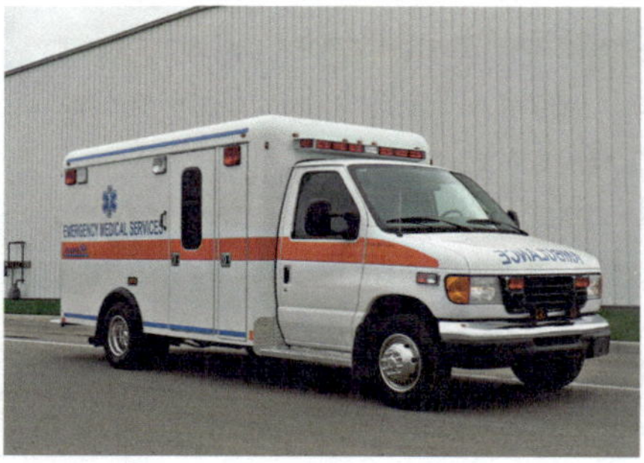

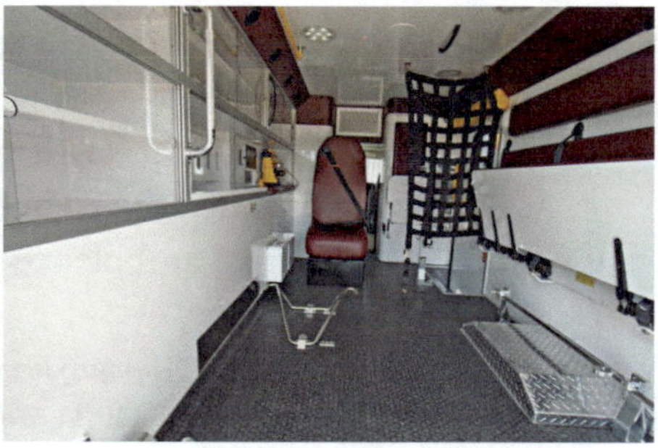

*While pictures of the original 2001 fleet purchase can't be located, this is one of the batch of Manitoba's 2005 Crestline Fleetmax units. (Courtesy of Crestline Coach)*

two newest ambulances continued to receive staffing funding via the city. This gave Winnipeg more staffed ambulances when needed. Since Murray's 1998 election, the city had acquired five additional ambulances and seventy new paramedic positions.[382]

Determining the sufficient number of ambulances is always relative. In December 2004, despite having twelve full-time units, on New Year's Eve[383] a patient with a broken leg as well as four other casualties were taken to hospital via fire department rescue squads. The issue was two-fold; while there was not always as many ambulances as needed for transport, a further problem was that with more firefighter-paramedics, firefighters don't want to wait for the extended periods of time needed for an ambulance. Given the perceived ongoing need to be available for quick responses to fires, they didn't want to keep fire apparatus out of service. This is an ongoing issue with many combined fire-EMS services—despite a dual role, firefighters tend to view their *primary* role as providing fire suppression. Ambulance shortages became acute during the summer of 2005 as Winnipeg navigated a serious heatwave. On one particularly hot day, despite having nineteen ambulances on duty (twelve full-time, five peak-period, and two special run units), Winnipeg EMS still couldn't keep up with the volume of calls.[384]

As a result of not always having adequate units to respond, the following month (August 2005), a medical priority dispatch system was introduced in an effort to ensure that units were always available to respond to emergency calls. Under medical priority dispatch, there are three levels of calls: emergency, non-urgent, and ambulance transport. The goal was to ensure that there are always three ambulances available for true emergency medical calls. When there were only five ambulances available, inter-facility hospital transfers were suspended. When Winnipeg was down to three available ambulances, non-urgent calls receive a response by a firefighter-paramedic, with an ambulance only being dispatched upon the firefighter-paramedic's request.

As the city approached the end of the first decade of the new century, the problem that actual ambulance numbers were not relevant couldn't

---

382 "Ambulances aren't new." *Winnipeg Free Press.* January 28, 2003.

383 David Kuxhaus. "Ambulance shortage 'a recipe for disaster'." *Winnipeg Free Press.* January 4, 2005.

384 Patti Edgar. "Hot weather put pressure on paramedics." *Winnipeg Free Press.* June 21, 2005.

have been more obvious. In 2006, WFPS was up to thirteen full-time and eight peak-time ambulances,[385] with another full-time unit added during the summer of 2007; thanks to an extra $3.8 million in provincial funding.[386] Winnipeg now had the same number of ambulances that Calgary found worked well in 1998. Despite the additional vehicles, the EMS-paramedics' union, now the Professional Paramedic Association of Winnipeg, continued to claim that there were insufficient ambulances in the city. This captures the challenge of any kind of emergency service supply. As a politician or administrator, you want to have as low a cost as possible; ultimately as few vehicles and staff as possible while maintaining reasonable service levels. At the same time, residents want as many units as possible (without actually paying for them) so they can get help quickly.

## Major Incident Response Vehicle

Over the 2008 and 2009 period, WFPS acquired a couple of additions which, if not enhancing EMS services directly, were additional resources. First off, in the fall of 2008, WFPS got its new Major Incident Response Vehicle or "MIRV."[387] Modeled after the Fire Department of New York's 2007 Major Emergency Response Vehicle, it was an eight-stretcher (five on standard patient transport stretchers and three on portable stretchers) ambulance based on an Eldorado city bus chassis.

Built by Saskatoon's Crestline Coach, and while not unique in Canada—either at the time, or now (Edmonton had operated an Orion bus-chassised ambulance since 1983, Toronto has had a variety of bus-based ambulances over the past forty years, and York Regional and Ottawa EMS now operate units similar to Winnipeg's) Winnipeg's was a bit different in that unlike Toronto and Edmonton, it wasn't a used, converted transit bus. It was built from the ground-up on a brand-new bus chassis as a fully functioning ambulance.

385 Bruce Owen. "Emergency response times a fiery election issue." *Winnipeg Free Press* July 13, 2006.

386 Bartley Kives. "Are enough ambulances on the road?" *Winnipeg Free Press.* August 15, 2007.

387 "'Jumbo ambulance' comes to Winnipeg." CBC News. June 26, 2008. https://www.cbc.ca/news/canada/manitoba/jumbo-ambulance-comes-to-winnipeg. Accessed March 5, 2024.

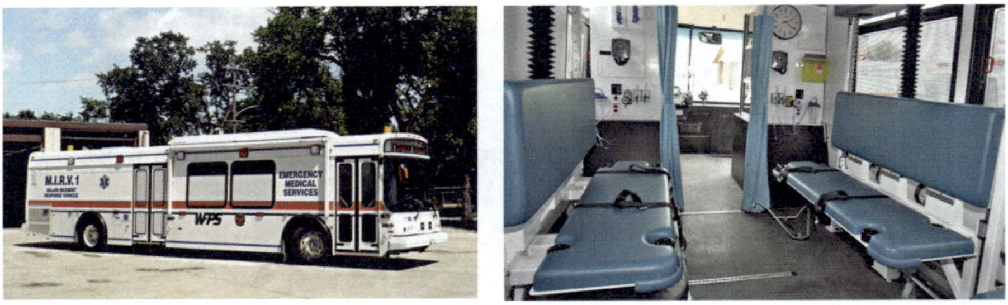

*The 2008 Crestline Eldorado Major Incident Response Vehicle. (Courtesy of Dave Stewardson, Crestline Coach)*

Strange as it may sound, other than having a large-capacity ambulance as an option for major incidents, when initially ordered, WFPS did not have a specific plan for the MIRV. It was recognized that it could be used for mass casualty situations; for evacuating large facilities such as nursing homes or apartment buildings; protracted incidents; bariatric transports; special events; Chemical, Biological, Radiological, Nuclear, Explosive (CBRNE) incidents; inter-facility transfer of multiple patients; and/or when rehabilitation was required for WFPS staff at incidents, but there wasn't a specific plan for its use. Conceptually, the city wanted something with more capacity than the original 1998 MIRVs built for the Pan Am Games.

The WFPS tried to figure out ways to use the MIRV to reduce the strain on regular ambulances—theorizing that it could replace a couple of ambulances. After using it for a while to pick up intoxicated/unconscious individuals along Main Street on Friday and Saturday nights, it eventually evolved into a response vehicle for major motor vehicle accidents and as a shelter for residents during winter apartment fires. While providing a potential transportation/onsite treatment option for multi-casualty emergencies, it was rarely used for its designed purpose. Showing its age, it was disposed of during the summer of 2024.

## Electronic Patient Care Reporting System

A second addition that was implemented during this period was the Electronic Patient Care Reporting (EPCR) system. The EPCR utilizes little tablet-style notebook computers—Panasonic Toughbooks. By helping to acquire and share patient information, the system saves significant time during each medical call. Each emergency medical response vehicle in Winnipeg carries an EPCR computer.

As soon as the first emergency responder arrives, whether a firefighter-paramedic or an EMS-paramedic, they immediately enter the patient's information and vital statistics into their computer. The data is simultaneously transmitted to the computers of EMS dispatchers, other responding EMS vehicles, and hospital emergency room staff. When transferring patients to other EMS providers, there's no need to provide a detailed explanation. All the needed data is entered into the EPCR and is ready for review by subsequent staff. Changes in the patient's condition are easy to identify, even by subsequent caregivers, as the system continuously upgrades the patient's vital signs.

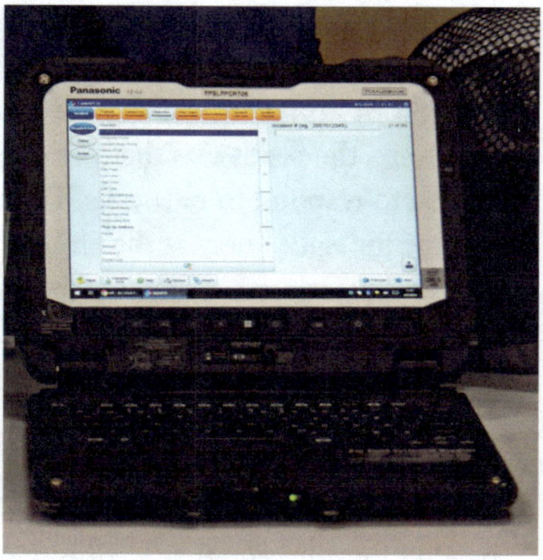

*The Electronic Patient Care Reporting Toughbook computer. (Courtesy of the author)*

By providing specific protocols for many situations, the system also takes the guesswork out of many uncommon scenarios for paramedics. This allows paramedics to follow along and provide proper care, even when not completely familiar with the patient's condition. In other, more complex situations, the tablets enable paramedics to get direct advice from emergency room physicians as they review the patient's statistics in real-time.[388] While initially ordered in 2006, the EPCR was finally fully operational and installed in all ambulances and first responder vehicles by April, 2008.[389]

## Wait Times Still an Issue

Despite technological advances and the introduction of community paramedics, hospital wait times provide one of the biggest obstacles to an efficient, manageable EMS. The simple reality is, despite technology, increased hospital wait times delay the hand-off of patients by paramedics

388 Mary Agnes Welch. "Computer to cut ambulance ride time." *Winnipeg Free Press.* February 13, 2006.

389 Joe Paraskevas. "Paramedic reports going electronic." *Winnipeg Free Press.* April 3, 2008.

to hospital staff. The WRHA exacerbated the situation in 2009 when a policy change had hospital emergency rooms giving the same triage to individuals brought by ambulance as those who came in on their own. Whether right or wrong, the result was that paramedics were left waiting at the hospital, unable to respond to new calls. This change in policy left two paramedics waiting for eight hours at the St. Boniface Hospital ER in February 2009.[390] As the year progressed, it got worse, with no ambulances being available in the city for thirty two cumulative hours in June, thirty seven hours in July, and twenty seven hours in August 2009.[391]

During the city's 2010 mayoral election, the EMS-paramedics' union, now the Manitoba Government Employees Union, launched a media campaign arguing that Winnipeg didn't have enough paramedics and needed an additional five ambulances. Mayoral incumbent Sam Katz responded by claiming Winnipeg had one of the fastest initial response times of major Canadian cities, and the problem was not the number of ambulances but the hospital wait times.[392]

Ultimately, the MGEU and Katz were both correct: It was a two-headed problem. The numbers speak for themselves. Between 2005 and 2010, there was a 17 percent increase in EMS call volumes; and between 2007 and 2010, there was a 44 percent increase in call processing times. In addition, between 2005 and 2009, there was a 37 percent increase in hospital turnaround times, and inter-facility transfers increased by 74 percent.[393] Put in plain language, there were a lot more calls for emergency medical help and it was taking longer to handle each call—a bit of an administrative mess for a cash-strapped city and province.

## Smaller Ambulances, More Tools

After receiving the new MIRV in 2008, new ambulances went from extremely big to small over the next few years. In 2009, Manitoba Health decided to try a smaller, more fuel-efficient ambulance style than the modular-style bodies used over the previous thirty years. As a result, it

---

390 "Waiting, waiting in the ER." *Winnipeg Free Press.* October 20, 2009.

391 Mary Agnes Welch. "No one to come to your rescue." *Winnipeg Free Press.* October 8, 2009.

392 Bartley Kives. "Katz: city's paramedics fastest." *Winnipeg Free Press.* September 21, 2010.

393 "Winnipeg Paramedics demand more ambulances." National Union of Public and General Employees. Press release. September 22, 2010.

had Crestline Ambulance create a Type I, van-styled prototype ambulance, based on a standard Mercedes Sprinter chassis; similar to the style used in many European countries. While they were maneuverable, fuel efficient, and very comfortable to drive, they were small, with low roofs and minimal equipment storage space.

For an emergency medical service that was moving toward a full ALS model—needing to carry a lot of equipment and a decent-sized area for patient care—the Mercedes Sprinter didn't work. While it potentially had enough room to be used as a non-emergency transfer ambulance, it did not have the needed space to provide an advanced life support level of care. The Sprinter was the first and last unit of its type tested by WFPS. During the same period, BC Ambulance also experimented with Mercedes Sprinter ambulances. While they acquired a fleet and put them in service for half a dozen years, BC Ambulance returned to modular bodies when the Sprinters began to wear out. It appears that the Sprinters are used extensively on the East Coast, but they primarily run BLS-based ambulances.

A reality in EMS is that they regularly get medical calls for patients who are "morbidly obese" or in everyday language, heavier than 350 pounds. For example, in 2009 alone, WFPS had 240 emergency calls involving obese or bariatric patients.[394] These calls create a two-sided problem for EMS. In treatment, all patients deserve respect and dignity. Still, the reality is that moving a patient who weighs hundreds of pounds more than usual can be dangerous and lead to severe injuries for paramedics.

In 2006, Manitoba Health attempted to remedy the problem providing WFPS with its first bariatric ambulance. While it was a start, it was not practical for Winnipeg. The five-piece ramp needed to be assembled and

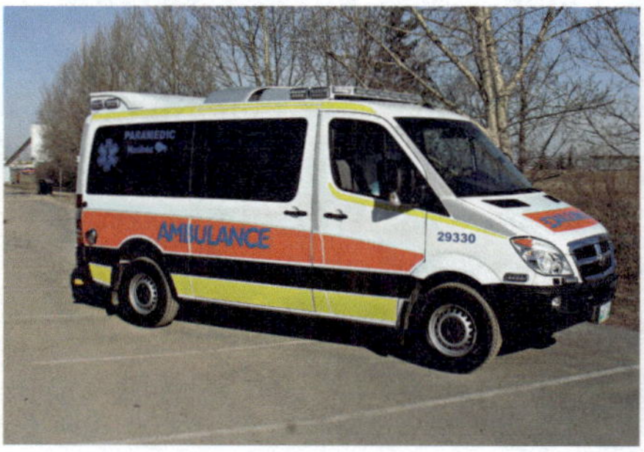


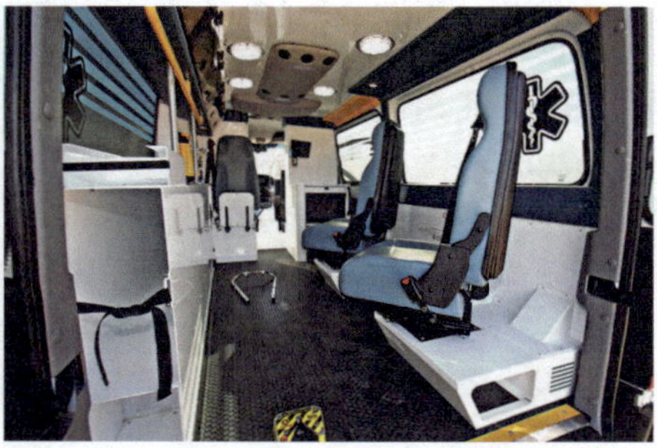

*2009 Crestline Mercedes Sprinter prototype ambulance. (Courtesy of Crestline Coach)*

394 "Message from Fire & Paramedic Chief Jim Brennan." *Lights & Sirens.* WFPS. June 2010: 1.

disassembled for each call, and the winch would slowly pull the stretcher up into the patient area. The problem was that the ambulance doors needed to be left open during the entire twenty-minute set-up/take-down process, making it uncomfortable and potentially unsafe for operation during winter pick-ups.[395] The time required to utilize the ramp also created a significant delay in transport during medical emergencies.

The arrival of the MIRV in 2008 provided a more efficient (and warm) means of transporting bariatric patients. Unfortunately, having a forty-foot-long bus-chassis ambulance pull up in front of a private residence was not too discreet for the patient and often created side-street maneuverability issues.

Fortunately, Manitoba Health's 2010 decision to have Crestline Ambulance custom-build a new bariatric ambulance addressed the problem. Under the direction of WFPS ambulance supervisor Stan Stone, Crestline took one of their intensive care ambulances, which had a body about fifteen centimeters wider and doors ten centimeters taller than a standard modular ambulance and installed a heavy-duty hydraulic ramp. The ramp automatically folds under the unit's floor at the flick of a switch, and both the ramp and the hydraulic stretcher can support 1,000 pounds, making it able to safely transport almost any patient. At first glance, it looks like an ordinary Winnipeg ambulance; not attracting the same attention as the MIRV. This causes less stress for patients.[396]

## Billing for Wait Times

While the WFPS had been gradually increasing its ambulance fleet and making inroads to decrease the need for ambulances, it finally acknowledged that the ultimate cause of the ambulance supply problem was the tie-up at hospital ERs. By early 2011, on many days. up to one-third of Winnipeg's ambulances were parked and waiting to unload patients. The issue reached a breaking point in April of 2011. The WFPS borrowed a trick from British Columbia Ambulance Service and started billing hospitals $130 an hour for paramedics left waiting in hospitals for more than ninety minutes. After sending out 414 bills for the month, WFPS put the

395 Stan Stone. "New Bariatric Ambulance." *Lights & Sirens*. WFPS. June 2010: 3.

396 Melissa Martin. "New ambulance gives lift to morbidly obese patients." *Winnipeg Free Press*. April 3, 2010.

hospitals on notice that the accepted wait time would drop to sixty minutes in October 2011.[397]

Unexpected costs have a way of stimulating change. Being hit with $60,000 in ambulance bills made the WRHA more receptive to creative problem solving; in working with the WRHA, WFPS came up with several ways to reduce wait times. The underlying problem with hospital waits is that paramedics were not permitted to drop off their patients until there had been an assessment by an emergency room physician. As of May 2011, several new initiatives were introduced to address the problem. First, a new policy permitted paramedics to hand off patients to other paramedics—enabling one set of paramedics to wait at the hospital, supervising patients, instead of two or three. Second, paramedics were permitted to hand off their patients to respiratory therapists before seeing a physician. Third, in some cases, the triage nurse could determine that an ambulance patient could be left in the waiting room without paramedic supervision. Finally, thanks to extra funding from the province, a paramedic was stationed at the Main Street Project—Winnipeg's Community Health Centre for its severely marginalized downtown population—on a 24/7 basis to deal with minor injuries. This reduced the number of people who actually needed to get transported to hospital.[398]

Unfortunately, these initiatives didn't address the real underlying problem—not enough money for emergency health care in Winnipeg. For most of the city's history, the problem kept being shoveled from one pile to another. By January 2014, the average patient off-load waits at hospital ERs were up to 83.3 minutes, up from the 2012 average off-load times of 74.6 minutes.[399]

At the risk of understatement, this was a difficult period financially for Manitoba, and it was reflected in Winnipeg's EMS. By 2015, Manitoba's ambulance fees highest in Canada, with a ride in Winnipeg being $512 for a city resident and $818 for visitors. For comparison purposes, Ontario was charging $45 for ambulance trips at the time.[400] The chal-

397 Jen Skerritt. "City hospitals billed $60,000." *Winnipeg Free Press.* May 21, 2011.
398 Jen Skerritt. "City hospitals billed $60,000." *Winnipeg Free Press.* May 21, 2011.
399 Larry Kusch. "Emergency room off-load times soar." *Winnipeg Free Press.* June 4, 2014.
400 Vera-Lynn Kubinec & Joanne Levasseur. "No free ride: Ambulance bills in Manitoba highest in Canada." CBC News. February 11, 2015. https://www.cbc.ca/news/canada/manitoba/no-free-ride-ambulance-bills-in-manitoba-highest-in-canada-1.2947262 Accessed: December 16, 2023.

lenge was, increasing fees and passing the cost on to the user didn't solve the problem. With half of user fees going unpaid, the increased fees mainly help to cover the fees not paid by users who couldn't afford the service charges in the first place.

In 2016, as per its funding agreement, the WRHA gave the city $20.6-million for EMS, of which $9.46-million was for firefighter-paramedics.[401] While it was helpful to have funding for the first responder/fire portion of Winnipeg's EMS, the reality is, most EMS calls require either an ambulance, an ALS paramedic, or both. As a result, the province was still not providing adequate financial support for the core of EMS.

Despite rising costs, and increasing hospital wait times, as the city and the province couldn't agree on new funding levels, the province froze the 2017 and 2018 provincial payments at the forementioned 2016 levels. This left Winnipeg with a $2-million shortfall for 2017 and a $4.6-million shortfall for 2018.[402] In response, city council turned to its fairly routine response and threatened to divest EMS services to the province, and asked WFPS Chief John Lane to outline options. Without giving away any secrets, considering the earlier discussion about Lane giving the appearance of siding with firefighters and not always supporting EMS-paramedics, it's not hard to guess Lane's recommendations.

## More Training, ERs Closing

In the midst of Lane reviewing the issue of Winnipeg divesting ambulance services and making recommendations, two other factors intervened that significantly affected the delivery of Winnipeg's EMS.

First off, Winnipeg's EMS-paramedics had started to get significantly higher levels of training. Many were being trained to the advanced life support level, and then received higher levels of specialized training, such as community paramedicine, tactical paramedicine, or paramedic specialist/critical care paramedicine. This enabled many of Winnipeg's EMS-paramedics to provide hospital-level treatment without needing to transport many non-emergency patients to the hospital. Due to this increase in training, from

401 Aldo Santin. "City works out kinks over future of ambulance funding." *Winnipeg Free Press.* March 15, 2018.

402 Aldo Santin. "Paramedic transfer would save city $3M: chief." *Winnipeg Free Press.* April 12, 2018.

2013 to 2017, the number of patients assessed or treated on scene increased by 57 percent from 16,366 to 23,716.[403] Unfortunately, due to restrictions in funding, with a few exceptions, most of the city's ALS paramedics were in ambulances; in 2019, 77 percent of ambulances were ALS.[404] As a result, ALS paramedics are also responsible for patient transportation. The province was, and still is to this day, generally reluctant to fund sole paramedics in chase cars. This is the key means of enabling an EMS-paramedic to work independent of the transport side of EMS and provide direct health care services to patients on site, including in people's homes.

This leads to the second factor that negatively affected Winnipeg's EMS; hospital emergency departments closings. In 2019, the WRHA closed the emergency departments at Victoria, Concordia, and Seven Oaks hospitals, and converted their facilities to urgent care clinics. As a step above walk-in medical clinics, urgent care clinics provide treatment for urgent but non-life-threatening conditions, such as: dehydration; severe cuts, and broken or sprained limbs. These are medical issues which often don't require an ambulance and/or can be fully dealt with by firefighter-paramedics.

At the same time, the province kept the emergency departments at St. Boniface, Health Sciences Centre, and Grace Hospitals. With the number of emergency departments in the city cut in half, ambulances were regularly redirected to other, less busy ERs. For example, between January and September 2019, the Health Sciences Centre made 1,242 ambulance redirects. These numbers were significantly higher than in previous years, the closest being 1,292 in 2016. Similarly, St. Boniface Hospital doubled its redirects; between January and September 2019 it made 300 redirects, compared to 158 redirects in 2018.[405]

At the risk of stating the obvious, when ALS paramedics are sidetracked by driving seriously ill or injured patients between hospitals, they can't also be doing house calls and treating patients on scene. While PCP-level firefighter-paramedics do a superb job of deciding when a

403 Tom Brodbeck. "Paramedics reduce need for trips to ER." *Winnipeg Free Press.* July 11, 2019.

404 Tom Brodbeck. "Paramedics reduce need for trips to ER." *Winnipeg Free Press.* July 11, 2019.

405 Stephanie Tsicos. "'Extremely frustrating': Winnipeg's two largest hospitals seeing increase in hospital diversions." *CTV News Winnipeg.* November 8, 2019.

person doesn't require medical aid, and they're great at stopping the clock on many medical emergencies until ALS paramedics can arrive, they don't have the skills or the tools to definitively treat many medical issues onsite.

Many jurisdictions, including British Columbia, get around this problem by having ambulances staffed by primary care paramedics, and ALS paramedics arriving in either non-transport ambulances or SUVs. This enables ALS paramedics to treat on the scene without necessarily transporting, and transport ambulances to take patients to the hospital without unnecessarily tying up ALS paramedics. The irony is this is the model that Winnipeg used in the early days of the paramedic program. However, as the numbers of ALS paramedics increased, the decision was made to assign them to ambulances. Over time this has resulted in ALS paramedics either transporting patients between hospitals, or waiting at hospitals to hand off their patients. The complexities were magnified (with increased numbers of seriously sick Winnipeggers) during the COVID-19 pandemic.

There were multiple requests made for additional ambulances and more staff, once the COVID-19 pandemic was underway. For example, in the fall of 2020, Chief Lane requested ten more ambulances and 120 new EMS-paramedics.[406] After seven years of negotiating, in May 2023, Manitoba Shared Health and Winnipeg finally hammered out a new agreement. Under the five-year contract, the province agreed to supply two additional ambulances and twenty new paramedics. While not the numbers requested over the previous umpteen years, it gave the city seventeen full-time ambulances, eleven peak-time ambulances, and two community paramedic or EPIC units.[407]

## The Twenty-First Century: Training and Specialized Services

As the new century emerged, the WFPS began working toward a fully integrated service—with cross-trained firefighters and paramedics.

Recognizing that increased medical training was needed, the WFPS began developing a system that would provide Winnipeggers with better

406 Joyanne Pursaga. "On the Hot Seat." *Winnipeg Free Press*. August 19, 2021.

407 Swidda Rassy. "Ambulance wait times increasing in Winnipeg." City News. April 12, 2023. https://winnipeg.citynews.ca/2023/04/12/ambulance-wait-times-increasing-in-winnipeg/. Accessed September 28, 2024.

EMS services. As a result, while Dr. Linda Nugent was still at the helm as medical director, Dr, Robert Grierson was hired in 2002 as the assistant medical director. This gave WFPS two highly competent physicians to design and coordinate emergency medical services.

In terms of staff skill-level, starting in 2001 most new WFPS hires—150 in the first two years—were graduates of the Manitoba Emergency Services College in Brandon and cross trained as firefighters and primary care paramedics.[408] While it seemed prudent at the time, because firefighters and EMS-paramedics had different pay scales, hiring staff who could work in either branch didn't evolve as well as intended.

Nevertheless, with a second physician onboard, things started moving almost immediately in 2002. First, the fire-medic position was created in the fire suppression branch. While essentially a firefighter on a first response fire vehicle who had scaled-down primary care paramedic (PCP) training, within a couple of years the training was expanded to provide firefighters with full PCP training.

Second, in 2002, the WFPS had its advanced life support training program certified by the Canadian Medical Association and began running inhouse training. The first certified ALS paramedics graduated in 2002.

## What's in a Name?

The titles of Winnipeg's emergency medical staff have changed many times during the fifty years of Winnipeg's public ambulance service. Starting as "ambulance attendants" and "drivers" in 1975, the name had evolved to Emergency Medical Technicians by the late 1970s/early 1980s. With the ALS pilot project in 1989, by the early 1990s, "paramedic" became the name of choice for Winnipeg EMS staff qualified to administer drugs. As the training for all levels of EMS staff increased, by the early 1990s, the term paramedic was generally used for all front-line EMS staff. The paramedics had a level of training structure of Level 1, Level 2, Level 2 Advanced, and Level 3.

On a formal level, in March 2020, the Paramedic Association of Canada introduced the National Occupancy Competency Profile for paramedics, which included their professional titles. It appears that from this point onwards, at least in Winnipeg, the standard name of choice for frontline EMS staff became "paramedic."

---

408 "Service's creation slow, methodical." *Winnipeg Free Press.* December 29, 2003.

It's important to note that in North America, there is little consistency in how the term "paramedic" is used. In Manitoba and British Columbia, despite different skillsets and different levels of qualifications, most prehospital emergency care professionals are called paramedics. In many US jurisdictions, Emergency Medical Technicians are equivalent to Manitoba's PCPs and paramedics are equivalent to Manitoba's ACPs. On Canada's East Coast, Emergency Medical Technicians are similar to Manitoba or BC's Emergency Medical Responders. The key point being that when comparing training and qualifications of prehospital emergency care staff, even between provinces, there is little consistency in job titles.

In 2002, in Winnipeg, the titles changed to Primary Care Paramedics, Intermediate Care Paramedics (PCPs who have completed their first year of training as Advanced Care Paramedics), and Advanced Care Paramedics. Many WFPS ACPs graduated from the WFPS' accredited training division, a three-year program involving hundreds of hours of clinical, didactic, and ambulance field training. Winnipeg EMS paramedics are trained in Advanced Life Support (ALS), Advanced Trauma Life Support (ATLS), Advanced Cardiac Life Support (ACLS), Prehospital Trauma Life Support (PHTLS), and Pediatric Advanced Life Support (PALS). Medical Supervisors (later named District Chiefs-Paramedic Operations) use chase vehicles to assist EMS-paramedics with pediatric and high-acuity calls.

In the process, Level 3 paramedics were given additional training in pediatrics, high risk transport, and dialysis. They were then renamed "Medical Supervisors" and grandfathered into being Critical Care Paramedics.

While the newly minted ALS paramedics were also trained in pediatrics, in actual practice, this was left in the medical supervisors' scope of practice. As the scope of practice has increased over the past twenty years, the basic skills needed for patients under the age of seventeen are being gradually incorporated into all levels of training.

In a nutshell, the skill sets for the different levels are as follows (updated to 2024 standards):

The Primary Care Paramedic (PCP) scope of practice means that PCPs must be able to:

- Assess and appropriately document vital signs.
- Maintain the upper airway with manual maneuvers and use an oropharyngeal airway and/or a nasopharyngeal airway as needed,
- Perform airway management including insertion of the I-gel supraglottic airway and insertion of an orogastric tube in conjunction with the I-gel supraglottic airway.
- Use tonsil tip, soft catheter, and bulb suction equipment.
- Perform chest auscultation and interpret breath sounds/air entry.
- Obtain an appropriate patient history using the SAMPLE medical assessment model.
- Perform basic assessment and care to patients with:
    - cardiovascular emergencies,
    - respiratory emergencies,
    - neurological emergencies,
    - environmental emergencies,
    - traumatic emergencies, and
    - obstetrical, neonatal, and pediatric emergencies.
- Perform three-lead cardiac monitoring and interpret basic cardiac dysrhythmia,
- Perform manual defibrillation,
- Perform twelve-lead ECG acquisition,
- Provide routine care during transport for common drainage or feeding tubes (excluding chest tubes),
- Manage emergency childbirth,
- Application of a Combat Application Tourniquet,
- Application of a SAM vented chest seal (a device for quickly sealing an open chest wound),
- Application of a SAM pelvic binder/sling,
- Complete the *Community Paramedic Specialty Training Program.*

- Complete either the *WFPS Orientation and Training for IV Access* or the *Tactical EMS Specialty Training Program*,
- Maintain peripheral intravenous locks or infusions without medications or blood products,
- Administer drugs including:
    - ASA
    - Epinephrine
    - Oral Glucose
    - Nitroglycerin
    - Nitro patch
    - Salbutamol
    - Naloxone
    - Olanzaphine (in consultation with an ACP, ACP-P, or DCPO only)
    - Epinephrine (able to administer pediatric dosages)
    - Salbutamol (able to administer pediatric dosages)
    - Naloxone (able to administer pediatric dosages)

The Intermediate Care Paramedic (ICP) scope of practice means that ICPs must be able to perform all PCP skills, plus care for adolescents (aged 10-16 years):

- Perform advanced airway management including foreign body removal,
- Perform continuous and tidal $CO_2$ monitoring (measuring the $CO_2$ level in the lungs),
- Administer Constant Positive Airway Pressure to CHF patients in respiratory distress,
- Perform 12 and 15 lead ECG acquisition and interpretation,
- Perform Valsalva maneuver,
- Initiate intravenous therapy,
- Maintain peripheral intravenous infusions with blood products,

- Initiate intraosseous infusions,
- Perform advanced assessment and care to patients with:
  - Cardiovascular emergencies,
  - Cardiac arrest,
  - Respiratory emergencies,
  - Neurological emergencies,
  - Environmental emergencies,
  - Traumatic emergencies, and
  - Adolescent emergencies.
- Administer additional drugs including:
  - 50% Dextrose
  - Amiodarone
  - Atropine
  - Midazolam
  - Dimenhydrinate (Gravol)
  - Diphenhydramine
  - Epinephrine
  - Lidocaine
  - Naloxone (Narcan)
  - Glucagon
- Maintain a pump containing:
  - Sodium Bicarbonate
  - Heparin
  - Lidocaine
  - Nitroglycerin

The Advanced Care Paramedic (ACP) scope of practice means they must be able to perform all PCP and ICP skills, plus care for adults, adolescents (aged 10-16 years), and pediatrics (aged 28 days—9 years):

- Use of dialysis fistula or subclavian dialysis catheter access for dialysis cardiac arrests,
- Use of magnet to temporarily suspend inappropriate therapy delivered by an implantable cardioverter-defibrillator,
- Provide advanced care to pediatrics (aged 28 days—9 years),
- Percutaneous needle cricothyrotomy,
- Needle chest decompression,
- Cardioversion,
- Transcutaneous pacing,
- Chemical sedation of agitated patients,
- Narcotic analgesia administration,
- Provide advanced care to patients with an ST Segment Elevation Myocardial Infarction (STEMI) including field administration of thrombolytic agents and/or direct referral to Cardiac Catheterization lab,
- They must also complete the *Community Paramedic Specialty Training Program* (Main Street Project or with the Emergency Paramedics in the Community program)
- Administer a full drug list for adults and adolescents including:
    - Fentanyl
    - Oxytocin
    - Topical lidocaine
    - Haloperidol
    - Furosemide
    - Midazolam
    - Insulin
    - Calcium Gluconate
    - Tenecteplase (STEMI—per-on-line medical direction)
    - Unfractionated Heparin (STEMI—per-on-line medical direction)

- Enoxaparin (STEMI—per-on-line medical direction)
- Clopidogrel (STEMI—per-on-line medical direction)
- Ticagrelor (STEMI—per-on-line medical direction)

• Administer a full drug list for pediatrics including:
  - Epinephrine
  - Lidocaine
  - Amiodarone
  - Sodium Bicarbonate
  - Atropine
  - 25% Dextrose
  - Glucagon
  - Midazolam
  - Fentanyl
  - Naloxone[409]

With both key programs up and running by 2004 (fire-medics and ALS training), Dr. Nugent left the city's employ and Dr. Grierson became Winnipeg's EMS Medical Director.

With a certified ALS program, Winnipeg could now move toward more specialization in EMS. As paramedicine has evolved over the past couple of decades, with the skill levels and the skill sets increasing, the role of paramedics has expanded in both directions. In Winnipeg and elsewhere, critical care paramedics are now helping to transport seriously ill patients—a job previously done by doctors and nurses. At the same time, both community paramedics and even ambulance-based ALS paramedics are providing on-site treatment for many minor illnesses and injuries, reducing the need for hospital visits. This is a national, and even world-wide trend. For example, during this period, Saskatchewan has been shifting its entire EMS model to a mobile health services model—recognizing that a lot of work done by paramedics in the street is replacing work previously done by family physicians and/or hospital emergency and outpatient departments.

409 WFPS. "Medical Scopes of Work." March 2024.

## Community Paramedics

As North America's demographics evolve, with seniors living longer, more people living with mental health issues, and more people living below the poverty line, the drain on emergency response and hospital services is prolific. For example, seniors (over age sixty) represent 14 percent of the current Canadian population. However, they use 40 percent of hospital services and account for 60 percent of paramedic responses in Canada. They also account for about 45 percent of provincial health spending.[410] As many of the calls from this segment are not emergency-related, community paramedics provide sound economics as an alternate means to deliver non-emergency healthcare in the community.

In a nutshell, community paramedics are advanced care paramedics with extra training in wound care, antibiotic treatment, vaccination delivery, and blood testing, as well as chronic disease management, prevention of illness, communicable diseases, and health restoration, As they are also often the initial point of contact in the health care system, they typically have a superior knowledge of community medical and mental health resources.

At time of writing, Winnipeg had four different community paramedic programs: Paramedics with the Emergency Paramedic in the Community (EPIC) program visit vulnerable patients where they are in their communities, helping to break down barriers to primary care. Community paramedics at the Main Street Project provide primary care to residents within the shelter system. The community paramedics at the Winnipeg Police Service's Central Processing Unit provide round-the-clock assessments of individuals entering and leaving the protective care facility. Finally, the Enhanced Low Acuity Triage (ELAT) program has community paramedics providing secondary 911 triage services to less serious, non-emergency callers who could benefit from non-ambulance transportation methods to hospital and/or more appropriate services in the community.

## Main Street Project

The Main Street Project was Winnipeg's first community paramedic project. Main Street Project is a community health centre that provides a wide range of health and safety services for the most severely marginalized

410 Michael Nolan, Tim Hillier, and Carmen D'Angelo. *Community Paramedicine in Canada.* Emergency Medical Services Chiefs of Canada. 2011: 59.

residents of Winnipeg. Of particular importance for EMS purposes, it also houses Winnipeg's Intoxicated Person's Detention Area, where residents are delivered when detained under the under the *Intoxicated Person Detention Act.* In 2002, Leon Elerman Bighetty died after police, assuming he was intoxicated, took him to the Main Street Project. He was eventually taken to hospital and found to have a head injury with internal bleeding. As a result of the head injury, he died six days later.

Bighetty's death led to a 2005 inquest report which recommend that staff at the Main Street Project have emergency medical responder (entry-level paramedic) training with a nurse practitioner on site. In 2009, primarily after a lot of fighting over who would pay for it, a pilot project was initiated with community paramedic Ryan Sneath on site.

The pilot project quickly demonstrated its value. Prior to the pilot project, the Main Street Project generated about 600 ambulance calls per year. With a community paramedic on site, this was reduced to 240 per year[411]. Since 2011, the Main Street Project's community paramedic desk has been staffed 24/7, with Winnipeg Regional Health Authority (WRHA) funding of $800,000 per year.

As a precursor to the community paramedic program, in 2007, the Downtown Winnipeg Business Improvement Zone (BIZ)—the corporation that promotes and markets Winnipeg's Downtown—acquired its own passenger transport vehicle and began taking intoxicated individuals to the Main Street Project for assistance and time in the Intoxicated Person's Detention Area. According to the *Winnipeg Free Press*, this reduced ambulance transports to the Main Street Project by about 2500 per year.[412] While the 2500 figure seems high, given that both EMS and police were delivering intoxicated people to the Main Street Project, I have not been able to get independent verification whether the 2500 is the number of people transported by EMS, the number transported by both police and EMS, or the number now transported by Downtown Winnipeg BIZ. However, even if the number includes both police and EMS deliveries, it is still an impressive reduction in call volume. It appears that Downtown Winnipeg BIZ eventually transferred its transportation service to the Main Street Project's "Van Patrol Outreach Program."

411 Larry Kusch. "EPIC CARE." *Winnipeg Free Press.* October 3, 2015.

412 Mary Agnes Welch. "No one to come to your rescue." *Winnipeg Free Press.* October 8, 2009.

## Primary Treatment and Referral Service Program

In 2009, the WFPS began experimenting with, and eventually using sole, mobile paramedics as a means of reducing ambulance usage. As mentioned earlier, with 911 calls, there's the roughly ten percent that are life threatening and need immediate response, and there's the 40 percent at the bottom whose concerns are often directed by 911 call takers to other services. However, the roughly 50 percent of calls in the middle need help, have legitimate health concerns, but don't always need a trip to the hospital.

This challenge was never more pronounced than during the 2009 H1N1 pandemic. Winnipeg EMS received dozens, and sometimes a couple of hundred calls per day from people who were quite sick and needed help.

The problem was, they didn't all need to go to the hospital. An idea was hatched to follow other North American jurisdictions, place a single community paramedic in a sedan, and have him or her respond to non-emergent H1N1 calls. The community paramedic would do on-scene assessments, provide medicine or other treatments as necessary, but only request an ambulance if truly needed.

Cities that use the community paramedic model have found that it significantly cuts down on the need for ambulances. Originally called the "Paramedics in Focus" program because it was envisioned that there would be up to four paramedic units driving Ford Focus compact sedans,[413] it evolved into the Primary Treatment and Referral Service (PTRS). Even though a local car dealership initially donated a Jeep Patriot and a Chevrolet HHR to the WFPS for the program,[414] the province declined to fund the program unless 911 call volumes were more than 300 per day for a three-day period. As the 911 medical calls remained at around 200 to 225 per day, funding was never provided.[415]

Nevertheless, the WFPS, using inhouse resources, created the program in a modified form.[416] In November and December of 2009, a

413 Mary Agnes Welch. "Sedans may replace ambulances." *Winnipeg Free Press.* October 16, 2009.

414 Mary Agnes Welch. "Local dealer donates cars for paramedics." *Winnipeg Free Press.* November 20, 2009.

415 "New paramedic units kept on hold for now." *Winnipeg Free Press.* November 27, 2009.

416 Christian Schmidt. "PTRS – Primary Treatment and Referral Service." *Lights and Sirens.* WFPS. June 2010: 3.

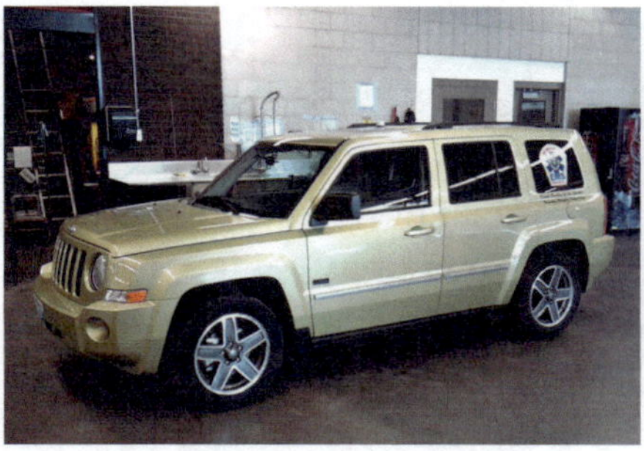

*The original PTRS response vehicle – a donated Jeep Patriot. (Courtesy of Brian Leach)*

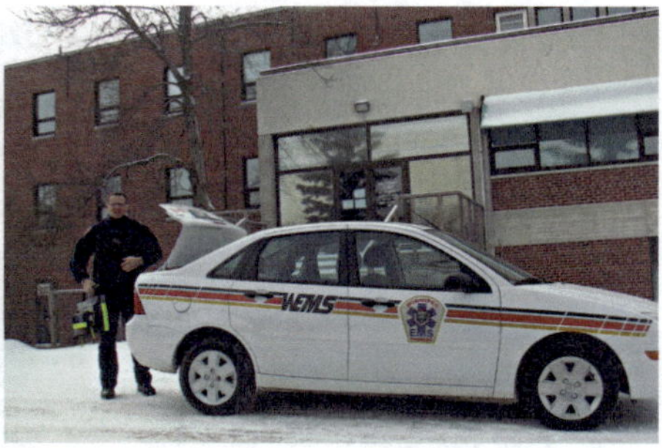

*The PTRS program eventually switched to using a Ford Focus. (Courtesy of WFPS).*

number of Intermediate Care Paramedics were given PTRS training—a two-day session where paramedics were trained to perform comprehensive health assessments using the Canadian Triage and Acuity Scale, and determine whether hospitalization was required.[417] Initially using the Jeep and the Chevrolet, eventually a Ford Focus was adapted for the program. While not used for triage as initially planned, WFPS ultimately initiated the program to respond to four distinct scenarios:

1. To relieve firefighter-paramedics who were on scene with a stable patient for more than thirty minutes but no ambulance was available.
2. When there were less than five available ambulances and the on-scene firefighter-paramedic requested an assessment of a stable patient.
3. Where a responding crew could not secure a scene involving a deceased casualty and were awaiting the arrival of police or a family member.
4. To relieve ambulance crews when they had excessive waits when dropping-off patients at overloaded hospital ERs.[418]

While not the community paramedic program envisioned, the PTRS program provided a means for a sole paramedic to reduce some of the existing strain. As staff resources permitted, the PTRS was used for three years until the 2013 EPIC pilot project received funding.

---

417 November 5, 2009 correspondence from Chris Bruce-Smith, WFPS to Bryan Leach.

418 WFPS, EOP – 1.23, "PTRS Deployment." December 3, 2010.

## Emergency Paramedic in the Community

After three years of negotiating, in 2013 the WRHA finally agreed to fund a pilot project, permitting community paramedics to provide assistance as originally envisioned. To the tune of $750,000 annually, the two-year Emergency Paramedic in the Community (EPIC) project was endorsed. Two of the Main Street Projects' paramedics were transferred to EPIC.

The pilot project targeted the top forty 911 callers, given that the top 1 percent of 911 callers account for 12 percent of paramedic responses.[419] The pilot also responded to calls for medical assistance when requested by residents of two inner city personal care homes and the Salvation Army building on Henry Avenue.

Winnipeg's 911 service responds to about 200 medical calls per day, but each of the top 40 users call almost every day, and paramedics respond to members of this high use group three to four times per day.[420] When one of the high users calls 911, an EPIC paramedic responds. If the patient's medical needs do not require transport to an Emergency Department, the EPIC paramedics assist onsite, providing a complete medical assessment. An ambulance only responds if requested by the EPIC paramedic.

Once the assessment is complete, arrangements are made to connect the patient with an appropriate community health resource such as home care, an Urgent Care Centre or Community Health Access Centre, and/or provide referrals for home care, primary care, or geriatric program assessment teams. The community paramedic also can provide assistance such as connecting with family doctors, arranging for pharmacy deliveries, and accessing adaptive equipment. Essentially the EPIC paramedic acts as a resource for getting the patient the services that are required—often when the patient doesn't know themselves what is needed. Once the needs of the patients are met, the EPIC program tracks these patients to ensure the resources put in place continue to be effective.

In addition, the EPIC program is proactive, following up on two to three firefighter or paramedic referrals per day, typically of people who, because of their economic and/or social situations, might end up frequently calling 911.

---

419 Larry Kusch. "EPIC CARE." *Winnipeg Free Press.* October 3, 2015.
420 Larry Kusch. "EPIC CARE." *Winnipeg Free Press.* October 3, 2015.

As the program "resulted in a 56% reduction in 911 calls by EPIC patients and a 62% reduction in ambulance transports to an Emergency Department,"[421] in 2015, the EPIC program was given permanent funding for one EPIC paramedic to be on shift from 7:00 a.m. to 7:00 p.m., seven days a week. In June 2019, provincial funding was provided for a second EPIC unit.

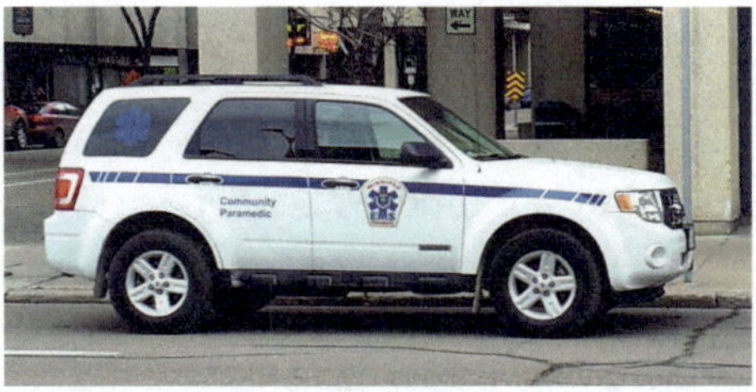

*Community Paramedic SUV. (Courtesy of Brian Leach)*

## COVID-19 PTRS Program

A slightly modified PTRS program was utilized in 2020 to provide non-emergent responses to COVID-19 related calls, and to assist firefighter-paramedics with COVID-19 related emergent calls when an ambulance was not available. With the 2020 version of PTRS, the unit responded with both a Primary Care Paramedic and an Advanced Care Paramedic.[422]

As a result of the pandemic, in May 2021 two additional EPIC units were funded by Shared Health to deal with COVID-19 related calls. Despite their need for responding to 911 over-users, the funding for these additional units was cut two years later, in 2023, as the COVID-19 pandemic was deemed over.

A PTRS pilot program was reinstituted again in September 2024, after the province cut back on the city's EPIC funding. In the 2024 reincarnation, the PTRS unit was staffed by two alternate-duty paramedics (EMS-paramedics whom, for health reasons, shouldn't be dragging heavy stretchers) and used to transport low acuity patients to Urgent Care Clinics and other, similar facilities.[423]

---

421 "Emergency Paramedic in the Community (EPIC) program to expand". Undated (2019) City of Winnipeg press release. https://www.winnipeg.ca/fr/node/30257. Accessed October 14, 2024.

422 WFPS, SOP – 1.19-O-PTRS. March 27, 2020

423 Marc Savard. 'PTRS Pilot Launch." WFPS memo. September 25, 2024.

## Winnipeg Police Central Processing Unit (CPU)

Community paramedics are assigned to the Central Processing Unit (the jail) of Winnipeg Police Service (WPS), on a round-the-clock, seven-day-a-week schedule. The paramedic assesses each individual being incarcerated, ensuring clients in remand are safe through medical monitoring and clearance, and are not negatively affected by underlying medical conditions.

## Enhanced Low Acuity Triage

In May 2021, WFPS launched the Enhanced Low-Acuity Triage (ELAT) or "EPIC 9" pilot project. At the emergency communications centre, 911 calls are screened by call-takers. Those that meet certain conditions—low risk/non-emergency—are transferred to an onsite Advanced Care Paramedic who completes a more in-depth medical assessment for low acuity patients. This helps WFPS determine if patients with low-acuity concerns can safely benefit from a different mode of transport to a hospital rather than an ambulance. The program started on May 23, 2021, and between May 23—Sept 9, out of 1,508 calls referred to the ELAT paramedic, 493 callers were deemed non-emergency, and 263 callers were sent to hospital by taxi instead of an ambulance.[424] This significantly reduced the number of required ambulance responses, and a decision was made to make referrals to an ELAT paramedic a permanent part of the dispatch process.

By 2024, medical calls to Winnipeg's 911 system were increasing by approximately 7 percent per year. In 2018 WFPS had 81,241 medical-related calls, increasing to 109,558 in 2023.[425] Being impossible to keep up with this kind of demand, in October 2024, WFPS adopted, and began phasing in a new five level Medical Priority Dispatch System (MPDS) which permits a much wider range of responses.

Traditionally, 911 medical calls are either "Priority One" (with lights and sirens) or "Priority Two" (no lights and sirens). The Canadian Triage and Acuity Scale, as developed by the Canadian Association of

---

424 Gabrielle Piche. "Paramedic calls 911 on city's ambulance services." *Winnipeg Free Press.* September 22, 2021.

425 Canadian Association of Emergency Physicians. *The Canadian Prehospital Acuity Scale – Educational Program.* March 2014. Alana Cole. "With 911 call volumes rising, Winnipeg Fire Paramedic Service develops new 5-priority dispatch system." CBC News. https://www.cbc.ca/news/canada/manitoba/911-call-volumes-dispatch-system. Accessed January 21, 2025.

Emergency Physicians, on which the MPDS is based, breaks emergency medical calls into five levels:

- Category 1 Severely ill, requires resuscitation
- Category 2 Requires emergent care and rapid medical intervention
- Category 3 Requires urgent care
- Category 4 Requires less-urgent care
- Category 5 Requires non-urgent care[426]

Under the new MPDS, the two lowest priority calls are referred to an ELAT paramedic, and can be referred to other community-based services. In the system developed for Winnipeg, set to be formally released in 2025, lower priority calls will be dispatched to non-EMS groups such as the Downtown Community Safety Partnership (DCSP), a safety/heath patrol and transport program which provides safety patrols and non-emergency first aid/health responses in Winnipeg's downtown area. The DCSP is a program established in April 2020 as a partnership between the Province of Manitoba, City of Winnipeg, Downtown Winnipeg BIZ, WFPS, WPS, and True North Sports and Entertainment. Through the use of an ELAT community paramedic, non-emergency medical calls are being dealt with in a more appropriate fashion.[427]

Enhanced Low-Acuity Triage is not a new concept in Canada. Since 2013, recognizing that most 911 medical calls are not medical emergencies, Nova Scotia's Emergency Medical Service's Clinical Support Desk has been using Advanced Care Paramedics or Acute Care Registered Nurses to assess and make alternate recommendations for non-emergency transport.[428] This was the first time this type of system was developed in Canada.

---

426 Elyse Skura. "The ambulance dispatch system was recommended 20 years ago. It's finally coming online", *CBC News.* March 21, 2024. Accessed January 21, 2025, https://www.cbc.ca/news/canada/ottawa/ottawa-ambulance-dispatch-paramedic-change-new-1.7151140.

427 Iris Dyck. "A common goal of care: Changes and partnerships at the WFPS", *Global News.* May 23, 2024. Accessed January 21, 2025: https://globalnews.ca/news/10520707/changes-partnerships-wfps/

428 Nova Scotia Paramedics Union. "Clinical Support Desk." https://web.archive.org/web/20141019203958/http://nspu.ca/roles-of-paramedics/clinical-support-desk. Accessed January 23, 2025.

After Winnipeg adopted the ELAT system, in February 2023, Alberta EMS followed suit. Utilizing a "shared response team" of registered nurses, non-emergency 911 EMS calls started being referred to nurses for assessment of potential alternate (non-ambulance) response options. Alberta Health claims that this referral system will reduce emergency ambulance calls in Alberta by approximately 40,000 per year.[429]

## Paramedics Active in Community Education and Response

During the 1999 Pan Am Games, the WFPS's paramedic bike squad demonstrated potential long-term benefits for the city.[430] As a result, in 2002, it was formalized as the Paramedics Active in Community Education and Response (PACER) program. It currently has roughly twenty paramedics involved—two paramedics plus a third alternate for each platoon. The program uses mountain bikes, each carrying a scaled-down version of a primary care paramedic's response gear. The program runs on the weekend day shifts each year during the summer, weather and resources permitting.

From PACER's formal creation in 2002 until the shop's closing in 2016, Gooch's Bicycle and Hobby Shop—an institution in the Winnipeg cycling community—donated the two bikes as well as the necessary annual maintenance and service.

The primary purpose of PACER is to provide medical care at major city events, such as the Canada Day celebrations, the Teddy Bears' Picnic, the Osborne Street Festival, the Fringe Festival, the Children's Festival, Kids of Mud Races, and the Dragon Boat Races. The bikes' maneuverability and high visibility makes them perfect for moving quickly through large crowds. This enables PACER paramedics to respond to incidents to assess, stabilize, and treat the patient until an ambulance arrives for transport.

In 2010, the program expanded to provide coverage on various bike trails around the city, as well as The Forks Skate Park, giving

---

429 Alberta Health Services. "HCAP: Faster response times for 911 calls." https://www.alberta.ca/release.cfm?xID=86476C49212DC-E6F5-3BF8-D7D8B610B541C0B7. Accessed January 26, 2025.

430 Chuck Tinguely. "Paramedics Active in Community Education and Response (PACER) Program." *Lights & Sirens.* WFPS. June 2010: 10.

rapid medical response while encouraging safe riding techniques and the use of property safety equipment. The program also assists the Main Street Project paramedics by interacting with people experiencing homelessness in the downtown area. Their role combines emergency medical response and public education; directly connecting with Winnipeggers at public events and in the downtown area to provide public safety information.

## Advanced Care Paramedic Practitioners

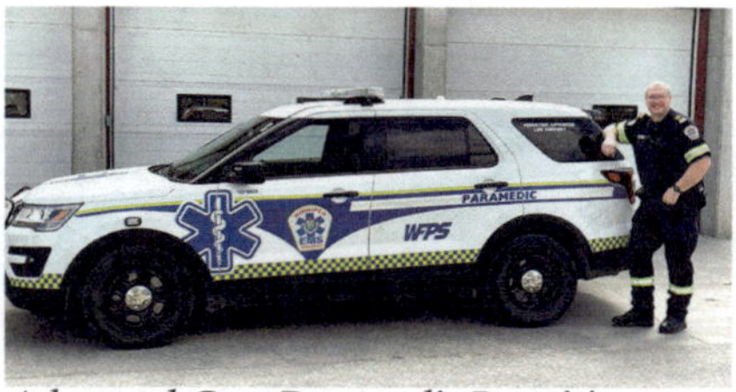

*Advanced Care Paramedic Practitioner Russ McKenzie and an ACP-P's non-transport "chase car." (Courtesy of WFPS)*

Since Winnipeg's first Advanced Life Support Pilot Project in 1986, EMS Supervisors, now called District Chiefs, Paramedic Operations (DCPO), have received additional training for more serious medical calls. In 2002, when the WFPS enhanced its EMS training protocols, supervisory staff acquired skills equivalent to critical care paramedics—the highest recognized paramedic level in Canada. While necessary, this often led to overload for supervisors, as they were required to provide both shift and on-scene management as well as the new, specialized medical skills.

During the 2016-2017 opioid crisis, and the subsequent COVID-19 pandemic, EMS across Canada found that their resources were being stretched like never before. As a result, many ambulance services, including Winnipeg's, introduced a new position of paramedic specialist, or as they're called in Winnipeg, an "Advanced Care Paramedic Practitioner" (ACP-P). The ACP-Ps have the same training as a DCPO, without management duties. The ACP-Ps respond to complex calls where regular paramedic crews need specialized advice or help with problem solving.

Currently, the ACP-P/DCPOs have the following skill sets which enable them to respond to calls involving children and infants, and those requiring advanced life support, respiratory or cardiac procedures, including all of the skills of a PCP, ICP, and ACP, plus:

- Perform an orotracheal intubation of an unconscious/semi-conscious patient.
- Perform topicalization of the upper airway with local anesthetic.
- Remove orotracheal or nasotracheal tube from a patient meeting extubation criteria.
- Provide advanced care to neonates (0-28 days) including:
  - Intraosseous (IO) cannulation,
  - Intranasal drug administration, and
  - Insertion of the i-gel supraglottic airway,
- Advanced obstetrical emergency management for breach and shoulder dystocia management (newborns being birthed in unnatural positions and probably stuck), including:
  - Loveset maneuver
  - Mauriceau maneuver
  - Rubin maneuver
  - Wood's corkscrew maneuver
- Palliative Care Program/Protocol—the *Learning Essential Approaches to Palliative* care training.
- Venipuncture blood draws as requested by the Winnipeg Police Service for evidence collection.
- A variety of specialized medications for neonatal patients (aged 0-28 days).[431]

Responding in either ambulances or SUV "chase cars", depending on staffing needs on a given day, ACP-Ps monitor all EMS dispatches for calls that may need specific assistance, assist with the transfer of high-risk patients between care facilities, respond to calls from ACPs requesting a higher level of skills, and are automatically dispatched to all calls involving:

- assaults/sexual assaults with multiple victims,
- breathing problems where a tracheostomy is required.

431 WFPS "Medical Scopes of Work". March 2024: 9.

- heart problems—especially those involving an Automated Implantable Cardioverter Defibrillator,
- pregnancy/childbirth/miscarriages involving high risk complications and third-trimester hemorrhaging, and
- car accidents with multiple casualties.[432]

## Tactical Emergency Medical Services

High risk police situations pose a challenge for EMS. Whether it be bomb threats, barricaded suspects, hostage takings, or similar scenarios, there are often associated injuries. The challenge is, for safety reasons, police are often hesitant to permit regular paramedics into the "hot zone" to provide medical care. Surprisingly, many of the related injuries (90 percent[433]) occur during the specialized training for handling these kinds of incidents.

This creates a problem. If there aren't paramedics present, it means that members of the specialized police team dealing with the issue, be it the tactical squad, the bomb squad, the crowd control squad, etc., get diverted to deal with the injury, putting the rest of the team at risk.

In Canada over the past fifteen years, three distinct models have emerged to address this issue. With the RCMP, officers with previous EMS experience are recruited as members of the force's Emergency Medical Response Team.[434] Members are located across the country and respond whenever there's a potential high risk police situation within the RCMP's jurisdiction. Some Canadian municipal police departments, such as Victoria, BC, follow a similar model and have members of their tactical team trained to provide emergency care. The downside of this model is that advance care paramedics are not immediately available in a crisis situation.

A second model was developed by the Ontario Provincial Police's Tactics and Rescue Unit (TRU). Off-duty ALS paramedics from the Ontario Emergency Medical Service are contracted by the OPP.[435]

432 WFPS Communications Centre. "International Academies of Emergency Dispatch System Policies – Policy 41 ACP-P". June 28, 2020.

433 Online interview with Shane Cooke, September 27, 2020.

434 Deidre Seiden. "The Paramedic Advantage." *RCMP Gazette*. Vol 76, No. 4 (2014).

435 Deidre Seiden. "The Paramedic Advantage." *RCMP Gazette*. Vol 76, No. 4 (2014).

They're given tactical training, enabling them to work with TRU and bomb squad officers. The advantage of the TRU model is that tactical paramedics work full-time providing emergency care, and come as licensed, practicing ALS Paramedics. The downside is, their OPP tactical work is a part-time, on-call job, so they are not always available when needed.

A third model was developed in 1996, as a joint project by Toronto Police's Emergency Task Force (Toronto's "SWAT team"—the ETF) and the Toronto Ambulance Service. With the ETF model, a group of Toronto paramedics were given tactical training by the Toronto Police ETF. The tactical paramedics in Toronto work regular ambulance duty shifts (with tactical gear—military-style shirt/pants, gloves, ballistic helmets, ballistic/bullet-proof vests, and medical backpacks - in their ambulance), and when needed by the ETF, they respond as part of the tactical team. There really isn't a disadvantage to this model. The tactical paramedics, being paramedics in their "day jobs," are routinely practicing emergency care. As well, being on duty (and there are tactical paramedics assigned to every shift), they're always ready to respond.

This model has been copied in many cities across Canada, including Winnipeg. In Winnipeg, shortly after the formation of WPS' full-time Tactical Support Team (TST), tactical officer Shane Cooke, a former WFPS paramedic, was tasked with designing a tactical paramedic program. After looking at programs across the country, it became apparent that the cooperative model, as created by Toronto, had significant advantages.[436]

By 2011, the WPS was actively having discussions with WFPS about developing a Tactical Emergency Medical Support Service (TEMS) for Winnipeg. Cooke, along with WFPS's Dave Johnston, began developing the unit. With the help of members of the Calgary and Ottawa police tactical teams, WPS created a formal program for Winnipeg, where tactical paramedics were recruited from amongst existing WFPS paramedics and trained for two weeks alongside new TST members.

The biggest obstacles to getting TEMS implemented, as has been seen through much of Winnipeg EMS's history, was a combination of political apathy and money. While WFPS Chief Shoemaker had a pass-

---

436 Online interview with S. Cooke, September 27, 2020.

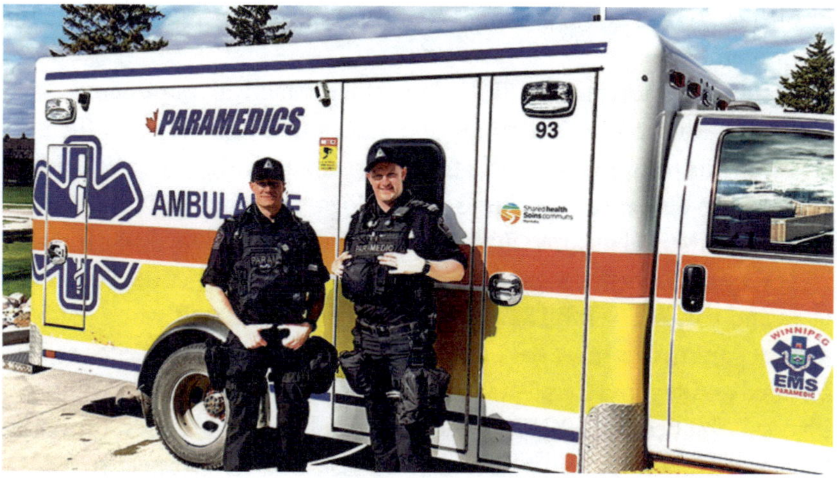

*Tactical paramedics Mark Lebtag and Matt Hiebert - WFPS Tactical Emergency Medical Services. (Courtesy of WFPS)*

ing interest in the idea,[437] through multiple changes of administration in both WFPS and WPS, there was no mutual interest in TEMS until John Lane became the WFPS chief in 2014. While there was the usual question about how Winnipeg would pay for the program, fortunately the Province's Criminal Forfeiture and Seizure Program provided an initial grant for TEMS and continues to come to the rescue with annual grants for most of TEMS' equipment.[438]

Since its formation in 2014, the tactical paramedic program—which runs out of the WFPS EMS Station No. 30 on Osborne Street—has expanded from the initial fourteen to twenty two advanced care paramedics. In its first year, while it responded to 286 calls (of which 232 were training or preplanned events), TEMS only treated fifteen patients, of which fourteen were minor injuries.[439] TEMS' advantage, and the way it benefits Winnipeg the most, is that it permits onsite advanced-level emergency care to be immediately available as opposed to being several blocks and many minutes away. It also provides immediate assistance to members of the TST in treating minor issues, such as dehydration

437 Interview with Bryan Leach, October 22, 2024

438 Online interview with S. Cooke, September 27, 2020.

439 Kim Kaschor. "What exactly does Winnipeg's tactical emergency medical unit do?" CBC News. August 4, 2015. https://www.cbc.ca/news/canada/manitoba/what-exactly-does-winnipeg-s-tactical-emergency-medical-unit-do-1.3178287, Accessed: August 8, 2017.

or blisters, which could quickly expand into more serious problems for team members.

Besides supporting the TST, Winnipeg's tactical paramedics also respond with the WPS's bomb squad and canine unit. In 2020, the unit expanded its training, with help from the staff at Bridgewater Veterinary Hospital, to also care for injured police dogs.[440]

Unlike other subgroups within WFPS, the selection of tactical paramedics is very role-specific. Selection process is a joint effort between both services and parallels WPS' TST selection process. WFPS staff who qualify as tactical paramedics must have a minimum five years of experience and be certified as Advanced Care Paramedics. They need to pass the Peace Officers Physical Abilities Test (POPAT); the physical obstacle course test for police tactical members. After passing the obstacle course, prospective TEMS members then have a day of real-life scenario-based testing. This process, while testing for various phobias, involves trained players performing life-like scenarios with mock injuries. These sessions are monitored and scored by both WPS and WFPS instructors. A final interview between staff from the TST and supervisory staff from each WFPS shift assesses each candidate's work ethic, leadership, teamwork, and decision-making qualities. Seniority is not a consideration in the selection process.[441]

By closely tying the TEMS members' selection to the same processes used for TST member selection, the WFPS has created a team that is accepted and works well with Winnipeg Police's tactical officers.

In comparison, in 2011 the BC Ambulance Service created its own TEMS unit. The selection process was determined through discussions with the paramedics' union, with seniority being a key consideration. The result was a highly trained service which police tactical teams around British Columbia will not utilize. While seeming obvious, the joint police-EMS selection process is crucial for success.

## Public Defibrillators

While not a service of Winnipeg's EMS, Manitoba's *Defibrillator Public Access Act* is a true game changer in terms of increasing the survival

440 Glen Dawkins. "Police, paramedics team up for emergency medical support for K9 cops." *Winnipeg Sun*. February 21, 2020. Online: https://winnipegsun.com/news/local-news/police-paramedics-team-up-for-emergency-medical-support-for-k9-cops.

441 Online interview with S. Cooke, September 27, 2020.

rate of people experiencing cardiac arrest in Winnipeg. Effective January 1, 2014, the legislation required all publicly accessed buildings, including schools, museums, cultural centres, community and fitness centres, curling clubs, golf courses, athletic and sports venues, casinos, shopping malls and airports, and train and bus stations to have AEDs installed by January 31, 2014, and locations registered with the Heart and Stroke Foundation and shared with 911 dispatchers.[442]

Now, when a person goes into cardiac arrest in Winnipeg, a call to 911 not only starts the process of emergency response, but the caller is provided with directions to the nearest AED. Accessing and using an AED before professional EMS help arrives is often the difference between life and death.

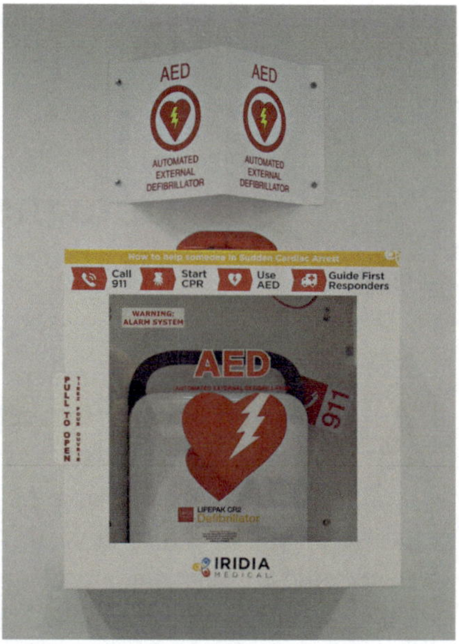


*Small, easy to use, fully automatic defibrillators are located in easily accessible public locations throughout Winnipeg. With voice prompts they can be used by anyone, even without training, to save a life. (Courtesy of the author)*

442 Larry Kusch. "Life-saving defibrillators for public spots." *Winnipeg Free Press.* December 6, 2012; and "Defibrillator law takes effect Jan. 1." *Winnipeg Free Press.* December 31, 2013.

# Into the Future

As we wind our way through 140 years of Winnipeg's EMS history, we reach today. EMS has been, and will continue to be, constantly evolving. As it moves from its current emergency response model to a mobile health or community services model, the changes will be phenomenal, yet again.

This raises the question: With the current evolution from a cold, uncomfortable, slow, horse-drawn hospital ambulance to a combined fire/EMS system where hospital-level care is only minutes away, have we created something good?

With respect to the WFPS, and the process it took to get here, it occurred to me that the answer can be found in one of my son's favorite childhood books: *Shark vs. Train* (Little, Brown Books for Young Readers, 2010). For those who haven't read it, it's a creative story which teaches about how everything is relative. In *Shark vs. Train*, two little boys are arguing about which toy is better. They put their two favorite toys into a series of contests. In some, for example diving underwater, the shark comes out on top. For others, such as pulling four carloads of coal up a steep hill, the train aces the shark. While it's written in a silly, funny, child-like format, it captures an important rule: *Context is everything.*

It's the same with the WFPS; whether the current system, with semi-merged services, is good or bad is completely contextual.

If the question is whether Winnipeg has a cost-efficient ambulance service, the answer is no, there are many models that can deliver EMS at a lower cost.

If the question is whether Winnipeg created a way to justify the continued funding of an expensive fire department, the answer is yes, the combined service creates a meaningful, productive role for firefighters when the actual number of structural fires is plummeting.

If the question is whether Winnipeg provides quick emergency medical response for its citizens, the answer is yes.

If the question is whether there is a better way to provide EMS, the answer is probably, but define *better*.

Irrespective of what question you ask about Winnipeg's EMS, one fact has remained constant throughout the past 140 years: when a Winnipegger is in medical distress, it doesn't matter whether it's day or night; rain or shine; flooded, snowy, or dry; hospital ERs are open or closed; the city or province is claiming to not have enough money for new ambulances; the casualty is on a quiet suburban street, in the middle of a crowded city park, or in a downtown office tower filled with active gunfire; there always have been and always will be dedicated professionals who arrive as quickly as they can and provide the best prehospital emergency care within their abilities; abilities that they continually strive to improve.

Who could ask for more?

## Where Are We Going in Canada?

As we reach the end of this ride through the history of EMS—in Winnipeg and elsewhere—it begs the question: Where are we going?

It's obvious that a key component of EMS—whether it be today, or 140 years ago—is people; dedicated, caring, creative people with an incurable desire to help others. The challenge is how that desire is directed.

Public EMS has evolved from essentially a hospital delivery service—designed to help bring business to a city's hospital—to an emergency response service, and sometimes, to an extension of the health care system.

Underlying this evolution, in Winnipeg and everywhere else in Canada, the age-old question remains: Who is going to pay for it? Despite there always being committed, caring people wanting to help their fellow citizens, for the past 140 years in Winnipeg, and even longer elsewhere, the issue of financing has been the decisive factor.

Funding for ambulances has been a problem since 1889 in Winnipeg, as demonstrated by the plethora of different people and agencies that have tried to deliver pre-hospital care. Even when Canada had a chance to rectify the problem in the 1960s with *Medical Care Act*, our country's precursor to the *Canada Health Act*, it ignored the issue of prehospital emergency care. Instead, Canada chose to focus on doctors and hospitals; only providing financial support for the medical services that doctors provide.

As a result, today where the *Canada Health Act* lets provinces select what medical services are provided to the public, the ultimate decision is left to the individual provinces' colleges of physicians. This ensures that the choices of what medical services are covered by public funds, for the most part, reflect the college members' biases. As prehospital emergency care is typically not within a physician's mandate, it's not a service considered worthy of public coverage anywhere in Canada, with the exception of Quebec.

To make the issue even more challenging, there is no clarity as to whether EMS is an emergency service or an extension of the public health service. EMS straddles both roles.

For the past fifty years (at time of writing) Winnipeg has provided a municipally run, partially public-funded, partially user-funded EMS. For the past thirty years, it has been operated in conjunction with Winnipeg's fire department. Is this the model that will continue?

A look at history will show that it's difficult to tell.

Is fifty years a reasonable amount of time to show a set pattern? Surprisingly, no! A look at the history of firefighting in North America very quickly dispels that myth. If you want to see the romance of firefighting, most involve images of horsedrawn fire apparatus—steamers and hook-and-ladder trucks, pulled by muscular horses, nostrils flaring, barreling toward an inferno.

The curious thing is, the use of horses in the firefighting industry came and went in a little over fifty years. In North America, we've had organized municipal fire departments for 350 years. Boston started their municipal fire service in 1679. Horses, as a means of pulling fire apparatus first made their appearance in New York in 1832. However, as firefighters were used to pulling apparatus by hand and didn't like having their manhood challenged by beasts, horses weren't widely accepted in the fire service until the 1850s/1860s. By the 1910s, horses were on their way out of the fire industry as

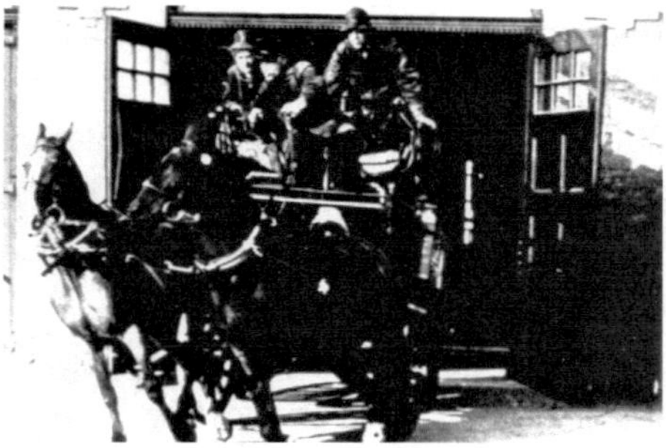

*While horses were used for a relatively short period during the history of emergency response, images such as these, showing horses barreling towards a raging inferno are often used to capture the romance of firefighting. (Courtesy of FFHSW)*

motorized apparatus became the norm. Fifty years, in the emergency response industry, or the health care industry for that matter, does not establish a pattern.

Can we get a sense of where Winnipeg EMS is going by looking at the rest of Canada? Probably not!

With Canadian cities watching their American counterparts, combined with the influence of the *White Paper*, the paramedic EMS model moved to Canada in the early 1970s. Calgary Fire Department set up their paramedic ambulance division in 1971. In 1974, Ottawa Ambulance Service became a public service when it was acquired by the Ministry of Health, and British Columbia Ambulance (a province-wide service) was created. The following year, both Toronto's Department of Ambulance Services and the Winnipeg Ambulance Service—exclusive suppliers of ambulance services for their respective jurisdictions—were created.

Fifty years later, the only major emergency medical services that have remained consistent are the British Columbia Ambulance Service, and the Toronto and Ottawa ambulance services—provincial service provided under contract by the respective cities. As discussed, the control and funding for Winnipeg's EMS has switched from the city to the province, with Winnipeg now providing the service under a service delivery contract to the province through a combined EMS-fire department. Manitoba now has a provincial ambulance service with two cities, Winnipeg and Brandon, opting to provide EMS under contract in conjunction with their fire departments. There were three cities, but as of February 1, 2025, Thompson gave up its contract to provide EMS, leaving only Brandon and Winnipeg as not being served directly by Manitoba EMS.

Without a definitive answer, a look at what's happening in the rest of Canada gives insight into where Winnipeg, and other cities, could potentially go. With EMS delivery changing so rapidly, the following is the most current possible summary of EMS across Canada. It illustrates the inconsistency of services from coast-to-coast.

In Western Canada, both British Columbia and Alberta have created provincial ambulance services. In BC, the province took over all of the separate ambulance service providers in 1975 and began providing direct services. It utilizes a combination of Emergency Medical Responders, Primary Care Paramedics, Advanced Care Paramedics, and Critical Care Paramedics.

In Alberta, the province created a provincial ambulance service—Alberta Health Services EMS—in 2009, providing direct EMS to all but about thirty municipalities and rural areas in the province. The remaining thirty communities provide EMS through their fire departments, via a contract agreement with the province; similar to the arrangement Manitoba has with the WFPS. Besides Winnipeg, Brandon (MB), and Kitimat (BC), these areas in Alberta appear to be the only other fire-based EMS providers in Canada.

Alberta's EMS staffing provides a combination of Emergency Medical Responders, Primary Care Paramedics, and Advanced Care Paramedics. While Alberta EMS has tactical paramedics, flight paramedics, community paramedics, and bicycle paramedics, they don't have critical care paramedics or paramedic specialists. Alberta EMS has a comprehensive Community Paramedic program—Mobile Integrated Healthcare—servicing Edmonton, Calgary, Medicine Hat, Lethbridge, Red Deer, Camrose, Grande Prairie, Peace River, and the surrounding areas.

Come spring 2025, Alberta reflects the pattern of ongoing change across Canada. As outlined below, in June 2024, Newfoundland established a provincial EMS and is moving to a private-sector managed service. EMS delivery in Thompson, Manitoba, in April 2025, has moved from a fire-based service to part of the provincial EMS. In Alberta, effective April 1, 2025, a new agency, Acute Care Alberta, separate from Alberta Health has evolved to manage and deliver EMS. Whether this remains a publicly managed agency, is contracted out to the private sector as in the Maritimes, or becomes a combination of the two is open to speculation.

Saskatchewan takes almost the opposite approach to British Columbia. While Saskatchewan Health Authority funds the province's ambulances, at time of writing, there are 106 different ambulance services, 51% contracted and 49% publicly run,[443] servicing the province's population of slightly over a million. This results in mainly Emergency Medical Responders (435) and Primary Care Paramedics (1273) providing services. Regina, Saskatoon, and 18 other areas have access to Advanced Life Support paramedics. Within the 51% of communities which are now contracting EMS, some, such as Moose Jaw, Saskatoon, and the rural areas around Saskatoon, are

443 Paramedic Services Chiefs of Saskatchewan. https://pscs.ca/about-semsa/about-us. Accessed January 26, 2025.

contracting with Medavie Health Services, a private ambulance service provider with its roots in the Maritimes.

Within Saskatchewan, the range of emergency medical services provided by the various private and public contracted providers include tiered BLS and ALS paramedic services (in Saskatoon and Regina), as well as specialized services including: flight paramedics (Saskatchewan Air Ambulance), tactical paramedics (Saskatoon and Regina), Community Paramedics in Cells (Saskatoon); the province-wide Health Bus, Heart Safe Program, and Saskatoon's "EMS Treatment and Referral pilot project," which extends paramedics' protocols for dealing with hypoglycemia, bleeding, and influenza-like illnesses,[444] so as to not require transport to a hospital ER.

In Ontario, managed by the Ministry of Health's Emergency Health Services Division, the province delivers EMS to roughly 16,000,000 residents through forty nine municipalities, counties, regional governments, and District Social Service Boards, as well as seven First Nations communities, as designated delivery agents. These agents provide the EMS directly or through contractors. As many of the delivery areas, especially in the southern part of the province, are heavily populated, the services provide a broad range of specialized paramedical responses.

While managed by the province's Ministry of Health and Social Services, EMS in Quebec is provided on a contract basis by a consortium of private companies, non-profit organizations, worker cooperatives, and in the Montreal/Laval area, a public sector company; *Urgences-sante* ("Health Emergencies"). Most EMS care in Quebec is at the BLS level, with the exception of *Urgences-sante* which also provides ALS paramedic services, a specialized team for the Montreal subway system, a bike team, and tactical paramedics. A unique part of Quebec's EMS is that because of the province's constitutional right to emergency care, there are a variety of insurance programs that ensure all Quebec residents can access EMS at no cost.

As for Nova Scotia, between 1994 and 2004, NS Emergency Health Services took over all private, local ambulance services (often operated

---

444 Laura Sciarpelletti. "Sask. Launches EMS treatment and referral project with aim of alleviating pressure on ERs." *CBC News.* January 11, 2023. https://www.cbc.ca/news/canada/saskatchewan/saskatchewan-health-authority-launches-ems-treatment-and-referral-pilot-project-in-saskatoon-1.6709161. Accessed January 26, 2025.

by funeral homes), and contracted all EMS in the province to a private company, Medavie Health Services. While primarily a PCP-based service, through Collaborative Emergency Centres across the province, paramedics also provide emergency room-type services. In 2023, in Halifax, Truro, Cape Breton, and Kentville, the province established the Single Paramedic Emergency ALS/BLS Response program. As roughly 30 percent of emergency calls are not transported to hospitals, sole paramedics respond in SUVs to less serious medical calls, such as chronic conditions, abdominal pain, minor injuries, and falls.[445]

New Brunswick, in 2007, consolidated all ambulance services in the province under Ambulance New Brunswick, and contracted out to a private company: Medavie Health Services NB. While primarily a BLS/PCP-based service, in 2017 the province started providing ALS paramedic services out of Moncton, Saint John, Fredericton and Bathurst, Ambulance New Brunswick has fifty-seven ALS paramedics[446] who respond in SUVs to assist Basic Life Support ambulances.

In 2006, Prince Edward Island took over the five existing ambulance services on the island, created Island EMS, and contracted out all EMS to a private company: Medavie Health Services. Besides the primary care ambulances, Island EMS also has five Community Paramedic SUVs, which can be cross tasked as emergency Advanced Care Paramedic Response Units, PEI also has the benefit of an active RCMP Emergency Medical Response Team—RCMP officers cross-trained with both special tactics and emergency medical care. As a result, the RCMP is able to bolster PEI's EMS by assisting with specialized issues, such as searches for lost persons,[447] mental health wellness checks, and providing tactical emergency medical services to Charlottetown Police's Priority Tactical Response and Containment Team.

In Newfoundland and Labrador, in June 2024, NL Health Services took over the operation of the sixty different ambulance services in their area. It was previously a blend of private and public providers. As of spring 2025, Medavie Health Services will be providing single

445 Nova Scotia Health. "Sending a SPEAR: Why dispatching a single paramedic can be the right answer to some 911 calls." Press release. October 18, 2023.

446 Department of Health, New Brunswick. "Advanced care paramedic program now available in more parts of the province." Press release. August 19, 2021.

447 Gavin Moore. "Three youth located safe after being lost in the woods, Tracadie Cross, PEI." News release. March 30, 2023.

provincial-wide EMS to Newfoundland. Hence, Newfoundland's EMS can best be described as *evolving*.

How does what the other provinces and territories are doing relate to the WFPS?

For the most part, there is a move toward provincially based ambulance services, with some publicly operated (BC, Alberta, Manitoba, with local exceptions), and some privately operated provincial services (New Brunswick, Nova Scotia, PEI, and soon, Newfoundland). Two provinces contract their EMS to local governments: Ontario and Quebec. Saskatchewan is a bit unique in that it funds a hundred or so different ambulance services, some public, some private, around the province.

In the United States, of the 200 most populated communities, 97 percent have the fire service delivering prehospital emergency medical service response. Additionally, the fire service provides critical advanced life support (ALS) response and care in ninety percent of the thirty most populated United States cities and counties.[448]

In Canada, the experience is the opposite. Besides Winnipeg, no other large Canadian city has EMS (besides first responder services) delivered by a fire department. There are smaller cities, such as Brandon, Manitoba, Kitimat, British Columbia, and a handful of Alberta communities, such as Lethbridge, Red Deer, Kitimat, Fort McMurray (Wood Buffalo), and Strathcona County. But otherwise, EMS is Canada delivered by a variety of provincial, municipal, and county emergency medical-based providers: some public and some contracted private.

How will this eventually affect Winnipeg's EMS? Ultimately, it depends on how, and if, Canada eventually amends the *Canada Health Act*. As physicians become less available—in 2024, 516,000 Torontonians didn't have access to a family physician and the number is expected to increase to one million by 2026[449]—it is falling more on EMS to bridge the gap. As a result, in many Canadian jurisdictions, the move in EMS is toward managing the steadily increasing number of

---

448 International Association of Fire Chiefs. "IAFC Position: Fire-based Emergency Medical Services." https://www.iafc.org/topics-and-tools/resources/resource/iafc-position-fire-based-emergency-medical-services. Accessed January 28, 2025.

449 Tara Anderson. *Toronto Paramedic Services – Rising Response Times Caused by Staffing Challenges and Pressures in the Healthcare System.* Auditor General – Toronto. 2024: 9.

non-emergent calls. Through increased screening of 911 calls, and subsequent referrals to community paramedics, outside services, alternate forms of transportation, and increasing paramedics' protocols to deal with more patients at the scene (without transporting to hospital and emergency rooms), it becomes possible to use paramedics to both decrease the number of ambulance trips and decrease the number of ER visits. The challenge is that in Winnipeg, the underlying reason for merging, or partially merging, fire and EMS was to save money. WFD has provided emergency medical response/first aid/resuscitation since 1928—just as it provides emergency response to car accidents, chemical spills, industrial entrapment, high angle scenarios, and a variety of other emergencies, and will likely always have this general emergency response role.

Whether WFPS is the appropriate provider of EMS on a broader scale really depends on how the *Canada Health Act* evolves. As much of EMS appears to be moving toward replacing physicians and hospitals, with paramedics providing non-emergent care, it comes down to cost. If *Canada Health Act* begins recognizing (and funding) EMS-paramedics as community health care providers, it will make little sense to have EMS services (beyond first responder-type services) provided by a fire department. WFD always has been, and absent a total transformation of the fire industry, always will be an emergency response service. This will make it more logical to have EMS-paramedics tied into the healthcare industry. On the other hand, if Canada continues to refuse to recognize that the EMS industry is replacing doctors and nurses and declines to provide proper funding for EMS under the *Canada Health Act*, keeping EMS as an emergency-based service under the WFPS may be the way that Winnipeg chooses to manage the costs.

The settlement of the debate by Winnipeg, and the rest of Canada, over whether EMS is funded primarily as an emergency response service or as a healthcare delivery service will ultimately determine who, or what, is the best provider of EMS in the city. Until that time, WFPS, as it delivers both fire as well as ambulance and paramedic services in Winnipeg, will continue to be a unique provider of EMS in Canada.

# Appendix A: Ambulance Stations

## 1975-1998

| | |
|---|---|
| EMS #1 | 161 Lipton @ Westminster (Wolseley)<br>Built 1913, originally WFD No. 14. 1975: EMS #1, Closed 1990 |
| EMS #1 | 726 Furby Street (Downtown)<br>Built: 1990, 1997: WFPS EMS No. 31 Current |
| EMS #2 | 325 Talbot Avenue<br>Built 1906, originally WFD No. 8. 1975: EMS #2, Closed: 1990. |
| EMS #2 | 2325 Grant Avenue, Fort Garry<br>Built: 1990 as EMS #2, 2002: WFPS EMS No. 32, Closed: 2012 |
| EMS #3 | 600 St. Mary's Road<br>Built 1914, originally St. Vital Police/Fire Station #1. 1975: EMS #3, Closed: 1998 |
| EMS #4 | 524 Osborne Street<br>Built 1913, originally WFD No. 15, EMS #4 (1975), then EMS #10 (1995), 1997: WFPS EMS No. 30, Current |
| EMS #4 | 701 Day Street, Transcona<br>Built 1985 as WFD No. 25. EMS #4 (Circa 1995 - joint fire/EMS). Current WFPS No. 25.<br>1066 Dorchester @ Wilton<br>(Built 1911, originally as WFD No. 12)—training only. |
| EMS #5 | McGregor & Liela Opened (1975), Closed (1990) |
| EMS #5 | 585 McGregor Street<br>Built 1990, 1997: WFPS EMS No. 35, Closed: 1998, moved to current WFPS Nos. 6 and 16 |

| | |
|---|---|
| EMS #6 | 525 Banting Drive @ Portage<br>Built 1972 (St James FD), EMS #6/WFD No. 20, (1977 circa).<br>1990: WFD No. 20 |
| EMS #6 | 2490 Portage Avenue (Silver Heights)<br>Built 1990: WFPS No. 20, Current |
| EMS #7 | 2340 Pembina Highway, Fort Garry (Victoria Hospital)<br>Circa 1975. Rebuilt 1989/90, 1998: WFPS EMS Station 37,<br>Closed 1998, moved to current WFPS No. 22. |
| EMS #8 | 640 Kimberly Avenue, East Kildonan<br>Circa 1975—joint station with WFD #8. EMS left in 1989.<br>Currently active fire station. |
| EMS #8 | 569 Watt Street Built 1989, 1997: EMS Station 38.<br>Closed 1998, moved to current WFPS No. 24. |
| EMS #9 | 799 Lilac Street<br>Built 1979 as EMS #9/WFD No. 3—joint fire/EMS, renovated 2021. 1998 WFPS No. 13.<br>2300 McPhillips Street (Seven Oaks General Hospital)<br>Circa 1996, closed 1998 |

## 1998 - Current

| | |
|---|---|
| WFPS No. 1 | 65 Ellen Street, Downtown (1965) |
| WFPS No. 5 | 845 Sargeant Avenue, West End<br>(1910, Reno 1982, Reno 2018) |
| WFPS No. 6 | 603 Redwood Avenue, North End (1998, Reno 2016) |
| WFPS No. 9 | 864 Marion Street, St. Boniface (1957, Reno 1975) |
| WFPS No. 10 | 1354 Border Street, St. James (1967, Reno 2016) |
| WFPS No. 11 | 1705 Portage Avenue, St. James (2015) |
| WFPS No. 12 | 1780 Taylor Avenue, River Heights (2012) |
| WFPS No. 13 | 799 Lilac Street, Fort Rouge (1979, Reno 2021) |
| WFPS No. 14 | 1057 St. Mary's Road, St. Vital (1957, Reno 1975) |
| WFPS No. 16 | 1001 McGregor Street, West Kildonan (1969, Reno 2018) |
| WFPS No. 17 | 1501 Church Avenue, North End (1963, Reno 2018) |
| WFPS No. 18 | 5000 Roblin Boulevard, Charleswood(2012) |
| WFPS No, 20 | 525 Banting Drive, Assiniboia(1972) |
| WFPS No. 21 | 1446 Regent Avenue West, Transcona (2007) |

| | |
|---|---|
| WFPS No. 22 | 1567 Waverley Street, Fort Garry(1977) |
| WFPS No. 24 | 1665 Rothesay Street, North Kildonan(1975) |
| WFPS No. 25 | 701 Day Street, Transcona(1985) |
| WFPS No. 27 | 27 Sage Creek Boulevard, Sage Creek (2012) |
| EMS No. 30 | 524 Osborne Street, Fort Rouge (1915, Reno 2021) |
| EMS No. 31 | 726 Furby Street, Downtown (1989) |
| EMS No. 36 | 2490 Portage Avenue, Silver Heights, (1990) |
| EMS No. 40 | 1030 Pacific Avenue, Downtown / North End (2010)<br>Storage/service only, not an active response station |

# Bibliography

## Books

Adsten, Peter. Crestline, *Building World Class Ambulances.* EMS Classics, 2008.

Anderson, Tara. *Toronto Paramedic Services—Rising Response Times Caused by Staffing Challenges and Pressures in the Healthcare System.* Auditor General—Toronto. 2024.

Artibise, Alan. *Winnipeg, An Illustrated History.* James Lorimer and Co., 1977.

Artibise, Alan F.J. *Winnipeg: A Social History of Urban Growth, 1874-1914.* McGill-Queen's University Press, 1975.

Barkley, Katherine Traver. *The Ambulance—The Story of Emergency Transportation of Sick and Wounded Through the Centuries.* Load-N-Go Press, 1978, 1990—reprint.

Bell, Ryan Corbett. *The Ambulance.* McFarland & Company, 2009.

Belton, G.P. *Organization Review Project.* Report, Fire Department, Ambulance Division. City of Calgary. 1982.

Bjarnason, Halldor K. *We Hold Thee Safe.* Firefighters Historical Society of Winnipeg, 2005.

Canadian Association of Emergency Physicians. *The Canadian Prehospital Acuity Scale—Educational Program.* March 2014.

Civil Defence Department. *Extracts from a brief submitted to the Manitoba Medical Association on ambulance services in Metropolitan Winnipeg.* Metropolitan Corporation of Greater Winnipeg, 1961.

Coulter, J.T. "Proposal for Fire/Ambulance Amalgamation." City of Winnipeg. April 22, 1980.

Duncan, Zoey. *Vital Signs.* Emergency Medical Services (EMS) Foundation, 2019.

Fellows, Bob, Graham Harris, Andrew Newton. *The History of the Paramedic Profession.* Self-published, 2024.

Finn, Lynea. *Paramedicine in Ottawa 1845-2001.* Self-published, 2017.

Gunderson, Harald. *A History of Funeral Service in Manitoba.* Manitoba Funeral Association, 2008.

Hanna, James A. *A Century of Red Blankets.* Boston Mills Press, 1982.

Hazzard, Kevin. *American Sirens.* Hachette Books, 2022.

*Healing & Hope: A History of Health Sciences Centre.* Health Sciences Centre, Winnipeg, 2009.

Katz, Samuel M. *Anytime Anywhere!* Pocket Books, 1997.

King, Martin. *Battlefield Medics: How Warfare Changed the History of Medicine.* Arcturus Publishing Limited, 2021.

Klein, Lynn. *The British Columbia Ambulance Service: Forty Years of Compassion and Care.* Self-published, 2018.

Matches, Alex. *The Rigs of Vancouver's Bravest.* Self-published, 2016.

McCall, Walter. *American Fire Engines Since 1900.* Crestline Publishing, 1976.

McCall, Walter M.P. *The American Ambulance 1900-2002.* Iconografix, 2003.

McCreery, Christopher. *The Maple Leaf and the White Cross.* Dundurn Press, 2008.

McPherson, Thomas A. *American Funeral Cars and Ambulances Since 1900.* Crestline Publishing, 1973.

McPherson, Thomas A. *Flxible Professional Vehicles: The Complete History.* Specialty Vehicle Press, 1993.

McPherson, Thomas A. *The Henney Motor Company—The Complete History.* Iconografix, 2009.

McPherson, Thomas A. *Miller-Meteor: The Complete Illustrated History.* Iconografix, 2010.

McPherson, Thomas A. *Superior: The Complete History. Specialty* Vehicle Press, 1995.

National Academy of Sciences and National Research Council. *Accidental Death and Disability: The Neglected Disease of Modern Society.* The National Academies Press, 1966,

Nemish, Vivian, and Peter Adsten. *The History of Saskatchewan Ambulance and Emergency Medical Services.* Saskatchewan Emergency Medical Services Association, 2016.

Newton, Bruce. *Accidents, Illness, and Sirens.* Grafo Print Media Inc., 2015.

Page, James O. *The Paramedics.* Backdraft Publications, 1979.

Paramedic Association of Manitoba. *Manitoba's Quiet Crisis.* May 2007.

Parker, Dave. *First Water, Tigers!* 2nd Ed. Victoria Fire Department Historical Society, 2008.

Paterson, J.E., et al., Ambulance and Fire Services Study, Quotation No. 590-80 "Emergency Medical System". December 19. 1980.

Plumbtree, Michael D. *Ambulances and Paramedics.* Self-published, 2011.

Rapport, Richard. *Seattle's Medic One.* The House Press, 2019.

Richardson, Gary R. *An Analysis of Fire Department and Ambulance Integration from a Process Perspective: Using Winnipeg Manitoba as a Case Study.* Department of Graduate Studies, University of Winnipeg. 1996.

Ring, Al; Ring, Bob. *Tucson Fire Department Emergency Medical Services.* Greater Tucson Fire Foundation. 2016.

*The Status of Women in the Civic Service.* City of Winnipeg, 1977.

Thompson, Susan A. *Her Worship.* Friesen Press, 2016.

Toews, Reg. *Manitoba EMS System Review.* Ministry of Health, Government of Manitoba. 2013: 21.

Winnipeg General Hospital. *Annual Report.* Multiple years.

Yardley, Richard, and Rozane Sutherland. *Emergency! Behind the Scene.* Jones and Bartlett Publishers, 2008.

## Articles/Periodicals

"$11,500 arrears claimed." *Winnipeg Free Press.* November 26, 1975.

"60 Veterans Allowed Taxi Cab Licenses." *Winnipeg Tribune.* July 30, 1946.

"A New Ambulance." *Winnipeg Free Press.* November 27, 1905.

"A new Focus." *Winnipeg Free Press.* October 17, 2008.

"Aged Patients Leave City in RCAF Planes." *Winnipeg Free Press.* May 15, 1950.

Alberta Health Services. "HCAP: Faster response times for 911 calls." https://www.alberta.ca/release.cfm?xID=86476C49212DC-E6F5-3BF8-D7D8B-610B541C0B7. Accessed January 26, 2025.

"Airlift Takes First Patients to Regina Refuge." *Winnipeg Free Press.* May 12, 1950.

"Ald. Blumberg Urges Better System of Caring For Accident Victims." *Winnipeg Free Press.* August 27, 1948.

"Aldermen Who Quit Early Draw Blast." *Winnipeg Free Press.* June 6, 1946.

"Almost half of Winnipeg ambulance bills went unpaid in 2022, report says", CBC News. May 1, 2023. https://www.cbc.ca/news/canada/manitoba/winnipeg-ambulance-costs-1.6828949. Accessed November 1, 2023.

"Ambulance cuts called medieval." *Winnipeg Free Press.* February 23, 1979.

"Ambulance, fire services link on Jan. 1." *Winnipeg Free Press.* October 13, 1982.

"Ambulance Payments Criticized, Defended." *Winnipeg Tribune.* December 10, 1959.

"Ambulance probe launched." *Winnipeg Free Press.* March 25, 1976.

"Ambulance purchase okayed by committee." *Winnipeg Free Press.* December 20, 1978.

"Ambulance Service Gets Aldermen In Argument." *Winnipeg Free Press.* January 31, 1946.

"Ambulance supervisors seek union." *Winnipeg Free Press.* June 17, 1976.
"Ambulances to get heart defibrillators." *Winnipeg Free Press.* November 28, 1984.
"Ambulances aren't new." *Winnipeg Free Press.* January 28, 2003.
Anderson, James C. "Prince Brothers Open Ambulance Service." *Winnipeg Tribune.* July 27, 1946.
"Another Four Institutions Still Battle To Halt Water." *Winnipeg Free Press.* May 6, 1950.
"Army Evacuates 659 Patients in 4 Institutions As Precaution." *Winnipeg Free Press.* May 8, 1950.
Asian Heritage Society of New Brunswick. "Chinese Labour on the Canadian Pacific Railway." at www.ahsnd.org. Accessed July 3, 2024.
"Automobile Ambulance for Winnipeg." *Manitoba Free Press.* June 3, 1911.
Bell, Jason. "Training draws fiery response." *Winnipeg Free Press.* December 29, 2005.
"Big Increase in Hospital Patients." *Manitoba Free Press.* January 10, 1916.
Billeck, Scott. "Three-digit emergency line in Winnipeg turns 60." *Winnipeg Sun.* June 21, 2019.
"Boy Critically Wounded in Play Duel." The *Winnipeg Tribune.* September 22, 1949.
Boyens, Ingeborg. "Departments to Justify Expenses." *Winnipeg Free Press.* November 3, 1978.
Brodbeck, Tom. "Paramedics reduce need for trips to ER." *Winnipeg Free Press.* July 11, 2019.
Brosnahan, Maureen. "Death of woman prompts new ambulance rules." *Winnipeg Free Press.* June 2, 1984.
Brosnahan, Maureen. "Fatal heart attack rate remains high." *Winnipeg Free Press.* April 26, 1984.
Brosnahan, Maureen. "Loose ambulance rules create risks." *Winnipeg Free Press.* October 14. 1980.
Brosnahan, Maureen. "MDs rap heart attach care." *Winnipeg Tribune.* February 15, 1980.
"Buy Auto Chassis." *Winnipeg Tribune.* April 28, 1917.
Campbell, Donald. "Ambulance workers rip firefighters over jaws of life." *Winnipeg Free Press.* April 2, 1990.
"City ambulance service wants extra $3 a ride." *Winnipeg Free Press.* April 10, 1976.
"Charity Ambulance Calls." The *Winnipeg Tribune.* September 12, 1912.
Chester. Margot. "City's "first responder' units go into service." *Winnipeg Sun.* September 15, 1982.

Christie, Alan. "Ambulance Owners Hit City Takeover." *Winnipeg Free Press.* June 11, 1975.
Christie, Alan. "Defence of private ambulances fails to convince civic committee." *Winnipeg Free Press.* June 30, 1976.
"City and General." *Manitoba Morning Free Press.* November 11, 1901.
"City Hospital at Parting of Ways Symington Says." *Winnipeg Tribune.* December 13, 1924.
"City paramedics win costly battle to form new union." *Winnipeg Free Press.* November 7, 1998.
"City to Guarantee Fees." *Manitoba Free Press.* December 7, 1912.
"City's 999 Only One On This Continent." *Winnipeg Free Press.* June 20, 1959.
City of Winnipeg History—Civic Emergency Program during the 1997 Flood, https://legacy.winnipeg.ca/History/flood/emergency_program/default.stm, Accessed December 31, 2023.
"City's Pleas for Money Net $55,000." *Winnipeg Free Press.* February 5, 1980.
Cleaver, E.C.. *City of Winnipeg Police Department.* Winnipeg, 1920.
Cole, Alana. "With 911 call volumes rising, Winnipeg Fire Paramedic Service develops new 5-priority dispatch system." *CBC News.* https://www.cbc.ca/news/canada/manitoba/911-call-volumes-dispatch-system. Accessed January 21, 2025.
Collison, John. "Emergency alert." *Winnipeg Sun.* August 8, 1995.
"Constables Ambulance Men." *Manitoba Free Press* Winnipeg. February 22, 1912.
"Coroner Announces Inquest Unnecessary." *Winnipeg Free Press.* December 1, 1922.
"Crashing the Party: Women of EMS." *feminem*, February 20, 2018, https://feminem.org/2018/02/20/crashing-party-women-ems. Accessed January 25, 2024.
Davis, Donald F. "The Canadian Taxi Wars, 1925-1950." *Urban History* Review. 27(1) (1998): 17.
Dawkins, Glen. "Police, paramedics team up for emergency medical support for K9 cops." *Winnipeg Sun.* February 21, 2020. Online: https://winnipegsun.com/news/local-news/police-paramedics-team-up-for-emergency-medical-support-for-k9-cops.
"Defibrillator law takes effect Jan. 1." *Winnipeg Free Press.* December 31, 2013.
Department of Health, New Brunswick. "Advanced care paramedic program now available in more parts of the province." Press release. August 19, 2021.
"Drank Carbolic Acid by Mistake." *Manitoba Free Press.* March 31, 1913.
Edgar, Patti. "City hears first of firefighters grievances." *Winnipeg Free Press.* October 1, 2004.

Edgar, Patti. "Fired up over merger." *Winnipeg Free Press.* March 6, 2004.
Edgar, Patti. "Firefighters claim a win in amalgamation fight." *Winnipeg Free Press.* March 8, 2005.
Edgar. Patti. "Firefighters' newsletter jokes 'unprofessional'." *Winnipeg Free Press.* September 23, 2004.
Edgar, Patti. "Firefighters try to extinguish merger." *Winnipeg Free Press.* February 21, 2004.
Edgar, Patti. "Hot weather put pressure on paramedics." *Winnipeg Free Press.* June 21, 2005.
Edgar, Patti; Kevin Rollason. "Fire hall fiasco divides unions." *Winnipeg Free Press.* September 22, 2004.
Egan, Paul. "Fire, paramedics a poor marriage?" *Winnipeg Free Press.* September 26, 2004.
Egan, Paul. "'Pussyfooting' blamed for poisonous relations." *Winnipeg Free Press.* September 25, 2004.
"Emergency Paramedic in the Community (EPIC) program to expand". Undated (2019) City of Winnipeg press release. https://www.winnipeg.ca/fr/node/30257. Accessed October 14, 2024.
"Exceptional Result in Examinations." *Manitoba Free Press.* February 22, 1913.
"Exonerate Driver Police Ambulance." *Manitoba Free Press.* July 30, 1915.
Fayerman, Pamela. "Fire crews seldom attend to medical calls, inquest told." *Winnipeg Free Press.* July 22, 1981.
Felding, Helen. "Union fights renaming fire dept." *Winnipeg Free Press.* September 8, 2000.
"Fire, ambulance, merger a step closer." *Winnipeg Free Press.* March 19, 1981.
"Fire Dept. Life Savers." *Winnipeg Tribune.* March 20, 1950.
"Fire Rescue Wagon Proves Life Saver." *Winnipeg Tribune.* March 16, 1950.
"Firemen Win." *Manitoba Free Press Winnipeg,* December 11, 1911.
Forbes, Steven. "Victim trapped extra 10 minutes." *Winnipeg Sun.* October 4, 1996.
"Fresh Feature to Monday's Fatality." *Manitoba Free Press.* July 28, 1915.
Gillespie, Darcy. "Paramedics to replace ambulance in Transcona." *Winnipeg Free Press.* February 9, 2000.
Giroday, Gabrielle. "Firefighters' union cites hectic year." *Winnipeg Free Press.* January 21, 2009.
Graham, Heidi. "Brawl rescue provokes spat within union." *Winnipeg Free Press.* March 21, 1986.
Graham, Heidi. "Use of pressure pants up to attendants, inquest told." *Winnipeg Free Press.* April 20, 1988.
Graham, Heidi. "Paramedic loss would be deadly, City woman warns." *Winnipeg Free Press.* March 30, 1992.

Guttormson, Kim. "Amalgamation cuts 61 jobs." *Winnipeg Free Press.* July 15, 1998.

Guttormson, Kim. "Casinos getting cardio-smart." *Winnipeg Free Press.* October 31, 1999.

Guttormson, Kim. "Councillors hear presentation on fire, ambulance merger." *Winnipeg Free Press.* July 16, 1998.

Guttormson, Kim. "Dept, merger sparks fiery debate." *Winnipeg Free Press.* July 7, 1998.

Guttormson. Kim. "Hamilton chief to merge City's fire, ambulance." *Winnipeg Free Press.* September 22, 1998.

"Head-On Collision Injures 11 Persons." *Winnipeg Free Press.* August 22, 1949.

Heart and Stroke Foundation. "The Amazing Story of CPR." at https://www.heartandstroke.ca/articles/the-amazing-story-of-cpr. Accessed August 30, 2024.

Hoffman, Michael. "A 'Quiet' Friday for the five-minute men." *Winnipeg Free Press.* June 20, 1979.

"Hospital Work." *Manitoba Daily Free Press.* February 7, 1890.

"Illegality Argument In Vain." *Winnipeg Free Press.* September 28, 1967.

"In Case of Accident." *Manitoba Daily Free Press.* June 10, 1891.

International Association of Fire Chiefs. "IAFC Position: Fire-based Emergency Medical Services." https://www.iafc.org/topics-and-tools/resources/resource/iafc-position-fire-based-emergency-medical-services. Accessed January 28, 2025.

"Johnstone quits ambulance post." *Winnipeg Free Press.* January 22, 1977.

"'Jumbo ambulance' comes to Winnipeg." CBC News. June 26, 2008. https://www.cbc.ca/news/canada/manitoba/jumbo-ambulance-comes-to-winnipeg. Accessed March 5, 2024.

"Jury on Double Killing." *Manitoba Free Press.* July 29, 1915.

Kaschor, Kim. "What exactly does Winnipeg's tactical emergency medical unit do?" CBC News. August 4, 2015. https://www.cbc.ca/news/canada/manitoba/what-exactly-does-winnipeg-s-tactical-emergency-medical-unit-do-1.3178287, Accessed: August 8, 2017.

Kao, Helen; Conant, Rebecca; Soriano, Theresa; McCormick, Wayne. "The Past, Present, and Future of House Calls.". *Clinics in Geriatric Medicine.* 25 (1) (February 2009): 19–34.

"Keep games out of paramedic decision." *Winnipeg Free Press.* March 14, 2015.

Kives, Bartley. "Are enough ambulances on the road?" *Winnipeg Free Press.* August 15, 2007.

Kives, Bartley. "Firefighters' deal with paramedics praised by mayor." *Winnipeg Free Press.* April 27, 2007.

Kives, Bartley. "Firefighters, paramedics deal to become official." *Winnipeg Free Press.* May 16, 2007.

Kives, Bartley. "Katz: city's paramedics fastest." *Winnipeg Free Press.* September 21, 2010.

Kowal, Joe. "Prepared to Move the sick, the infirm and the elderly to safety." https://legacy.winnipeg.ca/History/Flood/emergency_program/ambulance.stm. Accessed December 31, 2023.

Kubinec, Vera-Lynn; Joanne Levasseur. "No free ride: Ambulance bills in Manitoba highest in Canada." CBC News. February 11, 2015. https://www.cbc.ca/news/canada/manitoba/no-free-ride-ambulance-bills-in-manitoba-highest-in-canada-1.2947262 Accessed: December 16, 2023.

Kusch, Larry. "Emergency room off-load times soar." *Winnipeg Free Press.* June 4, 2014.

Kusch, Larry. "EPIC CARE." *Winnipeg Free Press.* October 3, 2015.

Kusch, Larry. "Life-saving defibrillators for public spots." *Winnipeg Free Press.* December 6, 2012

Kusch, Larry. "Tension Smoulders as Flames Fade." *Winnipeg Free Press.* December 23, 2017.

Kuxhaus, David. "Ambulance shortage 'a recipe for disaster'." *Winnipeg Free Press.* January 4, 2005.

Lane, John. "Winnipeg's integrated EMS-fire model is working." *Winnipeg Free Press.* March 19, 2015.

"Lecture to the CPR Employees." *Manitoba Daily Free Press.* February 8, 1893.

"Licensed Men Behind the Siren." *Winnipeg Tribune.* August 22, 1961.

"Man Brings Woman Back To Life Twice." The *Winnipeg Free Press.* December 19, 1966.

MacKenzie, Glen. "It's payback time, union members say." *Winnipeg Free Press.* May 17, 1999.

McArthur, Keith, et al. "Ambulance service cut blamed on underfunding." *Winnipeg Free Press.* May 14, 1999.

McArthur, Keith. "City's paramedics crying foul." *Winnipeg Free Press.* June 30, 1999.

MacArthur, Keith. "Emergency!" *Winnipeg Free Press.* January 11, 1998.

McArthur, Keith. "Paramedics turn up the heat on the City." *Winnipeg Free Press.* May 19, 1999.

McArthur, Keith. "Paramedics' dispute with City may be over soon." *Winnipeg Free Press.* July 3, 1999.

McArthur, Keith. "Paramedics in turmoil days before the strike vote." *Winnipeg Free Press.* May 15, 1999.

McArthur, Keith. "Road repairs may be put on back burner." *Winnipeg Free Press.* November 28, 1998.

McDougall, Glenn. "Doctors See Death Drama, Urge Need of City Safety." *Winnipeg Tribune.* October 24, 1949.
McIntyre, Mike. "City firefighters armed for war on heart attacks." *Winnipeg Free Press.* March 9, 1999.
McIntyre, Mike. "Sex at city fire hall alleged." *Winnipeg Free Press.* September 4, 2009.
McKinley, Patrick. "Ambulance plan gets yet another look." *Winnipeg Free Press.* February 2, 1983.
McKinley, Patrick. "Ambulance response satisfies City." *Winnipeg Free Press.* June 27, 1984.
McKinley, Patrick. "Budget proposal to cut 24 firefighters backed." *Winnipeg Free Press.* February 13, 1985.
McKinley, Patrick. "City Scraps Ambulance Amalgamation." *Winnipeg Free Press.* March 17, 1983.
McKinley, Patrick. "Report urges City scrap merger plan." *Winnipeg Free Press.* January 14, 1983.
McKinley, Patrick. "Troubled emergency service plan to start." *Winnipeg Free Press.* August 30, 1982.
Martin, Melissa. "New ambulance gives lift to morbidly obese patients." *Winnipeg Free Press.* April 3, 2010.
"Meanness." *Winnipeg Free Press.* April 29, 1961.
"Men Behind the Siren." The *Winnipeg Tribune.* August 22, 1961.
"Message from Fire & Paramedic Chief Jim Brennan." *Lights & Sirens.* WFPS. June 2010: 1.
Mitchell, Catherine. "Buses, bikes being outfitted for paramedics' use." *Winnipeg Free Press.* February 6, 1999.
"Modern Electric Ambulance for General Hospital." *Winnipeg Tribune.* January 20, 1912.
Moore, Gavin. "Three youth located safe after being lost in the woods, Tracadie Cross, PEI." News release. March 30, 2023.
"More Barriers in the Path of Criminals." *Manitoba Free Press.* July 4, 1913.
"Motorman hurt in Head-on Collision." *Manitoba Free Press* Winnipeg. January 19, 1912.
Muir, Shirley. "Hero's reward." *Winnipeg Sun.* March 23, 1986.
Necheff, Julia. "Ambulance speed, driver training unregulated, official says." *Winnipeg Free Press.* July 26, 1984.
"New Ambulances." *Winnipeg Free Press.* March 11, 2000.
"New Hospital Ambulance." ç. December 10, 1898.
"New paramedic units kept on hold for now." *Winnipeg Free Press.* November 27, 2009.
"New system would trace all 911 calls." *Winnipeg Free Press.* April 17, 1980.

Nicholson, Karen. "Manitoba History: A.C. Emmett and the Development of Good Roads in Manitoba." *Manitoba History*, Manitoba Historical Society, Number 27, Spring 1994.

Nolan, Michael; Tim Hillier; Carmen D'Angelo. *Community Paramedicine in Canada.* Emergency Medical Services Chiefs of Canada. 2011.

"Nothing Better than Winnipeg." *Manitoba Free Press* Winnipeg. October 16, 1911.

Nova Scotia Health. "Sending a SPEAR: Why dispatching a single paramedic can be the right answer to some 911 calls." Press release. October 18, 2023.

Nova Scotia Paramedics Union. "Clinical Support Desk." https://web.archive.org/web/20141019203958/http://nspu.ca/roles-of-paramedics/clinical-support-desk. Accessed January 23, 2025.

O'Brien, David. "Ambulances in trouble: mayor." *Winnipeg Free Press.* September 14, 1999.

O'Brien, David. "Faulty ambulances stay on road." *Winnipeg Free Press.* November 6, 1981.

O'Reilly, Edward. "Hospital Reminiscences." *WGH Nurses Alumni Journal.* 1929: 22.

O'Reilly, Edward B. "Hospital Reminiscences." *Nurses' Alumnae Annual.* 1937: 51.

"One Man Killed, Another May Die." *Manitoba Free Press.* July 27, 1915.

Ontario Paramedic Association. "History of Paramedics in Ontario." at: https://www.ontarioparamedic.ca/before-911/history-of-paramedics-in-ontario. Accessed July 1, 2024.

Owen, Bruce. "Emergency response times a fiery election issue." *Winnipeg Free Press* July 13, 2006.

Paramedic Chiefs of Saskatchewan. https://pscs.ca/about-semsa/about-us. Accessed January 26, 2025.

"Paramedic service tag $6.5 million." *Winnipeg Free Press.* September 10, 1991.

"Paramedics dispute staff shortage." *Winnipeg Free Press.* May 11, 2004.

"Paramedics left behind on amalgamation tour." CBC News, March 16, 2006. https://www.cbc.ca/news/canada/manitoba/paramedics-left-behind-on-amalgamation-tour-1.622975. Accessed March 5, 2024.

Paraskevas, Joe. "Paramedic's practical joke sparks probe." *Winnipeg Free Press.* December 14, 2006.

Paraskevas, Joe. "Paramedic reports going electronic." *Winnipeg Free Press.* April 3, 2008.

Pihichyn, Paul. "Better Training Urged For Ambulance Staff." *Winnipeg Free Press.* February 21, 1975.

"Police Ambulance on Reo Chassis sold to City." *Winnipeg Tribune.* June 30, 1917.

"Police Buy New Chassis." *Manitoba Free Press* Winnipeg. April 28, 1917.
"Police Probe." *Winnipeg Free Press.* March 5, 1940.
"Police Signal Service." *Manitoba Daily Free Press.* January 11, 1895.
"Probe Finds all Charges Not Proven." *Winnipeg Free Press.* October 1, 1940.
"Probe Hears Police Cars Used Privately." *Winnipeg Free Press.* May 11, 1940.
"Province Now In On Study." *Winnipeg Free Press.* June 27, 1969.
"Provincial Ambulance Plan Ready." *Winnipeg Free Press.* November 2, 1973.
Pursaga, Joyanna. "City officials urge ambulance service be transferred to provincial authority." *Winnipeg Free Press.* October 7, 2020.
Pursaga, Joyanne. "Dozens of firefighters drop paramedic role." *Winnipeg Free Press.* November 18, 2020.
Pursaga, Joyanne. "Fire chief announces retirement." *Winnipeg Free Press.* May 1, 2021.
Pursaga, Joyanne. "Firefighters union president won't seek re-election." *Winnipeg Free Press.* December 1, 2021.
Pursaga, Joyanne. "On the Hot Seat." *Winnipeg Free Press.* August 19, 2021.
Pursaga, Joyanne. "Paramedics, firefighters get say." *Winnipeg Free Press.* February 1, 2022.
Pursaga, Joyanne. "WFPS seeks to improve workplace with 'culture shift plan.'" *Winnipeg Free Press.* December 14, 2021.
Rassy, Swidda. "Ambulance wait times increasing in Winnipeg." City News. April 12, 2023. https://winnipeg.citynews.ca/2023/04/12/ambulance-wait-times-increasing-in-winnipeg/. Accessed September 28, 2024.
"Rescue staff seek divorce from union." *Winnipeg Free Press.* September 2, 1998.
"Rescue unit makes west safer." *Winnipeg Free Press.* August 7, 1988.
"Resuscitation Help Earns Chief's Praise." *Winnipeg Free Press.* January 9, 1969.
Retson, Don. "Ambulance response criticized." *Winnipeg Free Press.* June 22, 1984.
Retson, Don. "Heart victim's death linked to tight ambulance budget." *Winnipeg Free Press.* March 23, 1986.
Robson, Barbara. "Blood and Guts." *Winnipeg Free Press.* November 26, 1985.
Rodgers, Paul. "Hard-Luck Hero." *Winnipeg Sun.* March 20, 1986.
Rollason, Kevin. "Board proposes eliminating 102 fire, police jobs." *Winnipeg Free Press.* February 7, 1991.
Rollason, Kevin. "Council orders review of policy on use of extrication equipment." *Winnipeg Free Press.* January 8, 1991.
Rollason, Kevin. "Firefighters hope to extinguish cuts." *Winnipeg Free Press.* March 11, 1997.
Rollason, Kevin. "Responsibility for Jaws of Life to stay with ambulance crews." *Winnipeg Free Press.* June 25, 1991.
Rollason, Kevin; Alexandra Paul. "Fire hall anger bubbles over." *Winnipeg Free Press.* September 23, 2004.

Rubin, Joe. "Fire, ambulance merger could begin in August." *Winnipeg Free Press.* June 2, 1982.
"St. John Ambulance Branch is Formed." *Manitoba Free Press.* January 7, 1911.
Santin, Aldo. "Ambulance wants $100, even if nobody gets a ride." *Winnipeg Free Press.* November 4, 1996.
Santin, Aldo. "City cuts 18 middle-management jobs." *Winnipeg Free Press.* March 11, 1998.
Santin, Aldo. "City, province playing with lives, union says." *Winnipeg Free Press.* August 17, 1992.
Santin, Aldo. "City works out kinks over future of ambulance funding." *Winnipeg Free Press.* March 15, 2018.
Santin, Aldo. "Emergency Services Merger Set to Begin." *Winnipeg Free Press.* April 26, 1997.
Santin, Aldo. "Fire chief on the hot seat." *Winnipeg Free Press.* March 1, 2018.
Santin, Aldo. "Lifesavers Baffled." *Winnipeg Free Press.* August 17, 1992.
Santin, Aldo. "Merger Contract on Hold." *Winnipeg Free Press.* June 13, 1997.
Santin, Aldo. "Paramedic transfer would save City $3M: chief." *Winnipeg Free Press.* April 12, 2018.
Savard, Marc. 'PTRS Pilot Launch." WFPS memo. September 25, 2024.
"Say Police Ambulance Doing Private Work." *Winnipeg Free Press.* January 22, 1959.
Sciarpelletti, Laura. "Sask. Launches EMS treatment and referral project with aim of alleviating pressure on ERs." *CBC News.* January 11, 2023. https://www.cbc.ca/news/canada/saskatchewan/saskatchewan-health-authority-launches-ems-treatment-and-referral-pilot-project-in-saskatoon-1.6709161. Accessed January 26, 2025.
Schmidt, Christian. "PTRS—Primary Treatment and Referral Service." *Lights & Sirens.* WFPS. June 2010: 3.
Searle, Tyler. "Legal dispute between firefighter and paramedic dismissed." *Winnipeg Free Press.* December 11, 2022.
"Service's creation slow, methodical." *Winnipeg Free Press.* December 29, 2003.
"Shoemaker cautious about full-scale fire, ambulance merger." *CBC News.* May 24, 1999. https://www.cbc.ca/news/canada/shoemaker-cautious-about-full-scale-fire-ambulance-merger-1.177760. Accessed December 22, 2023.
"Signal System for Winnipeg Police." *Manitoba Free Press* Winnipeg. October 20, 1911.
"Silent Sirens." *Winnipeg Free Press.* May 13, 1966.
"Single ambulance, fire service urged." *Winnipeg Free Press.* March 4, 1981.
"Six Lives Lost in Saturday Night Fire—Five of Victims Buried Under Falling Walls." *Manitoba Free Press Winnipeg,* March 11, 1912.
Skerritt, Jen. "City hospitals billed $60,000." *Winnipeg Free Press.* May 21, 2011.

"Slayers, Bank Robbers Give City Wide Berth; Fatality Toll is Lower." *Winnipeg Free Press.* February 28, 1938.
Seiden, Deidre. "The Paramedic Advantage." *RCMP Gazette.* Vol 76, No. 4 (2014).
"Spivak's Motor Sales." *Winnipeg Tribune.* June 3, 1933.
"Stabbing sends police to hospital." *Winnipeg Free Press.* March 17, 1986.
"Staff shortage delays plan for additional ambulances." *Winnipeg Free Press.* May 8, 2004.
Stone, Stan. "New Bariatric Ambulance." *Lights & Sirens.* WFPS. June 2010: 3.
"Suppress the Gong." *Manitoba Daily Free Press*, February 7, 1889.
"Takeover urged for ambulances." *Winnipeg Free Press.* June 23, 1976.
Thampl, Radha Krishnan. "Proposal breathes life into program." *Winnipeg Free Press.* September 9, 1992.
"The Birth of the First Aid Kit": Johnson & Johnson Company website: https://ourstory.jnj.com/birth-first-aid-kit. Accessed October 2020.
"The CP Rail yards over the years", *Winnipeg Free Press.* July 6, 2012.
"The General Hospital." *Manitoba Daily Free Press.* March 10, 1899.
*The Generator.* Volume 14, Number 9, October 1972.
"The Hospital." *Manitoba Daily Free Press.* August 8, 1895.
"The Hospital Ambulance." *Manitoba Daily Free Press.* July 11, 1890.
"The Hospital Contracts." *Manitoba Morning Free Press.* April 18, 1899.
"The Jubilee Addition." *Winnipeg Daily Tribune.* October 6, 1899.
"The New Ambulance." *Manitoba Daily Free Press*, January 28, 1889.
"The Smallpox Cases." *Manitoba Daily Free Press.* April 29, 1900.
Thibault, Michael. "Ambulances busy, patients ride in rescue trucks." *Winnipeg Free Press.* February 12, 1995.
"Three Digit Emergency Dialing in Winnipeg." 2019 *Winnipeg Police Museum Annual Report*: 28.
Tinguely, Chuck. "Paramedics Active in Community Education and Response (PACER) Program." Lights & Sirens. WFPS. June 2010: 10.
Tsicos, Stephanie. "'Extremely frustrating': Winnipeg's two largest hospitals seeing increase in hospital diversions." *CTV News Winnipeg.* November 8, 2019.
Turner, Randy. "Plan cuts City 100 jobs." *Winnipeg Free Press.* February 17, 1997.
"Verdict of $12,000 for the Plaintiffs." *Manitoba Free Press*, Winnipeg. June 17, 1918.
"Verdict on Block Disaster Criticized." *Manitoba Free Press.* September 26, 1929.
"Vet Ambulance Seeking Grant." *Winnipeg Tribune.* December 31, 1948.
"Veteran Dead, Two Hurt In Car-Ambulance Crash." *Winnipeg Free Press.* January 20, 1951.
"Vets Ambulance for City Work." *Winnipeg Tribune.* July 10, 1959.
"Waiting, waiting in the ER." *Winnipeg Free Press.* October 20, 2009.

“Want Better Service.” *Manitoba Free Press.* December 5, 1912.
“Wants Ambulance.” *Manitoba Free Press* Winnipeg. April 6, 1912.
“Want Pay for Ambulance.” *Winnipeg Tribune.* October 17, 1912.
Weber, Terry. “MD quits ambulance advisory board.” *Winnipeg Free Press.* January 24, 1989.
Welch, Mary Agnes. “Computer to cut ambulance ride time.” *Winnipeg Free Press.* February 13, 2006.
Welch, Mary Agnes. “Local dealer donates cars for paramedics.” *Winnipeg Free Press.* November 20, 2009.
Welch, Mary Agnes. “Misdeeds at fire hall described.” *Winnipeg Free Press.* September 2, 2006.
Welch, Mary Agnes. “No one to come to your rescue.” *Winnipeg Free Press.* October 8, 2009.
Welch, Mary Agnes. “Paramedics not invited on mayor’s fire hall tour.” *Winnipeg Free Press.* March 15, 2006.
Welch, Mary Agnes. “Sedans may replace ambulances.” *Winnipeg Free Press.* October 16, 2009.
Welch, Mary Agnes. “Local dealer donates cars for paramedics.” *Winnipeg Free Press.* November 20, 2009.
Westaway, Nancy. “Ambulance service in critical condition: paramedics.” *Winnipeg Free Press.* January 4, 1998.
“What’s in a name?” *Winnipeg Free Press.* September 21, 2000.
Wild, Stevens. “Whole city covered by 10 to 15 vehicles.” *Winnipeg Free Press.* November 4, 1995.
“Winnipeg Paramedics demand more ambulances.” National Union of Public and General Employees. Press release. September 22, 2010.
“Winnipeg Police Ambulance.” *2020 Winnipeg Police Museum Annual Report:* 23.
“Work of the St. John Ambulance Association in Winnipeg.” *Manitoba Free Press*: Winnipeg. January 13, 1912.
Youngs, Fred. “Ambulance, fire merger at square one.” *Winnipeg Free Press*”. October 27, 1982.

# Index

Made in the USA
Monee, IL
05 November 2026

67808953R00155